Handbook of Experimental Pharmacology

Volume 293

The *Handbook of Experimental Pharmacology* is one of the most authoritative and influential book series in pharmacology. It provides critical and comprehensive discussions of the most significant areas of pharmacological research, written by leading international authorities. Each volume in the series represents the most informative and contemporary account of its subject available, making it an unrivalled reference source.

HEP is indexed in Medline/PubMed and Scopus.

Angélica Rueda • Madeline Nieves-Cintrón
Editors

Cardiovascular Alterations in Metabolic Diseases

Springer

Editors
Angélica Rueda
Department of Biochemistry
Campus Zacatenco, Cinvestav-IPN
Mexico City, Mexico

Madeline Nieves-Cintrón
Department of Pharmacology
University of California
Davis School of Medicine
Davis, CA, USA

ISSN 0171-2004 ISSN 1865-0325 (electronic)
Handbook of Experimental Pharmacology
ISBN 978-3-032-32139-8 ISBN 978-3-032-32140-4 (eBook)
https://doi.org/10.1007/978-3-032-32140-4

This Springer imprint is published by the registered company Springer Nature Switzerland AG
The registered company address is: Gewerbestrasse 11, 6330 Cham, Switzerland

Preface

The unprecedented rise in metabolic disorders, mainly obesity and diabetes, triggers a series of health problems that severely affect cardiovascular health. According to the World Health Organization, ischemic heart disease remains a leading cause of death worldwide, with metabolic disorders representing major contributing risk factors (WHO 2021; Martin et al. 2024). Metabolic syndrome and diabetes are among the most pressing public health challenges of our time, with prevalence rates doubling in recent decades and projections showing continued growth. Today, more than one in three adults globally are affected by metabolic syndrome, while over 537 million people live with diabetes (Noubiap et al. 2026). This rising burden underscores the urgent need to understand the molecular changes that drive cardiovascular disease in the context of metabolic disorders. Equally important is the implementation of effective interventions (such as healthier diets, regular physical activity, and reduced sedentary behavior) to prevent the progression of cardiometabolic diseases into advanced stages. Without such measures, patients face the risk of end-organ damage, including the kidneys, which contributes to the emergence of the cardiovascular-kidney-metabolic syndrome. This edition of the Handbook of Experimental Pharmacology examines the complex interplay among metabolic syndrome, diabetes, and cardiovascular dysfunction, offering insights into both underlying mechanisms and potential intervention strategies. The volume is also intended to serve as a pedagogical resource for understanding the fundamental mechanisms underlying cardiac and vascular dysfunction in metabolic syndrome and diabetes. The chapters progress from foundational concepts to specialized molecular mechanisms and translational perspectives. Beginning with experimental models of metabolic diseases (Chapter "Experimental Models for Studying Cardiovascular Dysfunction in Metabolic Syndrome") and population considerations such as sexual dimorphism in cardiometabolic syndrome (Chapter "Sexual Dimorphism in the Development of Cardiometabolic Syndrome"). The volume advances through pathophysiology, cellular remodeling mechanisms, and calcium signaling dysregulation (Chapters "Cardiac Cell Remodeling in Obesity and Diabetes", "Calcium Signaling Dysregulation in Diabetic Cardiomyopathy: Roles of STIM and Orai Channels", and "The SERCA Pump: A Key Molecular Target in Calcium Handling of Vascular Smooth Muscle Cells in Metabolic Syndrome"), followed by detailed discussions of mitochondrial dysfunction and oxidative stress, the role of innate immune receptors, and microRNAs (Chapters "Oxidative Modifications in Cardiac Mitochondrial and Ca^{2+} Handling Proteins in Obesity and Metabolic Syndrome: Antioxidant Alternatives", "Role of Innate Immune Receptors in Cardiac Damage Linked to Metabolic Disorders", and "Car diovascular Dysfunction in Type 2 Diabetes: The Role of MicroRNAs"). The final chapters focus on translational and clinical application, including biomarker discovery and the therapeutic impact of physical activity (Chapters "In Search of a Biomarker for Vasculopathy Associated with Metabolic Syndrome" and "Physical Activity and Its Impact on Cardiometabolic Disorders"). Together, these chapters offer a comprehensive perspective on the mechanism linking metabolic disorders to cardiovascular dysfunction. We are confident that this volume will deepen understanding of how metabolic syndrome and diabetes harm the cardiovascular system, while also encouraging further discussion and informed decision-making on the development of effective therapeutic interventions.

Mexico City, Mexico Angélica Rueda
Davis, CA, USA Madeline Nieves-Cintrón

References

Martin SS, Aday AW, Almarzooq ZI, Anderson CAM, Arora P, Avery CL, Baker-Smith CM, Barone Gibbs B, Beaton AZ, Boehme AK, et al (2024) Heart disease and stroke statistics: a report of US and Global Data from the American Heart Association. Circulation 149:e347–e913. https://doi.org/10.1161/CIR.0000000000001209

Noubiap JJ, Nansseu JR, Nyaga UF et al (2026) Worldwide trends in metabolic syndrome from 2000 to 2023: a systematic review and modelling analysis. Nat Commun 17:573. https://doi.org/10.1038/s41467-025-67268-5

WHO (2021) Diabetes. https://www.who.int/news-room/fact-sheets/detail/diabetes

Contents

Experimental Models for Studying Cardiovascular Dysfunction in Metabolic Syndrome

Jade L. Taylor, Eric A. Pereira da Silva, Hannah M. Voorhees, Maryann K. Ferrara, Sophia Salbato, Nuria Daghbouche-Rubio, Miguel Martín-Aragón Baudel, and Madeline Nieves-Cintrón

Contents

Abstract

Metabolic syndrome (MetS) encompasses an interconnected set of risk factors, including abdominal obesity, insulin resistance, hypertension, dyslipidemia, and systemic inflammation, all of which significantly increase the risk of cardiovascular diseases (CVDs). This chapter provides an overview of animal models used to study cardiovascular complications associated with MetS. We examine

J. L. Taylor · E. A. Pereira da Silva · H. M. Voorhees · M. K. Ferrara · S. Salbato · N. Daghbouche-Rubio · M. M.-A. Baudel · M. Nieves-Cintrón (✉)
Department of Pharmacology, University of California, Davis, CA, USA
e-mail: mcnieves@ucdavis.edu

A. Rueda, M. Nieves-Cintrón (eds.), *Cardiovascular Alterations in Metabolic Diseases*, Handbook of Experimental Pharmacology 293,
https://doi.org/10.1007/164_2026_800

commonly used models, including monogenic and polygenic rodent strains, diet-induced and chemically induced models, and large-animal systems, and discuss their strengths and limitations. The chapter then explores cardiac and vascular alterations in MetS and translation to humans. By integrating findings from diverse experimental models with human clinical data, the chapter aims to advance understanding of research on MetS-associated cardiovascular complications.

Keywords

db/db · Diabetes · GLP-1 · HFpEF · Hypertension · Myogenic tone · Obesity · SGLT2

1 Introduction

Metabolic syndrome (MetS) represents a significant public health challenge affecting approximately 20–40% of adults globally and increasing cardiovascular disease (CVD) risk (Gami et al. 2007; Guembe et al. 2020). MetS arises from the clustering of cardiometabolic risk factors, including central obesity, insulin resistance, hypertension, dyslipidemia, and chronic systemic inflammation, which synergize to exacerbate cardiovascular pathology (Alberti et al. 2009). Some definitions of MetS require central obesity (International Diabetes Federation) or insulin resistance (World Health Organization). Efforts to harmonize the definition of MetS allow diagnosis when any three of the five metabolic alterations are present, incorporating ethnic-specific waist circumference cutoffs (Alberti et al. 2009; Alberti et al. 2005). The biology underlying the cardiovascular complications of MetS is complex. Obesity-associated inflammation, oxidative stress, activation of the renin-angiotensin-aldosterone system (RAAS), and dysregulation of metabolic substrates interact synergistically to drive cardiac and vascular dysfunction. Understanding how these pathways interact to affect pathology and identifying mechanistic targets for therapeutic intervention requires experimental systems that can be carefully manipulated and monitored over time.

Preclinical animal models are key for the study of MetS-associated CVD. While no single model can fully recapitulate the spectrum of human MetS, the use of complementary systems enables mechanistic dissection across biological scales. Monogenic rodent models (e.g., ob/ob, db/db, Zucker obese) enable targeted investigation of specific pathways, such as leptin signaling defects. Polygenic models (e.g., SHR-SP obese, DS/obese, OLETF) more accurately represent the multifactorial genetic nature of MetS. Diet-induced models replicate environmental triggers, such as excess dietary fat, fructose, and cholesterol, which contribute to MetS. Large-animal models (pigs, rabbits, dogs, nonhuman primates) address critical limitations of rodent physiology, including differences in metabolism, coronary anatomy, and disease progression timescales, thus providing essential validation prior to clinical translation.

This chapter provides an overview of the diverse animal models currently used to study cardiovascular complications associated with MetS. The chapter first examines commonly used animal models of MetS, encompassing monogenic and polygenic genetic models, diet-induced models, chemically induced models, and large-animal systems. Next, it explores cardiac alterations in MetS, including the roles of chronic inflammation, oxidative stress, and metabolic dysfunction in pathological cardiac remodeling and functional impairment, particularly diastolic dysfunction. The discussion then addresses vascular dysfunction in MetS, spanning from large conduit arteries to the microcirculation. The chapter concludes with a perspective on the advantages and limitations of animal models of MetS and examples of the successful translation of preclinical research into clinical practice for glucose-lowering drugs, such as glucagon-like peptide-1 (GLP-1) receptor agonists and the sodium-glucose cotransporter 2 (SGLT2) inhibitors. By integrating findings from diverse experimental models with human clinical data, the chapter aims to advance understanding of research on MetS-associated cardiovascular complications.

2 Commonly Used Models in the Study of MetS-Associated Cardiovascular Complications

Monogenic and polygenic models that exhibit multiple features of MetS, including hypertension, obesity, insulin resistance, dyslipidemia, and systemic inflammation, have been developed through selective breeding for cardiometabolic traits in numerous small animal strains. These models are crucial for understanding the complex relationships between metabolic risk factors and evaluating potential therapeutic interventions. Diet-induced models are widely used to mimic human MetS and its associated complications. Some studies combine genetic and diet-induced models to accelerate disease progression or better replicate the multifaceted nature of MetS-induced cardiovascular complications. Furthermore, large-animal models, including dogs, rabbits, pigs, cats, and nonhuman primates, have played a crucial role in dissecting disease mechanisms and evaluating therapeutic strategies, thereby complementing findings from rodent studies and enhancing translational relevance. The following section provides an overview of commonly used models for studying MetS associated cardiovascular complications.

2.1 Monogenic Models

Ob/ob The obese mice were first observed spontaneously in 1949 at the Jackson Laboratory in Maine (Ingalls et al. 1950). The ob/ob mouse strain results from a nonsense mutation in the gene encoding the hormone leptin (*Lep^ob*), which prevents its production. Leptin, released from adipocytes, signals satiety to the brain, therefore suppressing appetite. In the absence of this signal, these mice exhibit hyperphagia, resulting in increased fat mass, larger adipocytes, and insulin resistance.

Db/db The db/db mice, a popular model of obesity and diabetes, were first described in 1966 as an inbred mouse strain exhibiting abnormal fat levels and hyperglycemia. Like the ob/ob mice, the db/db mice have impaired leptin signaling. However, in the db/db mutation, the phenotype arises from leptin receptor dysfunction rather than from impaired leptin production (Chen et al. 1996). The db/db mice show obesity, hyperglycemia, insulin resistance, dyslipidemia, and often hypertension (Hummel et al. 1972). They are widely used as preclinical models of MetS and T2DM, with phenotypes varying by age, sex, and strain background. For example, at 10–16 weeks of age, db/db mice on the C57BL/6 J background exhibit a MetS phenotype and are used in cardiometabolic research (Semeniuk et al. 2002).

Zucker Obese fa/fa Rats The Zucker obese (fa/fa) rats (initially described as Zucker fatty rats) arose spontaneously at the Lois and Theodore Zucker laboratory (Zucker and Zucker 1961). Obese rats started appearing in the litter at a 25% incidence. In the initial report, the phenotype was attributed to a single recessive gene; the lean control gene was designated Fa and the obese gene, fa (Zucker and Zucker 1961). Further genetic studies identified a missense mutation at position +269 in the leptin receptor that is responsible for the obese phenotype in these rats. The mutation results in reduced leptin affinity and responsiveness to exogenous leptin, as well as decreased receptor density. The Zucker obese rat is a commonly used genetic model that exhibits obesity, hyperinsulinemia, hypertriglyceridemia, and hypercholesterolemia; they are routinely normoglycemic and normotensive (Sultan et al. 2020). The Zucker obese rat was later bred to develop obesity and T2DM (Yokoi et al. 2013), giving rise to the *Zucker fa/fa diabetes mellitus rats (ZFDM)*. Like the Zucker obese rat, the ZFDM is a monogenic model of hyperphagia, obesity, and insulin resistance; however, the diabetic phenotype arises from selective breeding of Zucker obese rats with hyperglycemia and beta-cell failure, thereby contributing polygenically to diabetic progression.

Koletsky Rats Also known as Spontaneously Hypertensive Obese (SHROB) rats, they were first described in 1973. These rats result from breeding female Spontaneously Hypertensive Rats (SHR) with normotensive male Sprague-Dawley rats to study the blood pressure (BP) patterns of their offspring (Koletsky 1973). The obese phenotype arose spontaneously during selective breeding for the hypertensive phenotype in these crosses (Koletsky 1975). As in the Zucker obese rat, the obese phenotype in Koletsky rats results from a spontaneous mutation in the gene encoding the leptin receptor, although it has a different origin. In the Koletsky rat, a nonsense mutation introduces an early stop codon, resulting in a truncated protein and effectively producing a natural knockout of the leptin receptor (Koletsky 1975). The Koletsky rats exhibit simultaneous obesity, hypertension, hyperlipidemia, metabolic abnormalities, and atherosclerosis (Koletsky 1973; Tan et al. 1976). Moreover, these rats show inflammation, endothelial dysfunction, and insulin resistance (Molinar-Toribio et al. 2014). Under fasting conditions, the rats remain normoglycemic, making them among the earliest animal models of MetS.

Transgenic Models Several knockout and transgenic mouse models have been developed to study the roles of specific proteins in cardiovascular complications associated with MetS. Transgenic models typically target genes involved in lipid metabolism, inflammation, glucose regulation, and vascular function. For example, apolipoprotein E (ApoE)-deficient (ApoE−/−) mice were generated by gene targeting in embryonic stem cells (Piedrahita et al. 1992; Plump et al. 1992). ApoE is a key ligand for receptors in the low-density lipoprotein receptor (LDLR) family, which is essential for mediating hepatic uptake and redistributing cholesterol and other lipids to peripheral tissues, thereby maintaining lipid balance. ApoE−/− mice show hypercholesterolemia and develop atherosclerotic lesions across various arteries similar to those in humans, making them a common model for atherosclerosis (Plump et al. 1992; Zhang et al. 1992). Similarly, mice lacking the LDLR (responsible for the hepatic and peripheral uptake of low-density lipoprotein (LDL) particles) (Li et al. 2025; Sawhney and Madan 2024) display elevated cholesterol levels and develop atherosclerosis, although less severely than ApoE−/− mice. Crossbreeding LDLR and ApoE-knockout strains results in widespread atherosclerotic lesions with histopathological features similar to human disease; however, the severity and progression of atherosclerosis are not significantly greater than in ApoE−/− mice alone (Kampschulte et al. 2014; Langheinrich et al. 2007).

2.2 Polygenic Models

Spontaneously Hypertensive-Stroke Prone Obese Rat Model The Spontaneously Hypertensive rat (SHR) strain was first described in 1963 by Okamoto and Aoki. The strain was generated through the selective inbreeding of Wistar-Kyoto rats with elevated blood pressure (Okamoto and Aoki 1963; Okamoto et al. 1966). Continued selection for the hypertensive phenotype resulted in rats that exhibited higher heart rate (HR) and blood pressure at 4 weeks of age than control rats (Dickhout and Lee 1998). SHRs are, therefore, a commonly used rat model for studying hypertension and CVD (Lerman et al. 2019). Moreover, SHRs have been selectively bred with other strains, resulting in several strains with MetS traits (Koletsky 1973). Breeding of SHR littermates that exhibited stroke-like symptoms led to the development of *stroke-prone spontaneously hypertensive rats* (SHR-SP) (Okamoto et al. 1986). Crossing SHR-SP rats with Zucker obese rats (Hiraoka-Yamamoto et al. 2004) resulted in the development of the SHR-SP obese rat model, which exhibits obesity, hypertension, elevated cholesterol and triglycerides, and metabolic disorders (Hiraoka-Yamamoto et al. 2004).

Dahl/Salt-Sensitive Obese (DS/Obese) Rats Dahl/Salt-sensitive (DS) rats, reported in 1962, were produced through selective inbreeding of Sprague-Dawley rats. These rats become hypertensive when fed a diet containing 2–8% salt. They can be easily compared with normotensive rats fed a 0.4% salt diet (Dahl et al. 1962). Crossing DS and Zucker obese rats produced the DS/obese rats (Hattori et al. 2011). These rats have higher body weight, fat mass, and blood pressure than DS/lean rats, as well as

Table 1 Genetic and transgenic rodent models

Model	Origin/mutation	Phenotype/features
Ob/ob mice	Nonsense mutation in leptin gene (Lep^ob)	Obesity, insulin resistance
Db/db mice	Leptin receptor mutation (db)	Obesity, diabetes, glucose intolerance, hypertension, dyslipidemia
Zucker obese (fa/fa) rat	Missense mutation in leptin receptor (fa)	Obesity, hyperinsulinemia, hyperlipidemia, normoglycemia, normotensive
ZFDM rat	Derived from Zucker obese rat; bred for diabetes	Obesity, overt T2DM, β-cell failure
Koletsky rat	Nonsense mutation in leptin receptor	Obesity, hypertension, hyperlipidemia, atherosclerosis
ApoE−/− mice	Targeted deletion of ApoE gene	Hypercholesterolemia, atherosclerosis
LDLR−/− mice	Targeted deletion of LDL receptor gene	Hypercholesterolemia, mild atherosclerosis
SHR-SP obese rat	Cross SHR-SP × Zucker obese rat	Obesity, hypertension, dyslipidemia,
DS/obese rat	Cross DS × Zucker obese rat	Obesity, hypertension, hyperlipidemia, insulin resistance
OLETF rat	Spontaneous deletion in CCK-A receptor gene	Visceral obesity, insulin resistance, late-onset T2DM

higher cholesterol, triglycerides, and insulin concentrations (Murase et al. 2012). Additionally, DS/obese rats have been reported to develop hypertension even without a high-salt diet, unlike their lean counterparts (Hattori et al. 2011).

Otsuka Long-Evans Tokushima (OLETF) Rats The OLETF rat was established by researchers at Otsuka Pharmaceutical Co. in Tokushima, Japan, through the selective breeding of an outbred Long-Evans colony that naturally exhibited mild obesity and glucose intolerance (Kawano et al. 1992). By mating affected males with nondiabetic fertile females over several generations, a stable rat strain was developed that exhibits hyperphagia and key features of human MetS, including visceral obesity, insulin resistance, and late-onset T2DM (Kawano et al. 1992). The OLETF rat has a naturally occurring deletion in the cholecystokinin-A (CCK-A) receptor gene, resulting in impaired satiety signaling and chronic overeating (Moran and Bi 2006a, b; Moran et al. 1998). The polygenic background of OLETF rats, combined with progressive metabolic dysfunction similar to that observed in humans with cardiometabolic disease, makes them a valuable model for studying MetS-related CVD (Table 1).

2.3 Diet-Induced Models

Diet-induced models replicate key features of MetS, including obesity, insulin resistance, dyslipidemia, and, in some cases, hypertension. The diet regimen can be selected for its ability to reliably induce the desired disease phenotype or designed to mimic typical human consumption patterns, such as Western diets high in fat and sugar. A significant drawback of this dietary approach is the time and resources required to elicit metabolic alterations, which often require several weeks of dietary intervention (Wang and Liao 2012). The following section offers an overview of commonly used diet-induced models, including those that combine various dietary strategies to better reflect the multifactorial nature of human MetS.

High-Fat Diet A high-fat diet (HFD) is a commonly used model for studying diet-induced obesity, insulin resistance, T2DM, and cardiovascular complications. It consists of 40–60% of the food energy from fat, usually derived from lard, though palm and soybean oils are also used, depending on experimental goals. The ideal control diet should match the test diet in terms of protein and carbohydrate content. Common rat strains used for this model are Wistar and Sprague-Dawley (Marques et al. 2016). These models show increased weight gain, body fat mass, elevated leptin levels, leptin resistance, and insulin resistance (Marques et al. 2016). The C57BL/6 J mouse strain is highly susceptible to HFD-induced obesity and T2DM (Schreyer et al. 1998; Surwit et al. 1988), exhibiting increased insulin levels, insulin resistance, body weight, and cholesterol levels (Fraulob et al. 2010; Gallou-Kabani et al. 2007; Podrini et al. 2013).

Cafeteria Diet The foundational studies that led to the development of diet-induced obesity models using palatable food were conducted by Sclafani and Springer, who examined experimental obesity models and the similarities between hypothalamic-obese and diet-induced-obese rats (Sclafani and Springer 1976). A variety of supermarket foods, combined with laboratory chow and HFD, were used to induce dietary obesity (Sclafani and Springer 1976). The model later evolved into a model of human MetS, in which cafeteria-diet-fed rodents develop obesity, glucose intolerance, hyperinsulinemia, inflammation, and other MetS-relevant phenotypes (Sampey et al. 2011). The cafeteria diet model more closely mimics human eating habits by offering a variety of highly palatable foods (such as cookies, chips, and processed meats) rather than focusing on a single macronutrient (Lalanza and Snoeren 2021) and consistently shows higher energy intake and more severe insulin resistance compared to HFD models. However, effects on body weight and cholesterol vary between studies. This variability could arise from differences in diet composition (e.g., proportion of fats, refined carbohydrates, and dietary cholesterol) (Rothwell et al. 1982; Rothwell and Stock 1979; Zeeni et al. 2015). Feeding duration also modulates the phenotype, as insulin resistance and inflammation often emerge before maximal body weight gain (Gomez-Smith et al. 2016; Mucellini et al. 2014). Moreover, strain genetic makeup and sex-specific metabolic responses, such as lipid handling, further influence phenotype (Lai et al. 2014; Mn et al. 2017; Wang and Liao 2012). Commonly used strains include Wistar and Sprague-Dawley rats, as well as C57BL/6 J mice (Montgomery et al. 2013). BALB/c mice are also employed; although this strain generally exhibits resistance to diet-induced obesity, individual mice show significant variability and can be classified into obesity-prone and obesity-resistant groups (Boi et al. 2016).

Fructose, Sucrose, and High-Fat Diet Combining fructose or sucrose overload with HFD is a standard approach for modeling the Western diet in rodents. Fructose can be added directly through food pellets or drinking water (Sanchez-Lozada et al. 2007). In rats, a diet with 60% of total energy from fructose for just 2 weeks has been shown to increase blood pressure, insulin, and triglyceride levels, even without changes in body weight (Hwang et al. 1987). A more physiologically relevant model involves administering water containing 20% fructose for 8 weeks, resulting in significant weight gain (Mamikutty et al. 2014). Sucrose is a disaccharide composed of glucose and fructose and is a major dietary source of fructose in human diets. High-sucrose feeding is also widely used to model MetS (Nakayama et al. 2025). It is typically given by substituting complex carbohydrates in standard chow with 60–66% sucrose or by supplementing drinking water with 10–30% sucrose (Basaranoglu et al. 2013; Panchal et al. 2011). These dietary interventions exhibit MetS phenotypes, including increased body weight and visceral adiposity, fasting hyperinsulinemia, hypertriglyceridemia, impaired glucose tolerance and/or insulin resistance, and frequently elevated blood pressure (Cui et al. 2022; Sanchez-Lozada et al. 2007; Yang et al. 2012; Zhuhua et al. 2015).

2.4 Combined Models

The causes of cardiometabolic diseases, including T2DM and MetS, are multifactorial, involving both genetic predisposition and environmental factors such as diet, physical inactivity, and metabolic stressors. To better mimic the human condition, researchers have developed combined animal models that incorporate genetic susceptibility, dietary challenges, and chemical agents, such as streptozotocin (STZ). In the following section, we summarize commonly used combined models for studying the pathophysiology and cardiovascular complications associated with MetS.

Genetic and Diet Models Combining genetically predisposed animals with dietary interventions amplifies metabolic dysfunction and more faithfully captures the complexity of MetS and associated comorbidities. For instance, ob/ob and db/db mice on HFD or high-calorie diets exhibit more severe hepatic inflammation, necrosis, and fibrosis beyond their baseline metabolic dysfunction (Abe et al. 2019; Trak-Smayra et al. 2011). SHRs exhibit hypertension and insulin resistance but lack other features of MetS, such as obesity and dyslipidemia (Miesel et al. 2010; Wong et al. 2016). However, dietary interventions in SHR have been shown to reproduce MetS. SHRs on a high-fructose diet and an HFD have higher circulating very low-density lipoprotein (VLDL), LDL, and triacylglycerol (Lalanza and Snoeren 2021). SHRs fed a cafeteria diet develop obesity, insulin resistance, and elevated circulating triglycerides. Notably, SHRs on a cafeteria diet have been found to have higher blood pressure and heart rate than those on a regular chow diet

(Miesel et al. 2010). Transgenic models, such as ApoE−/− mice, have also been combined with dietary interventions to accelerate disease progression and investigate accelerated CVD within the context of metabolic dysfunction (King et al. 2010; Li et al. 2016).

Streptozotocin (STZ) & Diet STZ selectively targets pancreatic β-cells via the glucose transporter 2 (GLUT2), resulting in β-cell injury. STZ alone emulates insulin deficiency rather than MetS. However, by administering lower doses of STZ combined with high-fat or high-fructose diets, researchers can more accurately replicate the phenotypes of T2DM and MetS (Barriere et al. 2018; Mazzocco et al. 2025; Suman et al. 2016a). For example, Wistar rats fed a cholesterol-rich HFD for 3 weeks, followed by a single low dose of STZ (40 mg/kg), developed hyperglycemia, dyslipidemia (elevated triglycerides and LDL and lowered high-density lipoprotein), hypertension, and weight gain. Histological analysis also revealed inflammation, vascular edema, and aortic atherosclerotic plaques, particularly in SHR (Suman et al. 2016b). Another model, combining STZ (25 mg/kg) with an HFD and high-fructose diet (HFrD; 46.5% fructose, 25.7% lard) for 6 weeks, led to hyperglycemia, insulin resistance, and hypertriglyceridemia. However, body weight did not increase significantly. These models are valuable for studying the metabolic and cardiovascular complications of MetS, including vascular inflammation, myocardial fibrosis, and endothelial dysfunction (Table 2).

2.5 Large Animal Models

Large-animal models, such as dogs, rabbits, pigs, and nonhuman primates, are frequently used because of their similarity to human anatomy, bridging mechanistic studies in rodents and more translational preclinical research. For example, pig hearts closely resemble human hearts in size, coronary anatomy, and hemodynamics, and they share similar protein and lipid metabolic pathways, making them especially

Table 2 Diet-induced and combined models

Model	Origin/Intervention	Phenotype/Features
High-fat diet (HFD)	40–60% energy from fat (lard, palm, soy oil)	Obesity, insulin resistance, hyperlipidemia, hypercholesterolemia (esp. C57BL/6J mice)
Cafeteria diet	Palatable human foods (cookies, chips, processed meat)	Obesity, insulin resistance, hyperinsulinemia, inflammation, variable cholesterol
Fructose + HFD	Fructose (15–60%) + HFD (varied sources)	Obesity, insulin resistance, hypertension, NAFLD, T2DM
Genetic + diet	Ob/ob, db/db, SHR, ApoE−/− + diet	Exacerbated MetS features, hepatic inflammation, atherosclerosis
STZ + diet	Low-dose STZ + HFD/HFrD	T2DM, hyperglycemia, dyslipidemia, vascular inflammation, atherosclerosis, cardiac/renal dysfunction

valuable for cardiovascular research. In the following sections, we briefly discuss commonly used large-animal models for the study of MetS-associated cardiovascular complications.

Canine Dog models have been valuable for studying basic cardiovascular physiology and for advancing diabetes research. The classical model of experimental insulin-deficient diabetes was established in the 1920s by Banting and Best through pancreatectomy in dogs, which was crucial for the discovery of insulin and for studying the systemic effects of hyperglycemia (Banting et al. 1922). Dogs develop obesity and respond to HFD-induced obesity, developing human-like MetS (Partington et al. 2022). In canine models, obesity-associated inflammation is accompanied by cardiovascular dysfunction characterized by increased myocardial stiffness, impaired ventricular-vascular coupling, and elevations in systolic blood pressure (Partington et al. 2022; Tropf et al. 2017). However, dogs naturally resist atherosclerosis and need prolonged exposure to a high-fat, high-cholesterol diet (Mahley and Weisgraber 1974; Mahley et al. 1974; Moghadasian et al. 2001) or genetic modifications (Zhao et al. 2023), making them less suitable for studies on plaque formation and rupture.

Rabbit Rabbit models are widely used to study cardiovascular complications of MetS, as some physiological characteristics, especially lipid metabolism, closely resemble those observed in humans (Lozano et al. 2019). Unlike rodents, rabbits naturally carry most of their cholesterol in LDL, making them ideal for research on dyslipidemias and atherosclerosis. When fed high-fat, high-sucrose, or cholesterol-rich diets, rabbits develop key features of MetS, including insulin resistance, dyslipidemia, hypertension, and cardiac remodeling. (Alarcon et al. 2018; Sibouakaz et al. 2018). Rabbit models also exhibit elevated levels of inflammatory markers and oxidative stress, as observed in humans (Alarcon et al. 2018). These alterations lead to cardiovascular pathology, including aortic and coronary atherosclerosis, arterial stiffness, and cardiac hypertrophy with fibrosis (Alarcon et al. 2018; Ning et al. 2015; Zheng et al. 2009). Their responses to drugs such as statins (Bustos et al. 1998; Fukumoto et al. 2001; Oikonomidis et al. 2016; Zhang et al. 2016a) and antidiabetic medications (Gueguen et al. 2020; Marquie 1978) further confirm their utility in translational research. Overall, rabbit models offer a relevant and effective system for investigating the mechanisms and treatments of CVD associated with MetS.

Swine Pigs are often used in the study of cardiometabolic diseases because of their physiological, metabolic, and anatomical similarities to humans (Cluzel et al. 2022). Ossabaw, Yucatan, and Yorkshire pigs are commonly used as models to study cardiovascular complications associated with MetS (Charles et al. 2020; Low Wang et al. 2013; Panasevich et al. 2018). The Ossabaw miniature pig on a high-fat, high-cholesterol, and high-fructose diet consistently develops all major features of MetS, along with secondary conditions and hepatic steatosis (Bell et al. 2010; Panasevich et al. 2018), making it a useful model for translational research. Yorkshire pigs also develop all five human MetS criteria within approximately 12 weeks of HFD feeding, including obesity, dyslipidemia, insulin resistance, hypertension, and hyperglycemia, and are accompanied by cardiac comorbidities. Similarly, a 6-month high-fat, high-sugar diet in Yucatan micropigs led to hypertension, dyslipidemia, insulin resistance, and vascular dysfunction, including reduced flow-mediated vasodilation and impaired insulin signaling in the aorta (Low Wang et al. 2013), mirroring the early stages of human vascular disease. Swine models offer complementary platforms for investigating the progression of cardiometabolic disease, from early metabolic dysfunction to overt cardiovascular pathology, and for the evaluation of interventions with translational potential to clinical practice.

Nonhuman Primate (NHP) NHPs naturally develop components of MetS with aging or following exposure to high-fat, high-sugar diets, including central obesity, insulin resistance, dyslipidemia, hypertension, and atherosclerosis (Havel et al. 2017; Zhang et al. 2011). In a key study, NHPs fed a high-fructose diet for 6–12 months developed insulin resistance, central obesity, and dyslipidemia, with a subset progressing to T2DM. This model is valuable for studying the transition from MetS to T2DM and associated cardiovascular risks (Bremer et al. 2011). Close genetic, physiological, and behavioral similarities to humans allow for the study of chronic disease progression, including vascular remodeling, β-cell dysfunction, and systemic inflammation (Havel et al. 2017). Moreover, NHPs are key models in the late preclinical stages of therapeutic development for evaluating pharmacokinetics, safety, and efficacy in a metabolically relevant context (Gotfredsen et al. 2014; Kasichayanula et al. 2018; Knudsen 2010). Ethical concerns, as well as financial and husbandry requirements, limit their use (Table 3).

3 Cardiac Alterations

Individuals with MetS have a 2- to 3-fold increased risk of experiencing a cardiovascular event, and each additional MetS component can elevate the risk of major cardiovascular events, including myocardial infarction and stroke, by approximately 20–30% (Wilson et al. 2005). A meta-analysis of patients with stable coronary artery disease found that MetS increased cardiovascular mortality risk by approximately 19% and major adverse cardiovascular events by 17% (Su and Zhang 2023). Studies using animal models have facilitated the analysis of factors contributing to cardiac remodeling. Here we discuss recent findings.

3.1 Cardiac Structure and Remodeling

Inflammation and Oxidative Stress The following section provides an overview of inflammatory and oxidative pathways that contribute to cardiac remodeling in MetS (for a comprehensive examination see (Wenzl et al. 2021, and Gómez-Viquez, this volume). Each component of MetS is independently associated with chronic, low-grade systemic inflammation (Esposito and Giugliano 2004) and Val-Blasco,

Table 3 Large animal models

Model	Key features	Cardiovascular relevance	Limitations
Canine	Obesity, insulin resistance, hyperlipidemia, responds to HFD	Hypertension, inflammation-induced stiffness, and early MetS-related changes	Resistant to atherosclerosis. Prolonged/high-cholesterol diet or genetic manipulation required
Rabbit	LDL-dominant lipid transport, diet-induced MetS	Aortic/coronary atherosclerosis, cardiac remodeling, drug response (e.g., statins, anti-diabetics)	Less genetic manipulation flexibility than rodents
Swine	Human-like heart anatomy and metabolism; Ossabaw, Yorkshire, Yucatan breeds model full MetS with comorbidities	Vascular dysfunction, insulin signaling defects, cardiac and hepatic pathology	Cost, size, husbandry requirements
Nonhuman primate	Natural development of MetS with diet or age; exhibits obesity, insulin resistance, dyslipidemia, T2DM progression	Longitudinal studies of vascular remodeling, β-cell failure, atherosclerosis, systemic inflammation	Ethical concerns, cost, husbandry, limited availability

this volume). Collectively, these conditions facilitate the circulation of inflammatory cytokines, altered metabolic substrates, and immune dysregulation, highlighting the complex interplay underlying the pathogenesis of MetS (Wenzl et al. 2021). For example, inflammatory biomarkers such as C-reactive protein and interleukin-6 (IL-6) are elevated in both men and women with MetS (Brunner et al. 2002; Ridker et al. 2000) and in animal models (Bao et al. 2015; Martín-Cordero et al. 2011; Zhang et al. 2016b). Additionally, reduced circulating levels of the anti-inflammatory cytokine interleukin-10 (IL-10) have been observed in women with MetS (Esposito et al. 2003). These findings underscore the robust association between MetS and inflammation.

Obesity leads to the recruitment and hypertrophy of adipocytes (Verboven et al. 2018), which in turn increase the production of pro-inflammatory cytokines such as interleukin-1 (IL-1), IL-6, and tumor necrosis factor-alpha (TNF-α) (Uti et al. 2025). These cytokines recruit additional monocytes that infiltrate adipose tissue, which, in turn, release their own chemotactic and proinflammatory factors, thereby amplifying both local and systemic inflammation (Wenzl et al. 2021). Emerging evidence further suggests that diet-induced gut dysbiosis contributes to this systemic inflammatory burden through impaired intestinal barrier function and bacterial translocation, thereby activating the gut-heart axis and promoting myocardial inflammation, adverse cardiac remodeling, and cardiometabolic syndrome (Herisson et al. 2025).

Obesity and hypertension activate the Renin-Angiotensin-Aldosterone System (RAAS) in adipose tissue, leading to a significant secretion of angiotensinogen (Boustany et al. 2004; Manrique et al. 2009; Ornellas et al. 2018). Once cleaved, angiotensinogen is converted into angiotensin II, which, together with aldosterone, activates nuclear factor-kB (NF-κB) in cardiac fibroblasts. This activation promotes immune cell recruitment and contributes to cardiac remodeling (Lu et al. 2021).

Reactive oxygen species (ROS) are normal byproducts of cellular metabolism; however, excessive ROS production can cause oxidative stress, as seen in MetS (Gómez-Viquez, this volume). Adipocytes are significant sources of ROS, and their accumulation is linked to elevated circulating free fatty acid levels and oxidative stress (Cassis et al. 2008). Various animal models of obesity, including rodents and rabbits, have shown increased ROS production, findings that are recapitulated in obese patients (Aragno et al. 2009; Furukawa et al. 2004; Murase et al. 2012). This oxidative burden is further compounded by the RAAS, which also promotes ROS formation in adipocytes and cardiovascular tissue (Cassis et al. 2008). Angiotensin II can activate NADPH oxidase in the heart and vasculature (Dikalov and Nazarewicz 2013), contributing to ROS-related damage in salt-sensitive hypertension (Fujii et al. 2003; Matsui et al. 2008; Park et al. 2002). ROS activate redox-sensitive signaling pathways that induce metabolic alterations in the heart, driving remodeling and functional impairments (Wenzl et al. 2021). Together, chronic inflammation, oxidative stress, and hormonal imbalance converge to create a cardiac microenvironment primed for structural remodeling, hypertrophy, and fibrosis, which are key features of MetS-related cardiac disease.

Hypertrophy A strong association between MetS and left ventricular hypertrophy (LVH) has been consistently demonstrated in both clinical and preclinical studies (Li et al. 2013; Zhou et al. 2025). In this context, LVH represents a maladaptive response to increased myocardial workload and metabolic stress, characterized by left ventricular wall thickening, often accompanied by concentric remodeling that may reduce chamber compliance and diastolic function (Wenzl et al. 2021). Data from the Strong Heart Study indicate that individuals with MetS have a higher prevalence of LVH and an independently elevated risk of cardiovascular events compared with those without MetS, with LVH mediating a significant portion of the excess risk (de Simone et al. 2009). Even in patients with coexisting obesity and hypertension, the presence of MetS is associated with a 2.3-fold higher risk of LVH than in those lacking the full diagnostic criteria. This relationship is attenuated after adjustment for body mass index, suggesting that the impact of MetS on left ventricular (LV) parameters is partly driven by obesity severity (Guerra et al. 2011; Mulè et al. 2005).

Sex-specific differences in LV remodeling have been noted in clinical studies. In a study of nondiabetic hypertensive patients, women with MetS had a 24% greater LV mass and wall thickness than women without MetS. In contrast, men with MetS exhibited only a 9% increase compared with their counterparts. This difference did not reach significance in multivariate models, suggesting that MetS exercises a disproportionately greater influence on LV structure in women (Schillaci et al. 2006). Furthermore, women with MetS without established hypertension or T2DM showed a significantly higher prevalence of LV diastolic dysfunction compared to women without MetS, while no equivalent differences were observed in men. This pattern suggests that women may exhibit measurable subclinical ventricular dysfunction at an earlier stage of metabolic dysregulation, even before the development of overt comorbidities (Aijaz et al. 2008).

Animal models have been instrumental in recapitulating MetS-associated cardiac hypertrophy and investigating the underlying molecular mechanisms. Increases in heart or LV mass and LV wall thickness have been observed in several rat models, including the fructose-fed, salt overload, ZFDM, DS/obese, OLETF (Marino et al. 2023; Matsui et al. 2008; Murase et al. 2012; Otani et al. 2022; Zhang et al. 2018). Mice with diet and genetically induced metabolic dysfunction, including STZ-treated mice fed an HFD, obese db/db and ob/ob mice exposed to excess aldosterone, have also been described as showing LV remodeling (Alex et al. 2018; Hegyi et al. 2022; Zhao et al. 2016). LVH has also been observed in wild-type and transgenic mice with cardiac-specific L-type Ca^{2+} channel overexpression fed an HFD combined with nitric oxide synthase inhibition (L-NAME), as well as genetically hypertensive mouse strains (Li et al. 2023; Lira et al. 2023; Schiattarella et al. 2019; Sharma et al. 2023). Sex-dependent effects have also been reported in preclinical models, mirroring human studies: in the db/db model, females exhibited a 31.3% greater increase in cardiomyocyte size compared to age-matched db/db males (Alex et al. 2018). MetS-induced LVH is also well established in large animal models, including rabbits fed a high-fat or high-cholesterol diet (Carroll and Tyagi 2005; Nachar et al. 2019; Sibouakaz et al. 2018); pigs fed HFD (Li et al. 2017; Zhang et al. 2015), a high-fat/high-sucrose diet (Xia et al. 2015), or a western diet (Tang et al. 2025); and obese canines (Tropf et al. 2017). Clinical and preclinical data highlight the role of MetS as a major driver of pathological hypertrophy.

Fibrosis Adult cardiac fibroblasts are responsible for producing and maintaining the heart's extracellular matrix, particularly collagen types I and III, which are key to the preservation of myocardial structure and contractile force (Cavalera et al. 2014). Collagen I imparts tensile strength and rigidity, while collagen III contributes to elasticity and compliance. Enhanced fibroblast activation, altered collagen composition, and sustained inflammatory signals converge to increase extracellular matrix across multiple animal models and in humans with MetS (Cavalera et al. 2014; Mizushige et al. 2000; Yeo et al. 2025). Several MetS models, including Zucker obese rats, OLETF rats (Lee et al. 2012; Mizushige et al. 2000), BPH-STZ mice (Sharma et al. 2023), STZ mice fed a HFD (Marino et al. 2023; Zhang et al. 2018), db/db mice (Zhao et al. 2016), ob/ob mice (Zaman et al. 2004), and DS/obese rats, have shown enhanced total cardiac collagen content, often concomitant with increased collagen mRNA expression (Murase et al. 2012). Increased cardiac collagen deposition has also been described in both rabbit (Carroll and Tyagi 2005; Nachar et al. 2019; Sibouakaz et al. 2018; Zeng et al. 2017) and swine (Li et al. 2017; Tang et al. 2025; Xia et al. 2015) models of MetS. Human studies further support these findings. A global meta-analysis, conducted by Yeo et al. (2025), estimated that approximately one in three individuals with cardiometabolic conditions, including hypertension, T2DM, and obesity, develop myocardial fibrosis. Across conditions, hypertension showed the highest overall prevalence (35.7%), followed by T2DM (31.6%) and obesity/mixed populations (26.5%) (Yeo et al. 2025). These findings underscore the clinical relevance of fibrosis as a structural hallmark of MetS cardiomyopathy and highlight the crucial role of preclinical models in elucidating mechanisms.

3.2 Cardiac Function

Metabolic Substrate Utilization Cardiac metabolism and contractile function are interconnected; increased contractile demand elevates energy requirements, while alterations in substrate utilization can directly impact cardiac performance. Under resting aerobic conditions, the adult heart primarily relies on mitochondrial oxidative phosphorylation (OXPHOS) of fatty acids, which supplies approximately 60–90% of its ATP; the remainder is derived from carbohydrate oxidation, including glucose and lactate (Fukushima and Lopaschuk 2016; Mouton et al. 2020). The heart maintains metabolic flexibility to adapt to energy demands, such as increasing glucose oxidation during exercise; this adaptability is impaired in MetS. In patients with MetS, elevated circulating free fatty acids, combined with insulin resistance and impaired glucose utilization, result in a chronic shift toward fatty-acid-dependent OXPHOS (Fukushima and Lopaschuk 2016; Mouton et al. 2020). This metabolic shift has been consistently reproduced in rodent models of MetS. Ob/ob and db/db mice exhibit increased myocardial fatty acid oxidation and lipid accumulation (Buchanan et al. 2005; DeMarco et al. 2013; Dobrzyn et al. 2010). Similarly, Zucker obese, ZFDM, and OLETF rats exhibit elevated circulating free fatty acids that inhibit translocation of the glucose transporter GLUT4 to the cell membrane, thereby impairing glucose uptake and utilization (Lee et al. 2012; Semeniuk et al. 2002; van den Brom et al. 2009; Yokoi et al. 2013). In ZFDM rats, insulin-mediated myocardial glucose utilization is reduced by 66%, with a corresponding increase in reliance on fatty acid oxidation (van den Brom et al. 2009). Diet-induced MetS in pigs and dogs shows similar patterns of increased fatty acid oxidation and decreased glucose uptake (Henry et al. 2024). Despite increased cardiac fatty-acid-driven OXPHOS activity, excessive lipid accumulation promotes lipotoxicity and oxidative stress, contributing to a pro-inflammatory environment observed in MetS and potentially leading to further impaired myocardial function (Christoffersen et al. 2003; Fillmore et al. 2014; Hall et al. 2014).

The metabolic, structural, and functional consequences of MetS lead to cardiomyopathies and heart failure. Heart failure is a clinical syndrome characterized by structural or functional cardiac abnormalities that impair ventricular filling or ejection, leading to reduced cardiac output, elevated intracardiac filling pressures, reduced exercise tolerance, fatigue, peripheral edema, and pulmonary congestion

(Thorp and Filipp 2025). Cardiomyopathies associated with MetS most commonly present as heart failure with preserved ejection fraction (HFpEF), characterized by diastolic dysfunction and increased myocardial stiffness; however, in advanced stages or in the presence of ischemic injury, progression to heart failure with reduced ejection fraction (HFrEF), marked by impaired systolic function and reduced ejection fraction, may occur.

Systolic Dysfunction The phase of the cardiac cycle during which the heart (primarily the ventricles) contracts and ejects blood into the arterial circulation is known as systole. The amount of blood pumped during this phase is known as the ejection fraction (EF) and is used to assess systolic function. Systolic dysfunction occurs in approximately 24% of patients with T2DM (Fang et al. 2005). EF was negatively correlated to diastolic blood pressure in a cohort of patients, indicating that hypertension is associated with worse systolic function (Wu et al. 2024). This can be recapitulated in animal models, such as db/db, ob/ob, STZ mice, and rats fed a high-sucrose diet (Christoffersen et al. 2003; DeMarco et al. 2013; Vasanji et al. 2006; Wichi et al. 2007), which exhibit reduced EF and fiber shortening velocity. Reduced EF has also been observed in naturally diabetic cynomolgus monkeys and in monkeys fed a high-fat/high-sucrose diet (Gu et al. 2015; Zheng et al. 2021). Some of the same rodent models (STZ, db/db, and DS/obese rats), however, have also shown higher EF (Alex et al. 2018; Murase et al. 2012; Zhang et al. 2016b). A significantly elevated EF may indicate cardiac hypertrophy that impairs cardiac relaxation and filling (diastolic dysfunction) (Landucci et al. 2025).

Diastolic Dysfunction Diastole is the phase of the cardiac cycle when the ventricles relax and fill with blood from the atria. In diastolic dysfunction, the ventricles fail to relax properly, thereby impairing their ability to fill efficiently during diastole. Diastolic dysfunction affects approximately 60–75% of patients with diabetes, with prevalence rising significantly in patients with multiple comorbidities (Riehle and Bauersachs 2018). For example, patients with hypertension and MetS exhibit more severe diastolic dysfunction compared to those with hypertension alone. Similarly, obese individuals with hypertension have a more severe phenotype than in either condition individually (Kim et al. 2016; Mulè et al. 2005).

A key parameter of diastolic function, measured by echocardiography, is the E/A wave ratio, derived from transmitral Doppler flow patterns (Rajiah et al. 2023). The E wave represents early passive filling of the left ventricle, while the A wave reflects late filling due to atrial contraction (Fig. 1) (Oh et al. 2011; Rajiah et al. 2023). In healthy individuals, the E wave is typically larger than the A wave, resulting in a normal E/A ratio of about 1–1.5. In diastolic dysfunction, this pattern progresses through discernible stages. In Grade I (impaired relaxation), early filling is reduced, lowering the E wave, while atrial contraction compensates, increasing the A wave, resulting in a reversed E/A ratio ($E < A$). In Grade II (pseudonormalization), elevated left atrial pressure results in early filling, making the E/A ratio appear normal despite underlying dysfunction. In Grade III (restrictive filling), markedly elevated filling pressures cause the E wave to dominate ($E \gg A$), reflecting severe diastolic

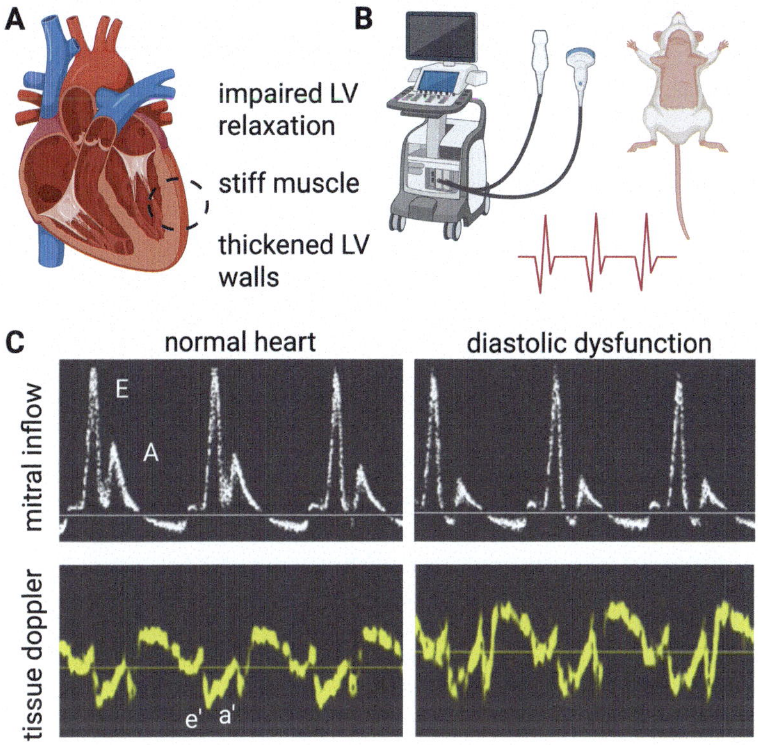

Fig. 1 Structural and functional analysis of left ventricular (LV) diastolic dysfunction using echocardiography. (**a**) Illustration showing key features of LV diastolic dysfunction, such as impaired myocardial relaxation, increased stiffness, and concentric wall thickening. (**b**) Experimental setup for transthoracic echocardiography in anesthetized mice to evaluate cardiac function. (**c**) Representative pulsed-wave Doppler (top) and tissue Doppler imaging (bottom) recordings from the apical four-chamber view of a normal heart (left) and a heart with diastolic dysfunction (right). Mitral inflow velocities (E and A waves) and septal annular velocities (e′ and a′) are displayed. Essential parameters for assessing diastolic function include the E/A and E/e′ ratios. (A and B created with Biorender)

impairment (Oh et al. 2011; Rajiah et al. 2023). Because pseudonormal patterns can mimic normal physiology, additional echocardiographic techniques—such as tissue Doppler imaging (TDI)—are often necessary. TDI measures the early diastolic mitral annular velocity (e'), which reflects the rate of myocardial relaxation (Oh et al. 2011; Rajiah et al. 2023). A reduced e' velocity combined with an elevated E/e' ratio indicates increased left ventricular filling pressures and helps distinguish pseudonormal from truly normal diastolic filling patterns.

Multiple animal models of MetS have been used to deepen the understanding of diastolic dysfunction. In genetically obese mice such as db/db and ob/ob (especially when combined with aldosterone-induced hypertension), echocardiographic findings include decreased E/A ratios, prolonged diastolic filling time, and increased left ventricular end-diastolic pressure (Alex et al. 2018; Christoffersen et al. 2003; DeMarco et al. 2013; Dobrzyn et al. 2010; Habibi et al. 2017; Hall et al. 2014; Hegyi et al. 2022; Semeniuk et al. 2002; Zhao et al. 2016). Similar findings have been reported in obese rat models, such as the Zucker obese and OLETF rats, in which prolonged diastolic filling time indicates impaired relaxation (Mizushige et al. 2000; Zhou et al. 2010). In ZFDM rats, age-dependent increases in end-diastolic volume and reduced e' velocity have been observed (Baynes and Murray 2009; van den Brom et al. 2009). This was accompanied by a reduction in maximal contraction force in isolated cardiomyocytes from this model (van den Brom et al. 2009).

Diet-induced models of MetS also replicate diastolic dysfunction. Diets high in fat, sucrose, or fructose independently impair diastolic parameters (Mostarda et al. 2012; Sankaralingam et al. 2014; Vasanji et al. 2006). When combined, these effects are often more pronounced, as seen in high-fat/high-sucrose and high-fat/high-fructose-fed mice (Croteau et al. 2020; Manrique et al. 2009). Increased E/e' ratios are also noted in high-cholesterol diet-fed rabbits and western diet-fed pigs (Nachar et al. 2019; Tang et al. 2025; Tropf et al. 2017). Diastolic dysfunction is also exacerbated in models combining HFD with low-dose STZ to mimic T2DM and models that combine HFD and chemical or surgical induction of hypertension. For example, HFD+ L-NAME and HFD-fed pigs that underwent unilateral renal artery stenosis surgery to make them hypertensive (Li et al. 2023; Lira et al. 2023; Schiattarella et al. 2019; Zhang et al. 2015).

3.3 Involvement of Sympathetic and Parasympathetic Innervation

The sympathetic nervous system acts on the heart via noradrenaline, primarily binding to β-1 adrenergic receptors and inducing a rise in heart rate. Concurrently, the binding of acetylcholine to parasympathetic muscarinic receptors in the heart has an inhibitory effect, decreasing the heart rate (Gordan et al. 2015). Cardiac dysfunction observed in MetS may be partially attributable to sympatho-vagal imbalance characterized by a shift toward sympathetic dominance and reduced parasympathetic (vagal) influence. Both humans with MetS and preclinical models of MetS show increased cardiac and vascular sympathetic tone and reduced vagal influence (Brito et al. 2008; Huggett et al. 2004). These alterations often precede the development of hypertension or diabetes (Canale et al. 2013; De Angelis et al. 2012). Autonomic imbalance results from central dysregulation, driven by insulin and leptin resistance, inflammation, and oxidative stress, as well as by impairment of peripheral arterial baroreceptor signaling and efferent vagal pathways (Canale et al. 2013; Harthmann et al. 2007).

3.4 Calcium Mishandling

Calcium cycling in cardiomyocytes is essential for excitation-contraction coupling. With each beat, a cardiomyocyte action potential triggers the opening of L-type calcium channels (LTCC), allowing calcium influx. LTCC-mediated calcium influx triggers further calcium release from the sarcoplasmic reticulum (SR) via ryanodine receptors (RyRs), leading to cardiomyocyte contraction. To terminate contraction and restore baseline levels, calcium is removed from the cytosol through sodium-calcium exchangers or reuptake into calcium stores by the sarco/endoplasmic reticulum calcium ATPase (SERCA) (Gilbert et al. 2020; see Avelino-Cruz, this volume). Animal models of MetS have provided key information showing that disruption of this tightly coordinated system contributes to contractile dysfunction, although the nature of the defects varies with disease stage. In STZ-treated rats and db/db mice, reduced calcium entry into cardiomyocytes has been observed at both the cellular and whole-heart levels (Bergh et al. 1988; Pereira et al. 2006). In a 15-week-old db/db mouse, whole-cell LTCC currents are blunted despite preserved single-channel activity, indicating that reduced channel number or membrane availability, rather than channel functionality, accounts for diminished channel density (Pereira et al. 2006). Subsequent work showed reduced LTCC protein expression in cardiomyocytes from db/db mice and ZFDM (Howarth et al. 2012; Lu et al. 2011b; Pereira et al. 2006). Emerging data from obesity and HFD models suggest that early MetS may not involve marked transcriptional downregulation of the LTCC but instead involves altered channel trafficking, membrane localization, or phosphorylation, consistent with preserved total protein but reduced function (Al Kury 2020; Aromolaran and Boutjdir 2017; Lu et al. 2011a). Thus, LTCC dysfunction in MetS appears to arise from reduced protein levels in advanced diabetes and from spatial/posttranslational modifications in earlier insulin-resistance states.

In addition to reduced Ca^{2+} entry, SR calcium content is reduced in both db/db mice (Pereira et al. 2006) and STZ-treated rats (Lacombe et al. 2007). This reduction could result from impaired calcium reuptake or increased calcium leak from the SR. Reduced SERCA expression has been consistently reported in several models, including db/db mice, Zucker obese rats, STZ rats, OLETF rats, sucrose-fed rats, and Western diet rats (Abe et al. 2002; Lacombe et al. 2007; Manrique et al. 2009; Pereira et al. 2006; Russ et al. 1991; Vasanji et al. 2006), suggesting compromised calcium reuptake. Accordingly, cardiomyocytes from db/db mice made hypertensive with aldosterone exhibit calcium transients with slower decay, consistent with slower SR reuptake (Hegyi et al. 2022). A reduction in RyR protein has also been reported in several models, including db/db mice, STZ mice fed an HFD, and STZ rats (Marino et al. 2023; Pereira et al. 2006). Despite fewer channels, the Ca^{2+} spark frequency was increased in STZ rats, suggesting that the functional channels may be leaky (Shao et al. 2007). Phosphorylation of RyR by CaMKII has been suggested to promote spontaneous Ca^{2+} events in a rodent model of early-stage diabetes and in models of MetS (Federico et al. 2017; Sommese et al. 2016). Disruption of myocyte calcium homeostasis, characterized by reduced SERCA expression, lower SR calcium content, and RyR2 dysregulation, has also been reported in diabetic and HFD canine models (Aromolaran and Boutjdir 2017; Dincer et al. 2006). In Ossabaw pigs with MetS, changes in calcium handling have been reported in coronary smooth muscle cells (Heaps et al. 2000; Hill et al. 2001). These studies underline the importance of calcium handling in MetS-related cardiomyopathy.

4 Vascular Dysfunction in MetS

MetS-associated vascular dysfunction contributes to hypertension and impaired tissue perfusion, and it also amplifies cardiac remodeling and end-organ damage. The vascular system consists of a branching network of large and small vessels that work together to regulate tissue perfusion, nutrient delivery, and hemodynamic stability. Large arteries, such as the aorta and its main branches, serve as conduit vessels that carry blood at high pressure and help control pulsatile blood flow. Small arteries, arterioles, and capillaries form the microcirculation, which regulates vascular resistance, facilitates gas and nutrient exchange, and actively responds to local metabolic demands.

Arteries are made up of three layers: the tunica intima, the tunica media, and the tunica adventitia. The tunica intima, the innermost layer, consists of endothelial cells that line the blood vessel lumen. These cells are essential for maintaining vascular health by regulating vasomotor tone, permeability, leukocyte adhesion, and preventing blood clots through the secretion of mediators such as NO and prostacyclin (Schreyer et al. 1998). In MetS, intimal dysfunction is characterized by reduced NO availability, oxidative stress, and heightened pro-inflammatory signaling, affecting both large vessels, such as the coronary and carotid arteries, and smaller vessels, including those in skeletal muscle, the kidneys, and the retinal arterioles. The tunica media primarily consists of vascular smooth muscle (VSMCs) embedded in an elastic, collagen-rich matrix. This layer regulates vessel diameter and compliance through coordinated contraction and relaxation. In large arteries, elastic fibers in the media help absorb the pulsatile pressure from the heartbeat. In contrast, in resistance arteries and arterioles, the smooth muscle plays a more prominent role, actively adjusting vascular tone. In MetS, VSMCs shift from a contractile to a synthetic phenotype, leading to matrix remodeling, collagen buildup, and elastin breakdown, which contribute to arterial stiffness and hypertrophy in both large and small vessels. The outermost layer, the tunica adventitia, contains fibroblasts, connective tissue, nerve endings, and, in larger vessels, the vasa vasorum, which supply nutrients to the adventitia and outer media layer of the vessel wall. In MetS-associated vascular disease, the adventitia may undergo fibrotic remodeling, exhibit sympathetic hyperactivity, and show infiltration by inflammatory cells, further worsening vascular damage (Kuppusamy et al. 2025; Kuwabara and Tallquist 2017; Zeng and Yang 2024).

The impact of MetS-associated vascular disease varies across the entire vascular tree. Large arteries are prone to atherosclerotic plaques and stiffening, while small resistance arteries exhibit reduced vasodilation and capillary rarefaction. The following sections discuss MetS-associated vascular dysfunction, drawing on evidence from preclinical models and clinical studies.

4.1 Conduit Arteries: Endothelial Dysfunction, Atherosclerosis, and Arterial Stiffness

Endothelial dysfunction is a key early event in conduit artery pathology in MetS, contributing to the development of atherosclerosis and arterial stiffening. Clinical studies have demonstrated impaired flow-mediated dilation and elevated circulating adhesion molecule levels, which are associated with insulin resistance, systemic inflammation, and adverse cardiovascular outcomes (Hingorani et al. 2000; Mahdi et al. 2020; Yang et al. 2024).

Metabolic stressors in MetS, including hyperglycemia, elevated free fatty acids, and oxidative stress, converge to reduce nitric oxide (NO) bioavailability. This occurs through uncoupling of endothelial nitric oxide synthase (eNOS), depletion of its cofactor, tetrahydrobiopterin (BH4), and increased scavenging of NO by ROS. In parallel, endothelial cells produce more vasoconstrictors such as endothelin-1 (ET-1) and thromboxane A2, further shifting the balance toward vasoconstriction and inflammation (Russo et al. 2002; Yang et al. 2024). Rodent models, including db/db, ob/ob, and Zucker obese rats, have been instrumental in defining these mechanisms. Studies in these models have identified NADPH oxidase activation, TNF-α-mediated inflammatory signaling, and oxidative stress-driven eNOS dysfunction as key contributors to impaired endothelium-dependent vasodilation (Bagi et al. 2003; Eringa et al. 2007; Lee et al. 2017; Pannirselvam et al. 2002; Shinozaki et al. 2004; Traupe et al. 2002; Winters et al. 2000; Youn et al. 2015).

Atherosclerosis is a chronic inflammatory disease of large arteries, and it is a significant cause of myocardial infarction, stroke, and peripheral arterial disease. Individuals with MetS have a higher risk of atherosclerotic lesions (Boudoulas et al. 2016). Endothelial dysfunction initiates this process by promoting lipid retention, leukocyte adhesion, foam cell formation, and sustained vascular inflammation (Gallo and Savoia 2024; Getz and Reardon 2012; Hwang et al. 1997; Yang et al. 2024). Genetically modified rodent models, particularly ApoE−/− and LDLR−/− mice, provide mechanistic insights into lesion development, immune cell recruitment, and inflammatory plaque remodeling (Wang et al. 2019; Zaragoza et al. 2011). However, these models rarely develop coronary artery disease or plaque rupture, which are hallmarks of advanced human disease.

Large-animal models overcome these constraints. Ossabaw pigs fed Western diets develop complex coronary plaques with necrotic cores, fibrous caps, and macrophage infiltration—closely mirroring human pathology (Dyson et al. 2006; Hamamdzic and Wilensky 2013). WHHL rabbits with LDLR deficiency develop aortic lesions characterized by calcifications and smooth muscle-derived foam cells (Ohtani et al. 2008; Shiomi and Ito 2009). These models demonstrate that advanced lesion structures and inflammatory characteristics are preserved in large species, making them key for preclinical drug and device testing and imaging.

Conduit artery dysfunction in MetS is also marked by increased arterial stiffness, commonly assessed by pulse wave velocity (PWV). Clinical studies have found that elevated PWV is an independent predictor of cardiovascular events in patients with hypertension and diabetes (Ben-Shlomo et al. 2014; Cruickshank et al. 2002). A longitudinal birth cohort study of 3,862 adolescents followed for 7 years (adjusting for age and multiple metabolic and lifestyle factors) found that increased arterial stiffness precedes the development of MetS, supporting a causal prognostic role (Agbaje 2023). Systematic reviews linking PWV to metabolic and cardiovascular outcomes also support these findings (Starzak et al. 2022; Stehouwer et al. 2008).

Mechanistic studies in animal models have provided insight into the cellular and molecular basis of stiffness. Rodent studies have shown that arterial stiffness can develop in response to high-fat or high-sucrose diets even in the absence of overt hypertension, suggesting that stiffness is not just a secondary consequence of elevated blood pressure (Weisbrod et al. 2013). Structural contributors include increased collagen deposition, elastin fiber fragmentation, and extracellular matrix remodeling (Kohn et al. 2015; Wesley et al. 2024). At the molecular level, advanced glycation end-products (AGEs), matrix metalloproteinases (MMPs), chronic low-grade inflammation, enhanced RAAS signaling, oxidative stress, and VSMC phenotypic switching from a contractile to a synthetic phenotype all contribute to reduced arterial compliance (Lacolley et al. 2017; Santana et al. 2014). Collectively, clinical studies and animal models support the roles of endothelial dysfunction, inflammation, and metabolic injury in promoting atherosclerotic lesion development and contributing to biomechanical stiffening of the arterial wall.

4.2 Small Resistance Arteries and Microcirculation

MetS-related pathology in small resistance arteries and the microcirculation directly affects tissue perfusion, nutrient exchange, and metabolic homeostasis. The microcirculation comprises small resistance arteries, arterioles, capillaries, and post-capillary venules, which function as an integrated network to regulate vascular resistance, blood flow, and exchange, as well as to support immune surveillance (Granger and Senchenkova 2010). Small resistance arteries, typically 100–300 μm in luminal diameter, have multiple layers of vascular smooth muscle and function as upstream regulators of microvascular flow. These arteries branch into arterioles, which typically range in diameter from 10 to 100 μm and are surrounded by 1–2 layers of VSMCs (Wenceslau et al. 2021). Through myogenic, endothelial, neural, and metabolic mechanisms, resistance arteries and arterioles adjust their caliber to match local blood flow to tissue demand, thereby contributing substantially to blood pressure regulation.

Capillaries are the primary sites for nutrient, gas, and hormone exchange. Structurally, they consist of a single layer of endothelial cells, a thin extracellular matrix called the basement membrane, pericytes, and a luminal endothelial glycocalyx. Pericytes are multifunctional cells that wrap around the microvascular wall (especially capillaries and post-capillary venules) and interact closely with endothelial cells to regulate functions such as blood flow, permeability, and endothelial phenotype. Downstream post-capillary venules, which contain many pericytes, serve as key sites for leukocyte adhesion, transmigration, and inflammatory signaling (Granger and Senchenkova 2010). Disruption of microvascular structure and function impairs vasodilation, barrier integrity, and tissue perfusion, thereby linking microvascular dysfunction to multi-organ metabolic dysregulation and elevated cardiovascular risk in MetS (Serne et al. 2007).

Resistant Artery Dysfunction on MetS In MetS, resistance arteries show impaired vasodilatory capacity, increased basal tone, and defective insulin delivery. Rodent models, such as db/db mice, Zucker obese rats, and GK rats, have shown impaired endothelium-dependent vasodilatory pathways, including acetylcholine- and insulin-mediated vasodilation, associated with reduced eNOS expression, BH4 depletion, increased oxidative stress, and elevated ET-1 signaling (Eringa et al. 2007; Pannirselvam et al. 2002; Shinozaki et al. 2004; Wallis et al. 2002; Witte et al. 2003). Endothelial ion channel dysfunction also contributes to impaired vasodilation in MetS and diabetes. STZ-treated rats show reduced expression of TRPV4 and SK/IK channels, impairing the TRPV4/SK/IK signaling axis that promotes endothelium-dependent hyperpolarization and vasodilation (Ma et al. 2013; Sonkusare et al. 2012). In db/db mice, reduced TRPV1 expression was associated with increased ROS production and endothelial dysfunction (Sun et al. 2013). Moreover, hyperglycemic conditions have been shown to increase store-operated Ca^{2+} entry (SOCE) by upregulating STIM and Orai channels in umbilical vein endothelial cells (HUVECs) and endothelial cells from patients with T2DM (Nieves-Cintron et al. 2021).

Endothelium-independent mechanisms, including alterations in VSMC Ca^{2+} handling and contractility, are also implicated in impaired resistance-artery function in MetS and diabetes. Central to VSMC function is precise spatiotemporal control of intracellular Ca^{2+} signaling. VSM Ca^{2+} homeostasis depends on the coordinated regulation of Ca^{2+} influx through plasma membrane voltage-dependent and receptor-operated channels, Ca^{2+} release from SR stores via RyR and inositol 1,4,5-trisphosphate receptors (IP_3Rs), and SR Ca^{2+} reuptake by sarco/endoplasmic reticulum Ca^{2+} ATPase (SERCA) (Tykocki et al. 2017). Ca^{2+} influx through plasma membrane L-type Ca^{2+} channels (Ca^{2+} sparklets), as well as IP_3R-mediated Ca^{2+} release, are linked to contraction. Meanwhile, subcellular Ca^{2+} release events generated by RyRs in the SR (Ca^{2+} sparks) activate closely apposed large-conductance Ca^{2+}-activated K^+ (BK_{Ca}) channels at the plasma membrane, promoting hyperpolarization and vasodilation (Nelson et al. 1995). In MetS and diabetes, the VSMC Ca^{2+} signaling network becomes dysregulated. Increased Ca^{2+} influx through voltage-gated Ca^{2+} channels elevates resting $[Ca^{2+}]_i$, thereby altering contractility and transcriptional regulation (Navedo et al. 2010; Nystoriak et al. 2017). Impaired SERCA expression (Rueda, this volume) and function reduce SR Ca^{2+} uptake, leading to Ca^{2+} store depletion and compensatory upregulation of SOCE pathways. While SOCE plays a minimal role in differentiated contractile VSMC, it becomes relevant during VSMC phenotypic switching from the contractile to the proliferative/synthetic state, a process that contributes to vascular remodeling in MetS (Brozovich et al. 2016; Trebak 2012). Altered RyR function disrupts Ca^{2+} spark generation, thereby impairing Ca^{2+} spark-BK_{Ca} coupling and reducing the hyperpolarization-mediated negative-feedback regulation of voltage-gated Ca^{2+} channel activity (Rueda et al. 2013). Collectively, these alterations contribute to abnormal vascular tone and reactivity.

A growing body of literature indicates that changes in the activity and expression of ion channels, including L-type Ca^{2+}, K_V, BK_{Ca}, K_{ATP}, RyR, and IP_3R, contribute to altered reactivity of resistance arteries in MetS and diabetes (Nieves-Cintron et al. 2021). For example, increased L-type Ca^{2+} activity and downregulation of BK_{Ca} and K_V channels contribute to increased vascular tone and hypertension in models such as HFD mice, STZ-treated mice, and rats (Nieves-Cintron et al. 2021). Similar findings are observed in swine models. In Ossabaw pigs, increased $Ca_V1.2$ phosphorylation and reduced BK_{Ca} β1 subunit expression led to heightened vascular contractility in resistance vessels (Berwick et al. 2013; Borbouse et al. 2009). Dysfunction of $K_V1.5$ and $K_V2.1$ in diet-induced obese pigs further supports a conserved mechanism of VSMC excitability and dysregulation (Mokelke et al. 2005; Yang et al. 2007). Notably, increased $Ca_V1.2$ activity and reduced BK_{Ca} activity have also been observed in VSM from human patients with diabetes (Nieves-Cintron et al. 2017; Nystoriak et al. 2017). These parallel findings across species support the therapeutic potential of VSMC ion channels in MetS-related hypertension.

Capillary Rarefaction MetS is characterized by capillary rarefaction, defined as a reduction in functional capillary density. This phenomenon is observed across multiple tissues, including skeletal muscle, brown adipose tissue, the kidney, the brain, and the myocardium (Horton and Barrett 2021; Paavonsalo et al. 2020). Rodent models of MetS have been key in shedding light on mechanisms underlying capillary rarefaction, suggesting that MetS and diabetes induce structural and functional capillary loss through endothelial dysfunction, impaired angiogenic signaling, oxidative stress, inflammation, and altered endothelial-pericyte interactions (Paavonsalo et al. 2020; Sorop et al. 2017). Capillary rarefaction has also been described in large-animal models, including obese Ossabaw pigs with MetS, which exhibit coronary artery remodeling and capillary rarefaction that contribute to myocardial ischemia (Trask et al. 2012). Diabetic Yorkshire pigs exhibit retinal capillary loss and basement membrane thickening, paralleling the progression of human diabetic retinopathy (Lee et al. 2010). Clinical studies provide parallel evidence of rarefaction in humans with MetS (Horton and Barrett 2021).

Pericyte Loss and Basement Membrane Remodeling Capillary instability in MetS is further driven by pericyte dysfunction and remodeling of the basement membrane. Rodent models of MetS consistently exhibit pericyte dropout, hypertrophy, and impaired endothelial-pericyte communication, particularly in the retina, where classic lesions include acellular capillaries and pericyte ghosts (Engerman et al. 1962;

Steinle et al. 2009). Acellular capillaries are non-functional basement membrane tubes devoid of endothelial and pericyte cells, while pericyte ghosts are residual imprints along the capillary wall following pericyte death. These lesions are well documented in db/db mice, ZFDM rats, and OLETF rats, which exhibit progressive pericyte loss, basement membrane thickening, and reduced capillary density with disease progression (Curtis et al. 2009; Miyamura et al. 1999; Robinson et al. 2012; Simmonds et al. 2024). Pericyte loss and rarefaction are also seen in peritubular and glomerular capillaries in diabetic nephropathy. In skeletal muscle and myocardium, similar processes impair tissue perfusion and oxygen delivery (Mauricio et al. 2023).

Young Ossabaw pigs fed a Western diet for 10 weeks develop retinal pericyte ghosts, reduced pericyte-to-endothelial ratios, decreased capillary density, and marked thickening of the capillary basement membrane (Lim et al. 2018). In the brain, diabetes is associated with pericyte loss, which contributes to cerebral microvascular dysfunction and cognitive impairment (Li and Fan 2023; van Sloten et al. 2020). Related models also show similar patterns. For example, the HIP rat, a non-obese transgenic model that expresses human islet amyloid polypeptide (hIAPP), develops islet amyloid deposition, progressive β-cell failure, hyperglycemia, pericyte loss, and intra-islet capillary rarefaction as the animals age (Hayden et al. 2008, 2010). Ren2 rats (a hypertensive model overexpressing the mouse renin gene) also exhibit oxidative stress and remodeling of pancreatic islet pericytes (Hayden et al. 2007). Such parallels further reinforce the pathophysiological importance of endothelial-pericyte interactions in maintaining capillary integrity in MetS.

Together, resistance artery dysfunction, VSMC ion channel remodeling, capillary rarefaction, and pericyte-basement membrane pathology contribute to MetS-associated microvascular phenotype. These changes limit tissue perfusion, impair insulin and oxygen delivery, and promote end-organ damage. The consistency of these mechanisms across rodent, large-animal, and human studies underscores the vasculature as a critical contributing factor to cardiometabolic disease.

5 Perspective

Rodent models provide unparalleled access to molecular mechanisms through genetic manipulation and high-throughput experimental paradigms, revealing causal pathways linking metabolic dysfunction to cardiac remodeling and vascular impairment, thereby informing therapeutic development. Recent examples of therapeutic development in cardiometabolic disease include glucagon-like peptide-1 (GLP-1) receptor agonists and sodium-glucose cotransporter 2 (SGLT2) inhibitors. GLP-1 is an incretin hormone produced in the gut. It stimulates insulin secretion, suppresses glucagon release, slows gastric emptying, and reduces appetite. SGLT2 in the kidneys reabsorbs glucose from the filtrate back into the blood. SGLT2 inhibitors lower blood glucose levels by preventing reabsorption, thereby allowing glucose to be excreted in the urine. Studies in ApoE−/− and LDLr−/− mice demonstrated that GLP-1 receptor agonists (liraglutide and semaglutide) reduce atherosclerotic plaque development by downregulating inflammatory pathways, including leukocyte recruitment, adhesion, and extravasation (Rakipovski et al. 2018). Similarly, SGLT2 inhibitors have been shown to reduce cardiac fibrosis by inhibiting the TGF-β/Smad pathway and by reducing oxidative stress and to improve cardiac energy metabolism by enhancing mitochondrial ATP production and reducing oxidative stress in diabetic rodent models (Bugga et al. 2022; Tian et al. 2021; Verma et al. 2018). Vascular studies in multiple diabetic and MetS rodent models have shown that SGLT2 inhibitors improve endothelial function, reduce arterial stiffness, and enhance coronary microvascular function through AMP-activated protein kinase activation, eNOS phosphorylation, and NADPH oxidase suppression (Al Thani et al. 2023). Systematic reviews support these cardioprotective effects across diverse preclinical models (Alshnbari et al. 2020). While rodent studies, as described above, have identified multiple potential cardioprotective pathways, the precise mechanisms underlying the cardiovascular benefits of SGLT2 inhibitors and GLP-1 agonists in humans remain incompletely understood, highlighting the need for mechanistic studies across model systems (Al Thani et al. 2023). Moreover, important limitations, including species-specific differences in lipid metabolism, coronary artery structure, and disease progression, can be significant compared with humans.

Large-animal models, such as swine, dogs, rabbits and NHP, more closely approximate human cardiometabolic physiology, including lipoprotein profiles, vascular architecture, endothelial dysfunction, arterial remodeling, and capillary rarefaction. As such, these models offer invaluable opportunities to validate mechanisms and to preclinically test pharmacological and device-based interventions. For example, the porcine coronary artery model has been instrumental in the development and safety assessment of drug-eluting stents, which have been extensively tested in healthy and diabetic/hypercholesterolemic swine before their adoption in clinical practice (Llano et al. 2011; Schwartz et al. 2004; Schwartz et al. 2008). GLP-1 agonists and SGLT2 inhibitors have been tested in clinically relevant MetS and diabetic swine models, confirming cardioprotective mechanisms in a more human-relevant context, including improved myocardial function and coronary microvascular dynamics (Harris et al. 2025; Muir et al. 2026).

NHPs have been used to evaluate the metabolism, safety/toxicology, and pharmacokinetics of GLP-1 agonists and SGLT2 inhibitors, but not necessarily their cardiovascular efficacy, as assessed in clinical trials (Al Thani et al. 2023; Gotfredsen et al. 2014; Zhang et al. 2020). Both GLP-1 agonists and SGLT2 inhibitors have been successfully implemented in the clinics. The EMPA-REG OUTCOME trial showed a 38% reduction in cardiovascular death and a 35% reduction in heart failure hospitalizations in patients with T2DM treated with empagliflozin compared with placebo (Zinman et al. 2015). In the LEADER and SUSTAIN-6 trials, the GLP-1 receptor agonists liraglutide and semaglutide reduced the risk of major adverse cardiovascular events by 13% and 26%, respectively (Marso et al. 2016a, 2016b). Recent evidence has expanded therapeutic applications beyond diabetes: SGLT2 inhibitors demonstrate benefits in the acute HF setting and across the HF spectrum, including HFpEF (Anker et al. 2021; Voors et al. 2022), whereas GLP-1 receptor agonists provide cardiovascular protection in patients with obesity and CVD, independent of diabetes (Lingvay et al. 2024). The integrative use of animal models continues to advance our understanding of the complex relationship between MetS and CVD, providing a mechanistic framework for advancing therapeutic development.

References

Abe T, Ohga Y, Tabayashi N, Kobayashi S, Sakata S, Misawa H et al (2002) Left ventricular diastolic dysfunction in type 2 diabetes mellitus model rats. Am J Phys Heart Circ Phys 282(1): H138–H148. https://doi.org/10.1152/ajpheart.2002.282.1.H138

Abe N, Kato S, Tsuchida T, Sugimoto K, Saito R, Verschuren L et al (2019) Longitudinal characterization of diet-induced genetic murine models of non-alcoholic steatohepatitis with metabolic, histological, and transcriptomic hallmarks of human patients. Biol Open 8(5): bio041251. https://doi.org/10.1242/bio.041251

Agbaje AO (2023) Arterial stiffness preceding metabolic syndrome in 3,862 adolescents: a mediation and temporal causal longitudinal birth cohort study. Am J Physiol Heart Circ Physiol 324(6):H905–H911. https://doi.org/10.1152/ajpheart.00126.2023

Aijaz B, Ammar KA, Lopez-Jimenez F, Redfield MM, Jacobsen SJ, Rodeheffer RJ (2008) Abnormal cardiac structure and function in the metabolic syndrome: a population-based study. Mayo Clin Proc 83(12):1350–1357. https://doi.org/10.4065/83.12.1350

Al Kury LT (2020) Calcium homeostasis in ventricular myocytes of diabetic cardiomyopathy. J Diabetes Res 2020:1942086. https://doi.org/10.1155/2020/1942086

Al Thani NA, Hasan M, Yalcin HC (2023) Use of animal models for investigating Cardioprotective roles of SGLT2 inhibitors. J Cardiovasc Transl Res 16(5):975–986. https://doi.org/10.1007/s12265-023-10379-5

Alarcon G, Roco J, Medina M, Medina A, Peral M, Jerez S (2018) High fat diet-induced metabolically obese and normal weight rabbit model shows early vascular dysfunction: mechanisms involved. Int J Obes 42(9):1535–1543. https://doi.org/10.1038/s41366-018-0020-6

Alberti KG, Zimmet P, Shaw J, Group, I. D. F. E. T. F. C (2005) The metabolic syndrome–a new worldwide definition. Lancet 366(9491):1059–1062. https://doi.org/10.1016/S0140-6736(05)67402-8

Alberti KG, Eckel RH, Grundy SM, Zimmet PZ, Cleeman JI, Donato KA et al (2009) Harmonizing the metabolic syndrome: a joint interim statement of the international diabetes federation task force on epidemiology and prevention; National Heart, Lung, and Blood Institute; American Heart Association; world heart federation; international atherosclerosis society; and International Association for the Study of obesity. Circulation 120(16):1640–1645. https://doi.org/10.1161/CIRCULATIONAHA.109.192644

Alex L, Russo I, Holoborodko V, Frangogiannis NG (2018) Characterization of a mouse model of obesity-related fibrotic cardiomyopathy that recapitulates features of human heart failure with preserved ejection fraction. Am J Physiol Heart Circ Physiol 315(4):H934–h949. https://doi.org/10.1152/ajpheart.00238.2018

Alshnbari AS, Millar SA, O'Sullivan SE, Idris I (2020) Effect of sodium-glucose Cotransporter-2 inhibitors on endothelial function: a systematic review of preclinical studies. Diabetes Ther 11(9):1947–1963. https://doi.org/10.1007/s13300-020-00885-z

Anker SD, Butler J, Filippatos G, Ferreira JP, Bocchi E, Bohm M et al (2021) Empagliflozin in heart failure with a preserved ejection fraction. N Engl J Med 385(16):1451–1461. https://doi.org/10.1056/NEJMoa2107038

Aragno M, Meineri G, Vercellinatto I, Bardini P, Raimondo S, Peiretti PG et al (2009) Cardiac impairment in rabbits fed a high-fat diet is counteracted by dehydroepiandrosterone supplementation. Life Sci 85(1):77–84. https://doi.org/10.1016/j.lfs.2009.04.020

Aromolaran AS, Boutjdir M (2017) Cardiac Ion Channel regulation in obesity and the metabolic syndrome: relevance to long QT syndrome and atrial fibrillation. Front Physiol 8:431. https://doi.org/10.3389/fphys.2017.00431

Bagi Z, Koller A, Kaley G (2003) Superoxide-NO interaction decreases flow- and agonist-induced dilations of coronary arterioles in type 2 diabetes mellitus. Am J Phys Heart Circ Phys 285(4): H1404–H1410. https://doi.org/10.1152/ajpheart.00235.2003

Banting FG, Best CH, Collip JB, Campbell WR, Fletcher AA (1922) Pancreatic extracts in the treatment of diabetes mellitus. Can Med Assoc J 12(3):141–146

Bao P, Liu G, Wei Y (2015) Association between IL-6 and related risk factors of metabolic syndrome and cardiovascular disease in young rats. Int J Clin Exp Med 8(8):13491–13499

Barriere DA, Noll C, Roussy G, Lizotte F, Kessai A, Kirby K et al (2018) Combination of high-fat/high-fructose diet and low-dose streptozotocin to model long-term type-2 diabetes complications. Sci Rep 8(1):424. https://doi.org/10.1038/s41598-017-18896-5

Basaranoglu M, Basaranoglu G, Sabuncu T, Senturk H (2013) Fructose as a key player in the development of fatty liver disease. World J Gastroenterol 19(8):1166–1172. https://doi.org/10.3748/wjg.v19.i8.1166

Baynes J, Murray DB (2009) Cardiac and renal function are progressively impaired with aging in Zucker diabetic fatty type II diabetic rats. Oxidative Med Cell Longev 2(5):328–334. https://doi.org/10.4161/oxim.2.5.9831

Bell LN, Lee L, Saxena R, Bemis KG, Wang M, Theodorakis JL et al (2010) Serum proteomic analysis of diet-induced steatohepatitis and metabolic syndrome in the Ossabaw miniature swine. Am J Physiol Gastrointest Liver Physiol 298(5):G746–G754. https://doi.org/10.1152/ajpgi.00485.2009

Ben-Shlomo Y, Spears M, Boustred C, May M, Anderson SG, Benjamin EJ et al (2014) Aortic pulse wave velocity improves cardiovascular event prediction: an individual participant meta-analysis of prospective observational data from 17,635 subjects. J Am Coll Cardiol 63(7): 636–646. https://doi.org/10.1016/j.jacc.2013.09.063

Bergh CH, Hjalmarson A, Sjögren KG, Jacobsson B (1988) The effect of diabetes on phosphatidylinositol turnover and calcium influx in myocardium. Horm Metab Res 20(7): 381–386. https://doi.org/10.1055/s-2007-1010842

Berwick CZ, Dick MG, O'Leary AH, Bender BS, Goodwill GA, Moberly PS et al (2013) Contribution of electromechanical coupling between KV and CaV1.2 channels to coronary dysfunction in obesity. Basic Res Cardiol 108(5). https://doi.org/10.1007/s00395-013-0370-0

Boi SK, Buchta CM, Pearson NA, Francis MB, Meyerholz DK, Grobe JL, Norian LA (2016) Obesity alters immune and metabolic profiles: new insight from obese-resistant mice on high-fat diet. Obesity (Silver Spring) 24(10):2140–2149. https://doi.org/10.1002/oby.21620

Borbouse L, Dick MG, Asano S, Bender BS, Dincer DU, Payne AG et al (2009) Impaired function of coronary BKCa channels in metabolic syndrome. Am J Phys Heart Circ Phys 297(5):H1629–H1637. https://doi.org/10.1152/ajpheart.00466.2009

Boudoulas DK, Triposkiadis F, Geleris P, Boudoulas H (2016) Coronary atherosclerosis: pathophysiologic basis for diagnosis and management. Prog Cardiovasc Dis 58(6):676–692. https://doi.org/10.1016/j.pcad.2016.04.003

Boustany CM, Bharadwaj K, Daugherty A, Brown DR, Randall DC, Cassis LA (2004) Activation of the systemic and adipose renin-angiotensin system in rats with diet-induced obesity and hypertension. Am J Physiol Regul Integr Comp Physiol 287(4):R943–R949. https://doi.org/10.1152/ajpregu.00265.2004

Bremer AA, Stanhope KL, Graham JL, Cummings BP, Wang W, Saville BR, Havel PJ (2011) Fructose-fed rhesus monkeys: a nonhuman primate model of insulin resistance, metabolic syndrome, and type 2 diabetes. Clin Transl Sci 4(4):243–252. https://doi.org/10.1111/j.1752-8062.2011.00298.x

Brito JO, Ponciano K, Figueroa D, Bernardes N, Sanches ÍC, Irigoyen MC, Angelis DK (2008) Parasympathetic dysfunction is associated with insulin resistance in fructose-fed female rats. Braz J Med Biol Res 41(9):804–808. https://doi.org/10.1590/s0100-879x2008005000030

Brozovich FV, Nicholson CJ, Degen CV, Gao YZ, Aggarwal M, Morgan KG (2016) Mechanisms of vascular smooth muscle contraction and the basis for pharmacologic treatment of smooth muscle disorders. Pharmacol Rev 68(2):476–532. https://doi.org/10.1124/pr.115.010652

Brunner EJ, Hemingway H, Walker BR, Page M, Clarke P, Juneja M et al (2002) Adrenocortical, autonomic, and inflammatory causes of the metabolic syndrome: nested case-control study. Circulation 106(21):2659–2665. https://doi.org/10.1161/01.cir.0000038364.26310.bd

Buchanan J, Mazumder PK, Hu P, Chakrabarti G, Roberts MW, Yun UJ et al (2005) Reduced cardiac efficiency and altered substrate metabolism precedes the onset of hyperglycemia and contractile dysfunction in two mouse models of insulin resistance and obesity. Endocrinology 146(12):5341–5349. https://doi.org/10.1210/en.2005-0938

Bugga P, Mohammed SA, Alam MJ, Katare P, Meghwani H, Maulik SK et al (2022) Empagliflozin prohibits high-fructose diet-induced cardiac dysfunction in rats via attenuation of mitochondria-driven oxidative stress. Life Sci 307:120862. https://doi.org/10.1016/j.lfs.2022.120862

Bustos C, Hernandez-Presa MA, Ortego M, Tunon J, Ortega L, Perez F et al (1998) HMG-CoA reductase inhibition by atorvastatin reduces neointimal inflammation in a rabbit model of atherosclerosis. J Am Coll Cardiol 32(7):2057–2064. https://doi.org/10.1016/s0735-1097(98)00487-2

Canale MP, Manca di Villahermosa S, Martino G, Rovella V, Noce A, De Lorenzo A, Di Daniele N (2013) Obesity-related metabolic syndrome: mechanisms of sympathetic overactivity. Int J Endocrinol 2013:865965. https://doi.org/10.1155/2013/865965

Carroll JF, Tyagi SC (2005) Extracellular matrix remodeling in the heart of the Homocysteinemic obese rabbit*. Am J Hypertens 18(5):692–698. https://doi.org/10.1016/j.amjhyper.2004.11.035

Cassis LA, Police SB, Yiannikouris F, Thatcher SE (2008) Local adipose tissue renin-angiotensin system. Curr Hypertens Rep 10(2):93–98. https://doi.org/10.1007/s11906-008-0019-9

Cavalera M, Wang J, Frangogiannis NG (2014) Obesity, metabolic dysfunction, and cardiac fibrosis: pathophysiological pathways, molecular mechanisms, and therapeutic opportunities. Transl Res 164(4):323–335. https://doi.org/10.1016/j.trsl.2014.05.001

Charles CJ, Lee P, Li RR, Yeung T, Ibraham Mazlan SM, Tay ZW et al (2020) A porcine model of heart failure with preserved ejection fraction: magnetic resonance imaging and metabolic energetics. ESC Heart Fail 7(1):92–102. https://doi.org/10.1002/ehf2.12536

Chen H, Charlat O, Tartaglia LA, Woolf EA, Weng X, Ellis SJ et al (1996) Evidence that the diabetes gene encodes the leptin receptor: identification of a mutation in the leptin receptor gene in db/db mice. Cell 84(3):491–495. https://doi.org/10.1016/s0092-8674(00)81294-5

Christoffersen C, Bollano E, Lindegaard ML, Bartels ED, Goetze JP, Andersen CB, Nielsen LB (2003) Cardiac lipid accumulation associated with diastolic dysfunction in obese mice. Endocrinology 144(8):3483–3490. https://doi.org/10.1210/en.2003-0242

Cluzel GL, Ryan PM, Herisson FM, Caplice NM (2022) High-fidelity porcine models of metabolic syndrome: a contemporary synthesis. Am J Physiol Endocrinol Metab 322(4):E366–e381. https://doi.org/10.1152/ajpendo.00413.2021

Croteau D, Qin F, Chambers JM, Kallick E, Luptak I, Panagia M et al (2020) Differential effects of Sacubitril/valsartan on diastolic function in mice with obesity-related metabolic heart disease. JACC: basic to translational. Science 5(9):916–927. https://doi.org/10.1016/j.jacbts.2020.07.006

Cruickshank K, Riste L, Anderson SG, Wright JS, Dunn G, Gosling RG (2002) Aortic pulse-wave velocity and its relationship to mortality in diabetes and glucose intolerance: an integrated index of vascular function? Circulation 106(16):2085–2090. https://doi.org/10.1161/01.cir.0000033824.02722.f7

Cui C, Wang C, Han S, Yu D, Zhu L, Jiang P (2022) Impact of a long-term high-fructose diet on systemic metabolic profiles of mice. FASEB Bioadv 4(8):560–572. https://doi.org/10.1096/fba.2021-00152

Curtis TM, Gardiner TA, Stitt AW (2009) Microvascular lesions of diabetic retinopathy: clues towards understanding pathogenesis? Eye (Lond) 23(7):1496–1508. https://doi.org/10.1038/eye.2009.108

Dahl LK, Heine M, Tassinari L (1962) Role of genetic factors in susceptibility to experimental hypertension due to chronic excess salt ingestion. Nature 194:480–482. https://doi.org/10.1038/194480b0

De Angelis K, Senador DD, Mostarda C, Irigoyen MC, Morris M (2012) Sympathetic overactivity precedes metabolic dysfunction in a fructose model of glucose intolerance in mice. Am J Physiol Regul Integr Comp Physiol 302(8):R950–R957. https://doi.org/10.1152/ajpregu.00450.2011

de Simone G, Devereux RB, Chinali M, Roman MJ, Lee ET, Resnick HE, Howard BV (2009) Metabolic syndrome and left ventricular hypertrophy in the prediction of cardiovascular events: the strong heart study. Nutr Metab Cardiovasc Dis 19(2):98–104. https://doi.org/10.1016/j.numecd.2008.04.001

DeMarco VG, Ford DA, Henriksen EJ, Aroor AR, Johnson MS, Habibi J et al (2013) Obesity-related alterations in cardiac lipid profile and nondipping blood pressure pattern during transition to diastolic dysfunction in male db/db mice. Endocrinology 154(1):159–171. https://doi.org/10.1210/en.2012-1835

Dickhout JG, Lee RM (1998) Blood pressure and heart rate development in young spontaneously hypertensive rats. Am J Phys 274(3):H794–H800. https://doi.org/10.1152/ajpheart.1998.274.3.H794

Dikalov SI, Nazarewicz RR (2013) Angiotensin II-induced production of mitochondrial reactive oxygen species: potential mechanisms and relevance for cardiovascular disease. Antioxid Redox Signal 19(10):1085–1094. https://doi.org/10.1089/ars.2012.4604

Dincer UD, Araiza A, Knudson JD, Shao CH, Bidasee KR, Tune JD (2006) Dysfunction of cardiac ryanodine receptors in the metabolic syndrome. J Mol Cell Cardiol 41(1):108–114. https://doi.org/10.1016/j.yjmcc.2006.04.018

Dobrzyn P, Dobrzyn A, Miyazaki M, Ntambi JM (2010) Loss of stearoyl-CoA desaturase 1 rescues cardiac function in obese leptin-deficient mice. J Lipid Res 51(8):2202–2210. https://doi.org/10.1194/jlr.M003780

Dyson MC, Alloosh M, Vuchetich JP, Mokelke EA, Sturek M (2006) Components of metabolic syndrome and coronary artery disease in female Ossabaw swine fed excess atherogenic diet. Comp Med 56(1):35–45

Engerman RL, Buesseler JA, Meyer RK (1962) Periodic acid-Schiff staining of retinal whole mounts. Arch Ophthalmol 68:62–65. https://doi.org/10.1001/archopht.1962.00960030066013

Eringa CE, Stehouwer ADC, Roos HM, Westerhof N, Sipkema P (2007) Selective resistance to vasoactive effects of insulin in muscle resistance arteries of obese Zucker (fa/fa) rats. Am J Physiol-Endocrinol Metab 293(5):E1134–E1139. https://doi.org/10.1152/ajpendo.00516.2006

Esposito K, Giugliano D (2004) The metabolic syndrome and inflammation: association or causation? Nutr Metab Cardiovasc Dis 14(5):228–232. https://doi.org/10.1016/s0939-4753(04)80048-6

Esposito K, Pontillo A, Giugliano F, Giugliano G, Marfella R, Nicoletti G, Giugliano D (2003) Association of low interleukin-10 levels with the metabolic syndrome in obese women. J Clin Endocrinol Metab 88(3):1055–1058. https://doi.org/10.1210/jc.2002-021437

Fang ZY, Schull-Meade R, Leano R, Mottram PM, Prins JB, Marwick TH (2005) Screening for heart disease in diabetic subjects. Am Heart J 149(2):349–354. https://doi.org/10.1016/j.ahj.2004.06.021

Federico M, Portiansky EL, Sommese L, Alvarado FJ, Blanco PG, Zanuzzi CN et al (2017) Calcium-calmodulin-dependent protein kinase mediates the intracellular signalling pathways of cardiac apoptosis in mice with impaired glucose tolerance. J Physiol 595(12):4089–4108. https://doi.org/10.1113/JP273714

Fillmore N, Mori J, Lopaschuk GD (2014) Mitochondrial fatty acid oxidation alterations in heart failure, ischaemic heart disease and diabetic cardiomyopathy. Br J Pharmacol 171(8):2080–2090. https://doi.org/10.1111/bph.12475

Fraulob JC, Ogg-Diamantino R, Fernandes-Santos C, Aguila MB, Mandarim-de-Lacerda CA (2010) A mouse model of metabolic syndrome: insulin resistance, fatty liver and

non-alcoholic fatty pancreas disease (NAFPD) in C57BL/6 mice fed a high fat diet. J Clin Biochem Nutr 46(3):212–223. https://doi.org/10.3164/jcbn.09-83
Fujii S, Zhang L, Igarashi J, Kosaka H (2003) L-arginine reverses p47phox and gp91phox expression induced by high salt in Dahl rats. Hypertension 42(5):1014–1020. https://doi.org/10.1161/01.Hyp.0000094557.36656.D0
Fukumoto Y, Libby P, Rabkin E, Hill CC, Enomoto M, Hirouchi Y et al (2001) Statins alter smooth muscle cell accumulation and collagen content in established atheroma of watanabe heritable hyperlipidemic rabbits. Circulation 103(7):993–999. https://doi.org/10.1161/01.cir.103.7.993
Fukushima A, Lopaschuk GD (2016) Cardiac fatty acid oxidation in heart failure associated with obesity and diabetes. Biochim Biophys Acta 1861(10):1525–1534. https://doi.org/10.1016/j.bbalip.2016.03.020
Furukawa S, Fujita T, Shimabukuro M, Iwaki M, Yamada Y, Nakajima Y et al (2004) Increased oxidative stress in obesity and its impact on metabolic syndrome. J Clin Invest 114(12): 1752–1761. https://doi.org/10.1172/jci21625
Gallo G, Savoia C (2024) New insights into endothelial dysfunction in Cardiometabolic diseases: potential mechanisms and clinical implications. Int J Mol Sci 25(5):2973. https://doi.org/10.3390/ijms25052973
Gallou-Kabani C, Vigé A, Gross MS, Rabès JP, Boileau C, Larue-Achagiotis C et al (2007) C57BL/6J and A/J mice fed a high-fat diet delineate components of metabolic syndrome. Obesity 15(8):1996–2005. https://doi.org/10.1038/oby.2007.238
Gami AS, Witt BJ, Howard DE, Erwin PJ, Gami LA, Somers VK, Montori VM (2007) Metabolic syndrome and risk of incident cardiovascular events and death: a systematic review and meta-analysis of longitudinal studies. J Am Coll Cardiol 49(4):403–414. https://doi.org/10.1016/j.jacc.2006.09.032
Getz SG, Reardon AC (2012) Animal models of atherosclerosis. Arterioscler Thromb Vasc Biol 32(5):1104–1115. https://doi.org/10.1161/atvbaha.111.237693
Gilbert G, Demydenko K, Dries E, Puertas RD, Jin X, Sipido K, Roderick HL (2020) Calcium signaling in cardiomyocyte function. Cold Spring Harb Perspect Biol 12(3). https://doi.org/10.1101/cshperspect.a035428
Gomez-Smith M, Karthikeyan S, Jeffers MS, Janik R, Thomason LA, Stefanovic B, Corbett D (2016) A physiological characterization of the cafeteria diet model of metabolic syndrome in the rat. Physiol Behav 167:382–391. https://doi.org/10.1016/j.physbeh.2016.09.029
Gordan R, Gwathmey JK, Xie LH (2015) Autonomic and endocrine control of cardiovascular function. World J Cardiol 7(4):204–214. https://doi.org/10.4330/wjc.v7.i4.204
Gotfredsen CF, Molck AM, Thorup I, Nyborg NC, Salanti Z, Knudsen LB, Larsen MO (2014) The human GLP-1 analogs liraglutide and semaglutide: absence of histopathological effects on the pancreas in nonhuman primates. Diabetes 63(7):2486–2497. https://doi.org/10.2337/db13-1087
Granger DN, Senchenkova E (2010) Inflammation and the microcirculation. Morgan & Claypool, San Rafael
Gu H, Liu Y, Mei S, Wang B, Sun G, Wang X et al (2015) Left ventricular diastolic dysfunction in nonhuman primate model of dysmetabolism and diabetes. BMC Cardiovasc Disord 15:141. https://doi.org/10.1186/s12872-015-0133-y
Gueguen C, Burke SL, Barzel B, Eikelis N, Watson AMD, Jha JC et al (2020) Empagliflozin modulates renal sympathetic and heart rate baroreflexes in a rabbit model of diabetes. Diabetologia 63(7):1424–1434. https://doi.org/10.1007/s00125-020-05145-0
Guembe MJ, Fernandez-Lazaro CI, Sayon-Orea C, Toledo E, Moreno-Iribas C, Cosials JB et al (2020) Risk for cardiovascular disease associated with metabolic syndrome and its components: a 13-year prospective study in the RIVANA cohort. Cardiovasc Diabetol 19(1):195. https://doi.org/10.1186/s12933-020-01166-6
Guerra F, Mancinelli L, Angelini L, Fortunati M, Rappelli A, Dessì-Fulgheri P, Sarzani R (2011) The association of left ventricular hypertrophy with metabolic syndrome is dependent on body mass index in hypertensive overweight or obese patients. PLoS One 6(1):e16630. https://doi.org/10.1371/journal.pone.0016630

Habibi J, Aroor AR, Sowers JR, Jia G, Hayden MR, Garro M et al (2017) Sodium glucose transporter 2 (SGLT2) inhibition with empagliflozin improves cardiac diastolic function in a female rodent model of diabetes. Cardiovasc Diabetol 16(1):9. https://doi.org/10.1186/s12933-016-0489-z

Hall ME, Maready MW, Hall JE, Stec DE (2014) Rescue of cardiac leptin receptors in db/db mice prevents myocardial triglyceride accumulation. Am J Physiol Endocrinol Metab 307(3):E316–E325. https://doi.org/10.1152/ajpendo.00005.2014

Hamamdzic D, Wilensky LR (2013) Porcine models of accelerated coronary atherosclerosis: role of diabetes mellitus and hypercholesterolemia. J Diabetes Res 2013:1–7. https://doi.org/10.1155/2013/761415

Harris DD, Broadwin M, Stone C, Sabe SA, Kanuparthy M, Nho JW et al (2025) Sex-specific improvements in myocardial function and angiogenesis with SGLT-2 inhibitor Canagliflozin in a swine model of metabolic syndrome. Int J Mol Sci 26(5). https://doi.org/10.3390/ijms26051887

Harthmann AD, De Angelis K, Costa LP, Senador D, Schaan BD, Krieger EM, Irigoyen MC (2007) Exercise training improves arterial baro- and chemoreflex in control and diabetic rats. Auton Neurosci 133(2):115–120. https://doi.org/10.1016/j.autneu.2006.10.004

Hattori T, Murase T, Ohtake M, Inoue T, Tsukamoto H, Takatsu M et al (2011) Characterization of a new animal model of metabolic syndrome: the DahlS.Z-Lepr(fa)/Lepr(fa) rat. Nutr Diabetes 1(1):e1. https://doi.org/10.1038/nutd.2010.1

Havel PJ, Kievit P, Comuzzie AG, Bremer AA (2017) Use and importance of nonhuman primates in metabolic disease research: current state of the field. ILAR J 58(2):251–268. https://doi.org/10.1093/ilar/ilx031

Hayden MR, Karuparthi PR, Habibi J, Wasekar C, Lastra G, Manrique C et al (2007) Ultrastructural islet study of early fibrosis in the Ren2 rat model of hypertension. Emerging role of the islet pancreatic pericyte-stellate cell. JOP 8(6):725–738. Retrieved from https://www.ncbi.nlm.nih.gov/pubmed/17993725

Hayden MR, Karuparthi PR, Habibi J, Lastra G, Patel K, Wasekar C et al (2008) Ultrastructure of islet microcirculation, pericytes and the islet exocrine interface in the HIP rat model of diabetes. Exp Biol Med (Maywood) 233(9):1109–1123. https://doi.org/10.3181/0709-RM-251

Hayden MR, Yang Y, Habibi J, Bagree SV, Sowers JR (2010) Pericytopathy: oxidative stress and impaired cellular longevity in the pancreas and skeletal muscle in metabolic syndrome and type 2 diabetes. Oxidative Med Cell Longev 3(5):290–303. https://doi.org/10.4161/oxim.3.5.13653

Heaps CL, Bowles DK, Sturek M, Laughlin MH, Parker JL (2000) Enhanced L-type Ca2+ channel current density in coronary smooth muscle of exercise-trained pigs is compensated to limit myoplasmic free Ca2+ accumulation. J Physiol 528(Pt 3):435–445. Retrieved from http://www.ncbi.nlm.nih.gov/entrez/query.fcgi?cmd=Retrieve&db=PubMed&dopt=Citation&list_uids=11060122

Hegyi B, Mira Hernandez J, Ko CY, Hong J, Shen EY, Spencer ER et al (2022) Diabetes and excess aldosterone promote heart failure with preserved ejection fraction. J Am Heart Assoc 11(23):e027164. https://doi.org/10.1161/jaha.122.027164

Henry JA, Couch LS, Rider OJ (2024) Myocardial metabolism in heart failure with preserved ejection fraction. J Clin Med 13(5). https://doi.org/10.3390/jcm13051195

Herisson FM, Cluzel GL, Llopis-Grimalt MA, O'Donovan AN, Koc F, Karnik K et al (2025) Targeting the gut-heart Axis improves cardiac remodeling in a clinical scale model of Cardiometabolic syndrome. JACC Basic Transl Sci 10(1):1–15. https://doi.org/10.1016/j.jacbts.2024.09.004

Hill BJ, Dixon JL, Sturek M (2001) Effect of atorvastatin on intracellular calcium uptake in coronary smooth muscle cells from diabetic pigs fed an atherogenic diet. Atherosclerosis 159(1):117–124. Retrieved from http://www.ncbi.nlm.nih.gov/entrez/query.fcgi?cmd=Retrieve&db=PubMed&dopt=Citation&list_uids=11689213

Hingorani DA, Cross J, Kharbanda KR, Mullen JM, Bhagat K, Taylor M et al (2000) Acute systemic inflammation impairs endothelium-dependent dilatation in humans. Circulation 102(9):994–999. https://doi.org/10.1161/01.cir.102.9.994

Hiraoka-Yamamoto J, Nara Y, Yasui N, Onobayashi Y, Tsuchikura S, Ikeda K (2004) Establishment of a new animal model of metabolic syndrome: SHRSP fatty (fa/fa) rats. Clin Exp Pharmacol Physiol 31(1–2):107–109. https://doi.org/10.1111/j.1440-1681.2004.03962.x

Horton WB, Barrett EJ (2021) Microvascular dysfunction in diabetes mellitus and Cardiometabolic disease. Endocr Rev 42(1):29–55. https://doi.org/10.1210/endrev/bnaa025

Howarth FC, Qureshi MA, Hassan Z, Isaev D, Parekh K, John A et al (2012) Contractility of ventricular myocytes is well preserved despite altered mechanisms of Ca2+ transport and a changing pattern of mRNA in aged type 2 Zucker diabetic fatty rat heart. Mol Cell Biochem 361(1–2):267–280. https://doi.org/10.1007/s11010-011-1112-y

Huggett RJ, Burns J, Mackintosh AF, Mary DA (2004) Sympathetic neural activation in nondiabetic metabolic syndrome and its further augmentation by hypertension. Hypertension 44(6): 847–852. https://doi.org/10.1161/01.HYP.0000147893.08533.d8

Hummel KP, Coleman DL, Lane PW (1972) The influence of genetic background on expression of mutations at the diabetes locus in the mouse. I. C57BL-KsJ and C57BL-6J strains. Biochem Genet 7(1):1–13. https://doi.org/10.1007/BF00487005

Hwang IS, Ho H, Hoffman BB, Reaven GM (1987) Fructose-induced insulin resistance and hypertension in rats. Hypertension 10(5):512–516. https://doi.org/10.1161/01.hyp.10.5.512

Hwang S-J, Ballantyne MC, Sharrett RA, Smith CL, Davis EC, Gotto MA, Boerwinkle E (1997) Circulating adhesion molecules VCAM-1, ICAM-1, and E-selectin in carotid atherosclerosis and incident coronary heart disease cases. Circulation 96(12):4219–4225. https://doi.org/10.1161/01.cir.96.12.4219

Ingalls AM, Dickie MM, Snell GD (1950) Obese, a new mutation in the house mouse. J Hered 41(12):317–318. https://doi.org/10.1093/oxfordjournals.jhered.a106073

Kampschulte M, Stockl C, Langheinrich AC, Althohn U, Bohle RM, Krombach GA et al (2014) Western diet in ApoE-LDLR double-deficient mouse model of atherosclerosis leads to hepatic steatosis, fibrosis, and tumorigenesis. Lab Investig 94(11):1273–1282. https://doi.org/10.1038/labinvest.2014.112

Kasichayanula S, Grover A, Emery MG, Gibbs MA, Somaratne R, Wasserman SM, Gibbs JP (2018) Clinical pharmacokinetics and pharmacodynamics of Evolocumab, a PCSK9 inhibitor. Clin Pharmacokinet 57(7):769–779. https://doi.org/10.1007/s40262-017-0620-7

Kawano K, Hirashima T, Mori S, Saitoh Y, Kurosumi M, Natori T (1992) Spontaneous long-term hyperglycemic rat with diabetic complications. Otsuka long-Evans Tokushima fatty (OLETF) strain. Diabetes 41(11):1422–1428. https://doi.org/10.2337/diab.41.11.1422

Kim J, Kim MG, Kang S, Kim BR, Baek MY, Park YM, Shin MS (2016) Obesity and hypertension in association with diastolic dysfunction could reduce exercise capacity. Korean Circ J 46(3): 394–401. https://doi.org/10.4070/kcj.2016.46.3.394

King VL, Hatch NW, Chan HW, de Beer MC, de Beer FC, Tannock LR (2010) A murine model of obesity with accelerated atherosclerosis. Obesity (Silver Spring) 18(1):35–41. https://doi.org/10.1038/oby.2009.176

Knudsen LB (2010) Liraglutide: the therapeutic promise from animal models. Int J Clin Pract Suppl (167):4–11. https://doi.org/10.1111/j.1742-1241.2010.02499.x

Kohn JC, Lampi MC, Reinhart-King CA (2015) Age-related vascular stiffening: causes and consequences. Front Genet 6:112. https://doi.org/10.3389/fgene.2015.00112

Koletsky S (1973) Obese spontaneously hypertensive rats--a model for study of atherosclerosis. Exp Mol Pathol 19(1):53–60. https://doi.org/10.1016/0014-4800(73)90040-3

Koletsky S (1975) Pathologic findings and laboratory data in a new strain of obese hypertensive rats. Am J Pathol 80(1):129–142. Retrieved from https://www.ncbi.nlm.nih.gov/pubmed/1171627

Kuppusamy M, Ottolini M, Chen YL, Daneva Z, Li J, Heng-Mae Cheung C et al (2025) Paracrine smooth muscle-to-endothelial signaling via TNF elevates blood pressure in obesity. Circ Res 137(6):812–828. https://doi.org/10.1161/CIRCRESAHA.124.326069

Kuwabara JT, Tallquist MD (2017) Tracking adventitial fibroblast contribution to disease: A review of current methods to identify resident fibroblasts. Arterioscler Thromb Vasc Biol 37(9): 1598–1607. https://doi.org/10.1161/ATVBAHA.117.308199

Lacolley P, Regnault V, Segers P, Laurent S (2017) Vascular smooth muscle cells and arterial stiffening: relevance in development, aging, and disease. Physiol Rev 97(4):1555–1617. https://doi.org/10.1152/physrev.00003.2017

Lacombe VA, Viatchenko-Karpinski S, Terentyev D, Sridhar A, Emani S, Bonagura JD et al (2007) Mechanisms of impaired calcium handling underlying subclinical diastolic dysfunction in diabetes. Am J Physiol Regul Integr Comp Physiol 293(5):R1787–R1797. https://doi.org/10.1152/ajpregu.00059.2007

Lai M, Chandrasekera PC, Barnard ND (2014) You are what you eat, or are you? The challenges of translating high-fat-fed rodents to human obesity and diabetes. Nutr Diabetes 4(9):e135. https://doi.org/10.1038/nutd.2014.30

Lalanza JF, Snoeren EMS (2021) The cafeteria diet: A standardized protocol and its effects on behavior. Neurosci Biobehav Rev 122:92–119. https://doi.org/10.1016/j.neubiorev.2020.11.003

Landucci L, Faxén UL, Benson L, Rosano GMC, Dahlström U, Lund LH, Savarese G (2025) Characterizing heart failure across the Spectrum of the preserved ejection fraction: does heart failure with Supranormal ejection fraction exist? Data from the Swedish heart failure registry. J Am Heart Assoc 14(6):e037502. https://doi.org/10.1161/jaha.124.037502

Langheinrich AC, Michniewicz A, Bohle RM, Ritman EL (2007) Vasa vasorum neovascularization and lesion distribution among different vascular beds in ApoE−/−/LDL−/− double knockout mice. Atherosclerosis 191(1):73–81. https://doi.org/10.1016/j.atherosclerosis.2006.05.021

Lee ES, Ma W, Rattigan ME, Aleshin A, Chen L, Johnson LL et al (2010) Ultrastructural features of retinal capillary basement membrane thickening in diabetic swine. Ultrastruct Pathol 34(1): 35–41. https://doi.org/10.3109/01913120903308583

Lee JE, Yi CO, Jeon BT, Shin HJ, Kim SK, Jung TS et al (2012) α-Lipoic acid attenuates cardiac fibrosis in Otsuka long-Evans Tokushima fatty rats. Cardiovasc Diabetol 11:111. https://doi.org/10.1186/1475-2840-11-111

Lee J, Lee S, Zhang H, Hill AM, Zhang C, Park Y (2017) Interaction of IL-6 and TNF-α contributes to endothelial dysfunction in type 2 diabetic mouse hearts. PLoS One 12(11):e0187189. https://doi.org/10.1371/journal.pone.0187189

Lerman LO, Kurtz TW, Touyz RM, Ellison DH, Chade AR, Crowley SD et al (2019) Animal models of hypertension: a scientific statement from the American Heart Association. Hypertension 73(6):e87–e120. https://doi.org/10.1161/HYP.0000000000000090

Li P, Fan H (2023) Pericyte loss in diseases. Cells 12(15). https://doi.org/10.3390/cells12151931

Li NY, Yu J, Zhang XW, Wang SX, Chang P, Ding Q et al (2013) Features of left ventricular hypertrophy in patients with metabolic syndrome with or without comparable blood pressure: a meta-analysis. Endocrine 43(3):548–563. https://doi.org/10.1007/s12020-013-9883-4

Li Y, C GZ, Wang XH, Liu DH (2016) Progression of atherosclerosis in ApoE-knockout mice fed on a high-fat diet. Eur Rev Med Pharmacol Sci 20(18):3863–3867. Retrieved from https://www.ncbi.nlm.nih.gov/pubmed/27735029

Li SJ, Liu CH, Chu HP, Mersmann HJ, Ding ST, Chu CH et al (2017) The high-fat diet induces myocardial fibrosis in the metabolically healthy obese minipigs-the role of ER stress and oxidative stress. Clin Nutr 36(3):760–767. https://doi.org/10.1016/j.clnu.2016.06.002

Li Y, Kubo H, Yu D, Yang Y, Johnson JP, Eaton DM et al (2023) Combining three independent pathological stressors induces a heart failure with preserved ejection fraction phenotype. Am J Physiol Heart Circ Physiol 324(4):H443–h460. https://doi.org/10.1152/ajpheart.00594.2022

Li Q, Tang M, Jin Y, Su G, Li Y, Ju K et al (2025) AAV8-LDLR gene therapy in Ldlr-KO and homozygous Ldlr p.W483X mice. Hum Gene Ther 36(13–14):976–988. https://doi.org/10.1089/hum.2024.164
Lim RR, Grant DG, Olver TD, Padilla J, Czajkowski AM, Schnurbusch TR et al (2018) Young Ossabaw pigs fed a Western diet exhibit early signs of diabetic retinopathy. Invest Ophthalmol Vis Sci 59(6):2325–2338. https://doi.org/10.1167/iovs.17-23616
Lingvay I, Deanfield J, Kahn SE, Weeke PE, Toplak H, Scirica BM et al (2024) Semaglutide and cardiovascular outcomes by baseline HbA1c and change in HbA1c in people with overweight or obesity but without diabetes in SELECT. Diabetes Care 47(8):1360–1369. https://doi.org/10.2337/dc24-0764
Lira JR, Guymon AL, Yang L, Sternburg JO, Giri S, Wang X (2023) The double-hit protocol induces HFpEF and impairs myocardial ubiquitin-proteasome system performance in FVB/N mice. Front Physiol 14:1208153. https://doi.org/10.3389/fphys.2023.1208153
Llano R, Winsor-Hines D, Patel DB, Seifert PS, Hamamdzic D, Wilson GJ et al (2011) Vascular responses to drug-eluting and bare metal stents in diabetic/hypercholesterolemic and nonatherosclerotic porcine coronary arteries. Circ Cardiovasc Interv 4(5):438–446. https://doi.org/10.1161/CIRCINTERVENTIONS.110.959957
Low Wang CC, Lu L, Leitner JW, Sarraf M, Gianani R, Draznin B et al (2013) Arterial insulin resistance in Yucatan micropigs with diet-induced obesity and metabolic syndrome. J Diabetes Complicat 27(4):307–315. https://doi.org/10.1016/j.jdiacomp.2013.02.009
Lozano WM, Arias-Mutis OJ, Calvo CJ, Chorro FJ, Zarzoso M (2019) Diet-induced rabbit models for the study of metabolic syndrome. Animals (Basel) 9(7). https://doi.org/10.3390/ani9070463
Lu Z, Ballou LM, Jiang YP, Cohen IS, Lin RZ (2011a) Restoration of defective L-type Ca2+ current in cardiac myocytes of type 2 diabetic db/db mice by Akt and PKC-iota. J Cardiovasc Pharmacol 58(4):439–445. https://doi.org/10.1097/FJC.0b013e318228e68c
Lu Z, Ballou LM, Jiang YP, Cohen IS, Lin RZ (2011b) Restoration of defective L-type Ca2+ current in cardiac myocytes of type 2 diabetic db/db mice by Akt and PKC-ι. J Cardiovasc Pharmacol 58(4):439–445. https://doi.org/10.1097/FJC.0b013e318228e68c
Lu W, Meng Z, Hernandez R, Zhou C (2021) Fibroblast-specific IKK-β deficiency ameliorates angiotensin II-induced adverse cardiac remodeling in mice. JCI Insight 6(18). https://doi.org/10.1172/jci.insight.150161
Ma X, Du J, Zhang P, Deng J, Liu J, Lam FF et al (2013) Functional role of TRPV4-KCa2.3 signaling in vascular endothelial cells in normal and streptozotocin-induced diabetic rats. Hypertension 62(1):134–139. https://doi.org/10.1161/HYPERTENSIONAHA.113.01500
Mahdi A, Tratsiakovich Y, Tengbom J, Jiao T, Garib L, Alvarsson M et al (2020) Erythrocytes induce endothelial injury in type 2 diabetes through alteration of vascular purinergic signaling. Front Pharmacol 11. https://doi.org/10.3389/fphar.2020.603226
Mahley RW, Weisgraber KH (1974) Canine lipoproteins and atherosclerosis. I. Isolation and characterization of plasma lipoproteins from control dogs. Circ Res 35(5):713–721. https://doi.org/10.1161/01.res.35.5.713
Mahley RW, Weisgraber KH, Innerarity T (1974) Canine lipoproteins and atherosclerosis. II Characterization of the plasma lipoproteins associated with atherogenic and nonatherogenic hyperlipidemia. Circ Res 35(5):722–733. https://doi.org/10.1161/01.res.35.5.722
Mamikutty N, Thent ZC, Sapri SR, Sahruddin NN, Mohd Yusof MR, Haji Suhaimi F (2014) The establishment of metabolic syndrome model by induction of fructose drinking water in male Wistar rats. Biomed Res Int 2014:263897. https://doi.org/10.1155/2014/263897
Manrique C, Lastra G, Gardner M, Sowers JR (2009) The renin angiotensin aldosterone system in hypertension: roles of insulin resistance and oxidative stress. Med Clin North Am 93(3): 569–582. https://doi.org/10.1016/j.mcna.2009.02.014
Marino F, Salerno N, Scalise M, Salerno L, Torella A, Molinaro C et al (2023) Streptozotocin-induced type 1 and 2 diabetes mellitus mouse models show different functional, cellular and molecular patterns of diabetic cardiomyopathy. Int J Mol Sci 24(2). https://doi.org/10.3390/ijms24021132

Marques C, Meireles M, Norberto S, Leite J, Freitas J, Pestana D et al (2016) High-fat diet-induced obesity rat model: a comparison between Wistar and Sprague-Dawley rat. Adipocyte 5(1): 11–21. https://doi.org/10.1080/21623945.2015.1061723

Marquie G (1978) Effect of metformin on lipid metabolism in the rabbit aortic wall. Atherosclerosis 30(3):165–175. https://doi.org/10.1016/0021-9150(78)90043-6

Marso SP, Bain SC, Consoli A, Eliaschewitz FG, Jodar E, Leiter LA et al (2016a) Semaglutide and cardiovascular outcomes in patients with type 2 diabetes. N Engl J Med 375(19):1834–1844. https://doi.org/10.1056/NEJMoa1607141

Marso SP, Daniels GH, Brown-Frandsen K, Kristensen P, Mann JF, Nauck MA et al (2016b) Liraglutide and cardiovascular outcomes in type 2 diabetes. N Engl J Med 375(4):311–322. https://doi.org/10.1056/NEJMoa1603827

Martín-Cordero L, García JJ, Hinchado MD, Ortega E (2011) The interleukin-6 and noradrenaline mediated inflammation-stress feedback mechanism is dysregulated in metabolic syndrome: effect of exercise. Cardiovasc Diabetol 10(1):42. https://doi.org/10.1186/1475-2840-10-42

Matsui H, Ando K, Kawarazaki H, Nagae A, Fujita M, Shimosawa T et al (2008) Salt excess causes left ventricular diastolic dysfunction in rats with metabolic disorder. Hypertension 52(2): 287–294. https://doi.org/10.1161/hypertensionaha.108.111815

Mauricio D, Gratacos M, Franch-Nadal J (2023) Diabetic microvascular disease in non-classical beds: the hidden impact beyond the retina, the kidney, and the peripheral nerves. Cardiovasc Diabetol 22(1):314. https://doi.org/10.1186/s12933-023-02056-3

Mazzocco YL, Bergero G, Del Rosso S, Cejas Gallardo ZM, Canalis AM, Baigorri RE et al (2025) A novel mouse model for studying complications related to type 2 diabetes using a medium-fat diet, fructose, and streptozotocin. Sci Rep 15(1):20861. https://doi.org/10.1038/s41598-025-04335-3

Miesel A, Müller H, Thermann M, Heidbreder M, Dominiak P, Raasch W (2010) Overfeeding-induced obesity in spontaneously hypertensive rats: An animal model of the human metabolic syndrome. Ann Nutr Metab 56(2):127–142. https://doi.org/10.1159/000278748

Miyamura N, Bhutto IA, Amemiya T (1999) Retinal capillary changes in Otsuka long-Evans Tokushima fatty rats (spontaneously diabetic strain). Electron-microscopic study. Ophthalmic Res 31(5):358–366. https://doi.org/10.1159/000055559

Mizushige K, Yao L, Noma T, Kiyomoto H, Yu Y, Hosomi N et al (2000) Alteration in left ventricular diastolic filling and accumulation of myocardial collagen at insulin-resistant prediabetic stage of a type II diabetic rat model. Circulation 101(8):899–907. https://doi.org/10.1161/01.cir.101.8.899

Mn M, Smvk P, Battula KK, Nv G, Kalashikam RR (2017) Differential response of rat strains to obesogenic diets underlines the importance of genetic makeup of an individual towards obesity. Sci Rep 7(1):9162. https://doi.org/10.1038/s41598-017-09149-6

Moghadasian MH, Frohlich JJ, McManus BM (2001) Advances in experimental dyslipidemia and atherosclerosis. Lab Investig 81(9):1173–1183. https://doi.org/10.1038/labinvest.3780331

Mokelke AE, Dietz JN, Eckman MD, Nelson TM, Sturek M (2005) Diabetic dyslipidemia and exercise affect coronary tone and differential regulation of conduit and microvessel K+ current. Am J Phys Heart Circ Phys 288(3):H1233–H1241. https://doi.org/10.1152/ajpheart.00732.2004

Molinar-Toribio E, Perez-Jimenez J, Ramos-Romero S, Lluis L, Sanchez-Martos V, Taltavull N et al (2014) Cardiovascular disease-related parameters and oxidative stress in SHROB rats, a model for metabolic syndrome. PLoS One 9(8):e104637. https://doi.org/10.1371/journal.pone.0104637

Montgomery MK, Hallahan NL, Brown SH, Liu M, Mitchell TW, Cooney GJ, Turner N (2013) Mouse strain-dependent variation in obesity and glucose homeostasis in response to high-fat feeding. Diabetologia 56(5):1129–1139. https://doi.org/10.1007/s00125-013-2846-8

Moran TH, Bi S (2006a) Hyperphagia and obesity in OLETF rats lacking CCK-1 receptors. Philos Trans R Soc Lond Ser B Biol Sci 361(1471):1211–1218. https://doi.org/10.1098/rstb.2006.1857

Moran TH, Bi S (2006b) Hyperphagia and obesity of OLETF rats lacking CCK1 receptors: developmental aspects. Dev Psychobiol 48(5):360–367. https://doi.org/10.1002/dev.20149

Moran TH, Katz LF, Plata-Salaman CR, Schwartz GJ (1998) Disordered food intake and obesity in rats lacking cholecystokinin A receptors. Am J Phys 274(3):R618–R625. https://doi.org/10.1152/ajpregu.1998.274.3.R618

Mostarda C, Moraes-Silva IC, Salemi VM, Machi JF, Rodrigues B, De Angelis K et al (2012) Exercise training prevents diastolic dysfunction induced by metabolic syndrome in rats. Clinics (Sao Paulo) 67(7):815–820. https://doi.org/10.6061/clinics/2012(07)18

Mouton AJ, Li X, Hall ME, Hall JE (2020) Obesity, hypertension, and cardiac dysfunction: novel roles of Immunometabolism in macrophage activation and inflammation. Circ Res 126(6): 789–806. https://doi.org/10.1161/circresaha.119.312321

Mucellini AB, Goularte JF, de Araujo da Cunha AC, Caceres RC, Noschang C, da Silva Benetti C et al (2014) Effects of exposure to a cafeteria diet during gestation and after weaning on the metabolism and body weight of adult male offspring in rats. Br J Nutr 111(8):1499–1506. https://doi.org/10.1017/S0007114513003838

Muir KC, Stone C, Harris DD, Kanuparthy M, Broadwin M, Hamze J et al (2026) Semaglutide augments vascular proliferation and cardiac performance in a large animal model of ischemic cardiomyopathy. Am J Physiol Heart Circ Physiol 330(3):H651–H663. https://doi.org/10.1152/ajpheart.00828.2025

Mulè G, Nardi E, Cottone S, Cusimano P, Volpe V, Piazza G et al (2005) Influence of metabolic syndrome on hypertension-related target organ damage. J Intern Med 257(6):503–513. https://doi.org/10.1111/j.1365-2796.2005.01493.x

Murase T, Hattori T, Ohtake M, Abe M, Amakusa Y, Takatsu M et al (2012) Cardiac remodeling and diastolic dysfunction in DahlS.Z-Lepr(fa)/Lepr(fa) rats: a new animal model of metabolic syndrome. Hypertens Res 35(2):186–193. https://doi.org/10.1038/hr.2011.157

Nachar W, Merlet N, Maafi F, Shi Y, Mihalache-Avram T, Mecteau M et al (2019) Cardiac inflammation and diastolic dysfunction in hypercholesterolemic rabbits. PLoS One 14(8): e0220707. https://doi.org/10.1371/journal.pone.0220707

Nakayama Y, Elliott KJ, Eguchi S (2025) Cardiovascular effects of sucrose in experimental animals and humans. Hypertension 82(11):1799–1808. https://doi.org/10.1161/HYPERTENSIONAHA.125.25720

Navedo MF, Takeda Y, Nieves-Cintron M, Molkentin JD, Santana LF (2010) Elevated Ca2+ sparklet activity during acute hyperglycemia and diabetes in cerebral arterial smooth muscle cells. Am J Physiol Cell Physiol 298(2):C211–C220. https://doi.org/10.1152/ajpcell.00267.2009

Nelson MT, Cheng H, Rubart M, Santana LF, Bonev AD, Knot HJ, Lederer WJ (1995) Relaxation of arterial smooth muscle by calcium sparks. Science 270(5236):633–637. Retrieved from http://www.ncbi.nlm.nih.gov/pubmed/7570021

Nieves-Cintron M, Syed AU, Buonarati OR, Rigor RR, Nystoriak MA, Ghosh D et al (2017) Impaired BKCa channel function in native vascular smooth muscle from humans with type 2 diabetes. Sci Rep 7(1):14058. https://doi.org/10.1038/s41598-017-14565-9

Nieves Cintron M, Flores-Tamez VA, Le T, Baudel MM, Navedo MF (2021) Cellular and molecular effects of hyperglycemia on ion channels in vascular smooth muscle. Cell Mol Life Sci 78(1):31–61. https://doi.org/10.1007/s00018-020-03582-z

Ning B, Wang X, Yu Y, Waqar AB, Yu Q, Koike T et al (2015) High-fructose and high-fat diet-induced insulin resistance enhances atherosclerosis in Watanabe heritable hyperlipidemic rabbits. Nutr Metab (Lond) 12:30. https://doi.org/10.1186/s12986-015-0024-3

Nystoriak AM, Nieves-Cintrón M, Patriarchi T, Buonarati RO, Prada PM, Morotti S et al (2017) Ser1928 phosphorylation by PKA stimulates the L-type Ca2+ channel CaV1.2 and vasoconstriction during acute hyperglycemia and diabetes. Sci Signal 10(463):eaaf9647. https://doi.org/10.1126/scisignal.aaf9647

Oh JK, Park SJ, Nagueh SF (2011) Established and novel clinical applications of diastolic function assessment by echocardiography. Circ Cardiovasc Imaging 4(4):444–455. https://doi.org/10.1161/CIRCIMAGING.110.961623

Ohtani H, Shingu T, Chayama K, Hayashi K (2008) Different role of macrophages and vascular smooth muscle cells in atherosclerotic lesions of Watanabe heritable hyperlipidemic (WHHL) rabbit between aorta and coronary artery. Hiroshima J Med Sci 57(2):53–60. Retrieved from https://www.ncbi.nlm.nih.gov/pubmed/18717187

Oikonomidis N, Kavantzas N, Korou LM, Konstantopoulos P, Pergialiotis V, Misiakos E et al (2016) Pre-treatment with simvastatin prevents the induction of diet-induced atherosclerosis in a rabbit model. Biomed Rep 5(6):667–674. https://doi.org/10.3892/br.2016.780

Okamoto K, Aoki K (1963) Development of a strain of spontaneously hypertensive rats. Jpn Circ J 27:282–293. https://doi.org/10.1253/jcj.27.282

Okamoto K, Tabei R, Fukushima M, Nosaka S, Yamori Y (1966) Further observations of the development of a strain of spontaneously hypertensive rats. Jpn Circ J 30(6):703–716. https://doi.org/10.1253/jcj.30.703

Okamoto K, Yamamoto K, Morita N, Ohta Y, Chikugo T, Higashizawa T, Suzuki T (1986) Establishment and use of the M strain of stroke-prone spontaneously hypertensive rat. J Hypertens Suppl 4(3):S21–S24. Retrieved from https://www.ncbi.nlm.nih.gov/pubmed/3465899

Ornellas F, Bringhenti I, Mattos B, Mandarim-de-Lacerda CA, Aguila MB (2018) Father's obesity programs the adipose tissue in the offspring via the local renin-angiotensin system and MAPKs pathways, especially in adult male mice. Eur J Nutr 57(5):1901–1912. https://doi.org/10.1007/s00394-017-1473-4

Otani K, Funada H, Teranishi R, Okada M, Yamawaki H (2022) Cardiovascular characteristics of Zucker fatty diabetes mellitus rats, an animal model for obesity and type 2 diabetes. Int J Mol Sci 23(8). https://doi.org/10.3390/ijms23084228

Paavonsalo S, Hariharan S, Lackman HM, Karaman S (2020) Capillary rarefaction in obesity and metabolic diseases—organ-specificity and possible mechanisms. Cells 9(12):2683. https://doi.org/10.3390/cells9122683

Panasevich MR, Meers GM, Linden MA, Booth FW, Perfield JW 2nd, Fritsche KL et al (2018) High-fat, high-fructose, high-cholesterol feeding causes severe NASH and cecal microbiota dysbiosis in juvenile Ossabaw swine. Am J Physiol Endocrinol Metab 314(1):E78–E92. https://doi.org/10.1152/ajpendo.00015.2017

Panchal SK, Poudyal H, Iyer A, Nazer R, Alam MA, Diwan V et al (2011) High-carbohydrate, high-fat diet-induced metabolic syndrome and cardiovascular remodeling in rats. J Cardiovasc Pharmacol 57(5):611–624. https://doi.org/10.1097/FJC.0b013e31821b1379

Pannirselvam M, Verma S, Anderson JT, Triggle RC (2002) Cellular basis of endothelial dysfunction in small mesenteric arteries from spontaneously diabetic (db/db−/−) mice: role of decreased tetrahydrobiopterin bioavailability. Br J Pharmacol 136(2):255–263. https://doi.org/10.1038/sj.bjp.0704683

Park JB, Touyz RM, Chen X, Schiffrin EL (2002) Chronic treatment with a superoxide dismutase mimetic prevents vascular remodeling and progression of hypertension in salt-loaded stroke-prone spontaneously hypertensive rats. Am J Hypertens 15(1 Pt 1):78–84. https://doi.org/10.1016/s0895-7061(01)02233-6

Partington C, Hodgkiss-Geere H, Woods GRT, Dukes-McEwan J, Flanagan J, Biourge V, German AJ (2022) The effect of obesity and subsequent weight reduction on cardiac structure and function in dogs. BMC Vet Res 18(1):351. https://doi.org/10.1186/s12917-022-03449-4

Pereira L, Matthes J, Schuster I, Valdivia HH, Herzig S, Richard S, Gómez AM (2006) Mechanisms of [Ca2+]i transient decrease in cardiomyopathy of db/db type 2 diabetic mice. Diabetes 55(3):608–615. https://doi.org/10.2337/diabetes.55.03.06.db05-1284

Piedrahita JA, Zhang SH, Hagaman JR, Oliver PM, Maeda N (1992) Generation of mice carrying a mutant apolipoprotein E gene inactivated by gene targeting in embryonic stem cells. Proc Natl Acad Sci USA 89(10):4471–4475. https://doi.org/10.1073/pnas.89.10.4471

Plump AS, Smith JD, Hayek T, Aalto-Setala K, Walsh A, Verstuyft JG et al (1992) Severe hypercholesterolemia and atherosclerosis in apolipoprotein E-deficient mice created by homologous recombination in ES cells. Cell 71(2):343–353. https://doi.org/10.1016/0092-8674(92)90362-g

Podrini C, Cambridge EL, Lelliott CJ, Carragher DM, Estabel J, Gerdin AK et al (2013) High-fat feeding rapidly induces obesity and lipid derangements in C57BL/6N mice. Mamm Genome 24(5–6):240–251. https://doi.org/10.1007/s00335-013-9456-0

Rajiah PS, Moore A, Broncano J, Anand V, Kolluri N, Shah DJ et al (2023) Diastology with cardiac MRI: A practical guide. Radiographics 43(9):e220144. https://doi.org/10.1148/rg.220144

Rakipovski G, Rolin B, Nohr J, Klewe I, Frederiksen KS, Augustin R et al (2018) The GLP-1 analogs Liraglutide and Semaglutide reduce atherosclerosis in ApoE(−/−) and LDLr(−/−) mice by a mechanism that includes inflammatory pathways. JACC Basic Transl Sci 3(6): 844–857. https://doi.org/10.1016/j.jacbts.2018.09.004

Ridker PM, Hennekens CH, Buring JE, Rifai N (2000) C-reactive protein and other markers of inflammation in the prediction of cardiovascular disease in women. N Engl J Med 342(12): 836–843. https://doi.org/10.1056/nejm200003233421202

Riehle C, Bauersachs J (2018) Of mice and men: models and mechanisms of diabetic cardiomyopathy. Basic Res Cardiol 114(1):2. https://doi.org/10.1007/s00395-018-0711-0

Robinson R, Barathi VA, Chaurasia SS, Wong TY, Kern TS (2012) Update on animal models of diabetic retinopathy: from molecular approaches to mice and higher mammals. Dis Model Mech 5(4):444–456. https://doi.org/10.1242/dmm.009597

Rothwell NJ, Stock MJ (1979) Regulation of energy balance in two models of reversible obesity in the rat. J Comp Physiol Psychol 93(6):1024–1034. https://doi.org/10.1037/h0077631

Rothwell NJ, Saville ME, Stock MJ (1982) Effects of feeding a "cafeteria" diet on energy balance and diet-induced thermogenesis in four strains of rat. J Nutr 112(8):1515–1524. https://doi.org/10.1093/jn/112.8.1515

Rueda A, Fernandez-Velasco M, Benitah JP, Gomez AM (2013) Abnormal Ca2+ spark/STOC coupling in cerebral artery smooth muscle cells of obese type 2 diabetic mice. PLoS One 8(1): e53321. https://doi.org/10.1371/journal.pone.0053321

Russ M, Reinauer H, Eckel J (1991) Diabetes-induced decrease in the mRNA coding for sarcoplasmic reticulum ca(2+)-ATPase in adult rat cardiomyocytes. Biochem Biophys Res Commun 178(3):906–912. https://doi.org/10.1016/0006-291x(91)90977-f

Russo G, Leopold AJ, Loscalzo J (2002) Vasoactive substances. Vasc Pharmacol 38(5):259–269. https://doi.org/10.1016/s1537-1891(02)00250-1

Sampey BP, Vanhoose AM, Winfield HM, Freemerman AJ, Muehlbauer MJ, Fueger PT et al (2011) Cafeteria diet is a robust model of human metabolic syndrome with liver and adipose inflammation: comparison to high-fat diet. Obesity (Silver Spring) 19(6):1109–1117. https://doi.org/10.1038/oby.2011.18

Sanchez-Lozada LG, Tapia E, Jimenez A, Bautista P, Cristobal M, Nepomuceno T et al (2007) Fructose-induced metabolic syndrome is associated with glomerular hypertension and renal microvascular damage in rats. Am J Physiol Renal Physiol 292(1):F423–F429. https://doi.org/10.1152/ajprenal.00124.2006

Sankaralingam S, Abo Alrob O, Zhang L, Jaswal JS, Wagg CS, Fukushima A et al (2014) Lowering body weight in obese mice with diastolic heart failure improves cardiac insulin sensitivity and function: implications for the obesity paradox. Diabetes 64(5):1643–1657. https://doi.org/10.2337/db14-1050

Santana AB, de Souza Oliveira TC, Bianconi BL, Barauna VG, Santos EW, Alves TP et al (2014) Effect of high-fat diet upon inflammatory markers and aortic stiffening in mice. Biomed Res Int 2014:914102. https://doi.org/10.1155/2014/914102

Sawhney JPS, Madan K (2024) Familial hypercholesterolemia. Indian Heart J 76 Suppl 1(Suppl 1): S108–S112. https://doi.org/10.1016/j.ihj.2023.12.002

Schiattarella GG, Altamirano F, Tong D, French KM, Villalobos E, Kim SY et al (2019) Nitrosative stress drives heart failure with preserved ejection fraction. Nature 568(7752):351–356. https://doi.org/10.1038/s41586-019-1100-z

Schillaci G, Pirro M, Pucci G, Mannarino MR, Gemelli F, Siepi D et al (2006) Different impact of the metabolic syndrome on left ventricular structure and function in hypertensive men and women. Hypertension 47(5):881–886. https://doi.org/10.1161/01.Hyp.0000216778.83626.39

Schreyer SA, Wilson DL, LeBoeuf RC (1998) C57BL/6 mice fed high fat diets as models for diabetes-accelerated atherosclerosis. Atherosclerosis 136(1):17–24

Schwartz RS, Chronos NA, Virmani R (2004) Preclinical restenosis models and drug-eluting stents: still important, still much to learn. J Am Coll Cardiol 44(7):1373–1385. https://doi.org/10.1016/j.jacc.2004.04.060

Schwartz RS, Edelman E, Virmani R, Carter A, Granada JF, Kaluza GL et al (2008) Drug-eluting stents in preclinical studies: updated consensus recommendations for preclinical evaluation. Circ Cardiovasc Interv 1(2):143–153. https://doi.org/10.1161/CIRCINTERVENTIONS.108.789974

Sclafani A, Springer D (1976) Dietary obesity in adult rats: similarities to hypothalamic and human obesity syndromes. Physiol Behav 17(3):461–471. https://doi.org/10.1016/0031-9384(76)90109-8

Semeniuk LM, Kryski AJ, Severson DL (2002) Echocardiographic assessment of cardiac function in diabetic db/db and transgenic db/db-hGLUT4 mice. Am J Physiol Heart Circ Physiol 283(3):H976–H982. https://doi.org/10.1152/ajpheart.00088.2002

Serne EH, de Jongh RT, Eringa EC, IJzerman RG, Stehouwer CD (2007) Microvascular dysfunction: a potential pathophysiological role in the metabolic syndrome. Hypertension 50(1):204–211. https://doi.org/10.1161/HYPERTENSIONAHA.107.089680

Shao CH, Rozanski GJ, Patel KP, Bidasee KR (2007) Dyssynchronous (non-uniform) Ca2+ release in myocytes from streptozotocin-induced diabetic rats. J Mol Cell Cardiol 42(1):234–246. https://doi.org/10.1016/j.yjmcc.2006.08.018

Sharma A, Choi JSY, Watson AMD, Li L, Sonntag T, Lee MKS et al (2023) Cardiovascular characterisation of a novel mouse model that combines hypertension and diabetes co-morbidities. Sci Rep 13(1):8741. https://doi.org/10.1038/s41598-023-35680-w

Shinozaki K, Ayajiki K, Nishio Y, Sugaya T, Kashiwagi A, Okamura T (2004) Evidence for a causal role of the renin-angiotensin system in vascular dysfunction associated with insulin resistance. Hypertension 43(2):255–262. https://doi.org/10.1161/01.hyp.0000111136.86976.26

Shiomi M, Ito T (2009) The Watanabe heritable hyperlipidemic (WHHL) rabbit, its characteristics and history of development: A tribute to the late Dr. Yoshio Watanabe. Atherosclerosis 207(1):1–7. https://doi.org/10.1016/j.atherosclerosis.2009.03.024

Sibouakaz D, Othmani-Mecif K, Fernane A, Taghlit A, Benazzoug Y (2018) Biochemical and ultrastructural cardiac changes induced by high-fat diet in female and male Prepubertal rabbits. Anal Cell Pathol (Amst) 2018:6430696. https://doi.org/10.1155/2018/6430696

Simmonds SJ, Grootaert MOJ, Cuijpers I, Carai P, Geuens N, Herwig M et al (2024) Pericyte loss initiates microvascular dysfunction in the development of diastolic dysfunction. Eur Heart J Open 4(1):oead129. https://doi.org/10.1093/ehjopen/oead129

Sommese L, Valverde CA, Blanco P, Castro MC, Rueda OV, Kaetzel M et al (2016) Ryanodine receptor phosphorylation by CaMKII promotes spontaneous ca(2+) release events in a rodent model of early stage diabetes: the arrhythmogenic substrate. Int J Cardiol 202:394–406. https://doi.org/10.1016/j.ijcard.2015.09.022

Sonkusare SK, Bonev AD, Ledoux J, Liedtke W, Kotlikoff MI, Heppner TJ et al (2012) Elementary Ca2+ signals through endothelial TRPV4 channels regulate vascular function. Science 336(6081):597–601. https://doi.org/10.1126/science.1216283

Sorop O, Olver TD, van de Wouw J, Heinonen I, van Duin RW, Duncker DJ, Merkus D (2017) The microcirculation: a key player in obesity-associated cardiovascular disease. Cardiovasc Res 113(9):1035–1045. https://doi.org/10.1093/cvr/cvx093

Starzak M, Stanek A, Jakubiak GK, Cholewka A, Cieslar G (2022) Arterial stiffness assessment by pulse wave velocity in patients with metabolic syndrome and its components: is it a useful tool in clinical practice? Int J Environ Res Public Health 19(16). https://doi.org/10.3390/ijerph191610368

Stehouwer CD, Henry RM, Ferreira I (2008) Arterial stiffness in diabetes and the metabolic syndrome: a pathway to cardiovascular disease. Diabetologia 51(4):527–539. https://doi.org/10.1007/s00125-007-0918-3

Steinle JJ, Kern TS, Thomas SA, McFadyen-Ketchum LS, Smith CP (2009) Increased basement membrane thickness, pericyte ghosts, and loss of retinal thickness and cells in dopamine beta hydroxylase knockout mice. Exp Eye Res 88(6):1014–1019. https://doi.org/10.1016/j.exer.2008.12.015

Su Y, Zhang X (2023) Association of Metabolic Syndrome with adverse outcomes in patients with stable coronary artery disease: A meta-analysis. Horm Metab Res 55(2):96–102. https://doi.org/10.1055/a-1946-4823

Sultan A, Singh J, Howarth FC (2020) Mechanisms underlying electro-mechanical dysfunction in the Zucker diabetic fatty rat heart: a model of obesity and type 2 diabetes. Heart Fail Rev 25(5): 873–886. https://doi.org/10.1007/s10741-019-09872-4

Suman RK, Mohanty IR, Borde MK, Maheshwari U, Deshmukh YA (2016a) Development of an experimental model of diabetes co-existing with metabolic syndrome in rats. Adv Pharmacol Sci 2016:9463476. https://doi.org/10.1155/2016/9463476

Suman RK, Ray Mohanty I, Borde MK, Maheshwari U, Deshmukh YA (2016b) Development of an experimental model of diabetes co-existing with metabolic syndrome in rats. Adv Pharmacol Sci 2016:9463476. https://doi.org/10.1155/2016/9463476

Sun J, Pu Y, Wang P, Chen S, Zhao Y, Liu C et al (2013) TRPV1-mediated UCP2 upregulation ameliorates hyperglycemia-induced endothelial dysfunction. Cardiovasc Diabetol 12:69. https://doi.org/10.1186/1475-2840-12-69

Surwit RS, Kuhn CM, Cochrane C, McCubbin JA, Feinglos MN (1988) Diet-induced type II diabetes in C57BL/6J mice. Diabetes 37(9):1163–1167. Retrieved from http://www.ncbi.nlm.nih.gov/entrez/query.fcgi?cmd=Retrieve&db=PubMed&dopt=Citation&list_uids=3044882

Tan E, Butkus A, Koletsky S (1976) Hepatic cholesterol metabolism in vitro in the obese spontaneously hypertensive, hyperlipemic and atherosclerotic rat. Exp Mol Pathol 25(2): 142–151. https://doi.org/10.1016/0014-4800(76)90024-1

Tang X-L, Alloosh M, Ou Q, Luo L, Agrawal DK, Kalra DK et al (2025) A new model of heart failure with preserved ejection fraction induced by metabolic syndrome in Ossabaw miniature swine. Basic Res Cardiol 120(3):559–578. https://doi.org/10.1007/s00395-025-01112-1

Thorp EB, Filipp M (2025) Contributions of inflammation to Cardiometabolic heart failure with preserved ejection fraction. Ann Rev Pathol Mech Dis 20:143–167. https://doi.org/10.1146/annurev-pathmechdis-111523-023405

Tian J, Zhang M, Suo M, Liu D, Wang X, Liu M et al (2021) Dapagliflozin alleviates cardiac fibrosis through suppressing EndMT and fibroblast activation via AMPKalpha/TGF-beta/Smad signalling in type 2 diabetic rats. J Cell Mol Med 25(16):7642–7659. https://doi.org/10.1111/jcmm.16601

Trak-Smayra V, Paradis V, Massart J, Nasser S, Jebara V, Fromenty B (2011) Pathology of the liver in obese and diabetic Ob/Ob and db/db mice fed a standard or high-calorie diet. Int J Exp Pathol 92(6):413–421. https://doi.org/10.1111/j.1365-2613.2011.00793.x

Trask AJ, Katz PS, Kelly AP, Galantowicz ML, Cismowski MJ, West TA et al (2012) Dynamic micro- and macrovascular remodeling in coronary circulation of obese Ossabaw pigs with metabolic syndrome. J Appl Physiol (1985) 113(7):1128–1140. https://doi.org/10.1152/japplphysiol.00604.2012

Traupe T, Lang M, Goettsch W, Münter K, Morawietz H, Vetter W, Barton M (2002) Obesity increases prostanoid-mediated vasoconstriction and vascular thromboxane receptor gene expression. J Hypertens 20(11):2239–2245. https://doi.org/10.1097/00004872-200211000-00024

Trebak M (2012) STIM/Orai signalling complexes in vascular smooth muscle. J Physiol 590(17): 4201–4208. https://doi.org/10.1113/jphysiol.2012.233353
Tropf M, Nelson OL, Lee PM, Weng HY (2017) Cardiac and metabolic variables in obese dogs. J Vet Intern Med 31(4):1000–1007. https://doi.org/10.1111/jvim.14775
Tykocki NR, Boerman EM, Jackson WF (2017) Smooth muscle ion channels and regulation of vascular tone in resistance arteries and arterioles. Compr Physiol 7(2):485–581. https://doi.org/10.1002/cphy.c160011
Uti DE, Atangwho IJ, Omang WA, Alum EU, Obeten UN, Udeozor PA et al (2025) Cytokines as key players in obesity low grade inflammation and related complications. Obesity Med 54: 100585. https://doi.org/10.1016/j.obmed.2025.100585
van den Brom CE, Huisman MC, Vlasblom R, Boontje NM, Duijst S, Lubberink M et al (2009) Altered myocardial substrate metabolism is associated with myocardial dysfunction in early diabetic cardiomyopathy in rats: studies using positron emission tomography. Cardiovasc Diabetol 8(1):39. https://doi.org/10.1186/1475-2840-8-39
van Sloten TT, Sedaghat S, Carnethon MR, Launer LJ, Stehouwer CDA (2020) Cerebral microvascular complications of type 2 diabetes: stroke, cognitive dysfunction, and depression. Lancet Diabetes Endocrinol 8(4):325–336. https://doi.org/10.1016/S2213-8587(19)30405-X
Vasanji Z, Cantor EJ, Juric D, Moyen M, Netticadan T (2006) Alterations in cardiac contractile performance and sarcoplasmic reticulum function in sucrose-fed rats is associated with insulin resistance. Am J Physiol Cell Physiol 291(4):C772–C780. https://doi.org/10.1152/ajpcell.00086.2005
Verboven K, Wouters K, Gaens K, Hansen D, Bijnen M, Wetzels S et al (2018) Abdominal subcutaneous and visceral adipocyte size, lipolysis and inflammation relate to insulin resistance in male obese humans. Sci Rep 8(1):4677. https://doi.org/10.1038/s41598-018-22962-x
Verma S, Rawat S, Ho KL, Wagg CS, Zhang L, Teoh H et al (2018) Empagliflozin increases cardiac energy production in diabetes: novel translational insights into the heart failure benefits of SGLT2 inhibitors. JACC Basic Transl Sci 3(5):575–587. https://doi.org/10.1016/j.jacbts.2018.07.006
Voors AA, Angermann CE, Teerlink JR, Collins SP, Kosiborod M, Biegus J et al (2022) The SGLT2 inhibitor empagliflozin in patients hospitalized for acute heart failure: a multinational randomized trial. Nat Med 28(3):568–574. https://doi.org/10.1038/s41591-021-01659-1
Wallis GM, Wheatley MC, Rattigan S, Barrett JE, Clark DHA, Clark GM (2002) Insulin-mediated hemodynamic changes are impaired in muscle of Zucker obese rats. Diabetes 51(12): 3492–3498. https://doi.org/10.2337/diabetes.51.12.3492
Wang CY, Liao JK (2012) A mouse model of diet-induced obesity and insulin resistance. Methods Mol Biol 821:421–433. https://doi.org/10.1007/978-1-61779-430-8_27
Wang Y, Dubland AJ, Allahverdian S, Asonye E, Sahin B, Jaw EJ et al (2019) Smooth muscle cells contribute the majority of foam cells in ApoE (apolipoprotein E)-deficient mouse atherosclerosis. Arterioscler Thromb Vasc Biol 39(5):876–887. https://doi.org/10.1161/atvbaha.119.312434
Weisbrod RM, Shiang T, Al Sayah L, Fry JL, Bajpai S, Reinhart-King CA et al (2013) Arterial stiffening precedes systolic hypertension in diet-induced obesity. Hypertension 62(6): 1105–1110. https://doi.org/10.1161/HYPERTENSIONAHA.113.01744
Wenceslau CF, McCarthy CG, Earley S, England SK, Filosa JA, Goulopoulou S et al (2021) Guidelines for the measurement of vascular function and structure in isolated arteries and veins. Am J Physiol Heart Circ Physiol 321(1):H77–H111. https://doi.org/10.1152/ajpheart.01021.2020
Wenzl FA, Ambrosini S, Mohammed SA, Kraler S, Lüscher TF, Costantino S, Paneni F (2021) Inflammation in metabolic cardiomyopathy. Front Cardiovasc Med 8:742178. https://doi.org/10.3389/fcvm.2021.742178
Wesley CD, Neutel CHG, De Meyer GRY, Martinet W, Guns PJ (2024) Unravelling the impact of active and passive contributors to arterial stiffness in male mice and their role in vascular aging. Sci Rep 14(1):18337. https://doi.org/10.1038/s41598-024-68725-9

Wichi R, Malfitano C, Rosa K, De Souza SB, Salemi V, Mostarda C et al (2007) Noninvasive and invasive evaluation of cardiac dysfunction in experimental diabetes in rodents. Cardiovasc Diabetol 6:14. https://doi.org/10.1186/1475-2840-6-14

Wilson PW, D'Agostino RB, Parise H, Sullivan L, Meigs JB (2005) Metabolic syndrome as a precursor of cardiovascular disease and type 2 diabetes mellitus. Circulation 112(20): 3066–3072. https://doi.org/10.1161/CIRCULATIONAHA.105.539528

Winters B, Mo Z, Brooks-Asplund E, Kim S, Shoukas A, Li D et al (2000) Reduction of obesity, as induced by leptin, reverses endothelial dysfunction in obese (Lepob) mice. J Appl Physiol 89(6):2382–2390. https://doi.org/10.1152/jappl.2000.89.6.2382

Witte K, Reitenbach I, Stolpe K, Schilling L, Kirchengast M, Lemmer B (2003) Effects of the endothelin A receptor antagonist Darusentan on blood pressure and vascular contractility in type 2 diabetic Goto-Kakizaki rats. J Cardiovasc Pharmacol 41(6):890–896. https://doi.org/10.1097/00005344-200306000-00009

Wong SK, Chin KY, Suhaimi FH, Fairus A, Ima-Nirwana S (2016) Animal models of metabolic syndrome: a review. Nutr Metab 13:65. https://doi.org/10.1186/s12986-016-0123-9

Wu Y, Chen C, Wei FF, Liang W, Dong Y, Liu C et al (2024) Associations between long-term averages of metabolic parameters in adulthood and cardiac structure and function in later life. Hypertens Res 47(2):496–506. https://doi.org/10.1038/s41440-023-01475-9

Xia J, Zhang Y, Xin L, Kong S, Chen Y, Yang S, Li K (2015) Global transcriptomic profiling of cardiac hypertrophy and fatty heart induced by long-term high-energy diet in Bama miniature pigs. PLoS One 10(7):e0132420. https://doi.org/10.1371/journal.pone.0132420

Yang Y, Jones WA, Thomas RT, Rubin JL (2007) Influence of sex, high-fat diet, and exercise training on potassium currents of swine coronary smooth muscle. Am J Phys Heart Circ Phys 293(3):H1553–H1563. https://doi.org/10.1152/ajpheart.00151.2007

Yang ZH, Miyahara H, Takeo J, Katayama M (2012) Diet high in fat and sucrose induces rapid onset of obesity-related metabolic syndrome partly through rapid response of genes involved in lipogenesis, insulin signalling and inflammation in mice. Diabetol Metab Syndr 4(1):32. https://doi.org/10.1186/1758-5996-4-32

Yang D-R, Wang M-Y, Zhang C-L, Wang Y (2024) Endothelial dysfunction in vascular complications of diabetes: a comprehensive review of mechanisms and implications. Front Endocrinol 15. https://doi.org/10.3389/fendo.2024.1359255

Yeo TM, Chin CWL, Seah CWA, Cheng LJ, Lin W, Dalakoti M et al (2025) Global prevalence of myocardial fibrosis among individuals with cardiometabolic conditions: a systematic review and meta-analysis. Eur J Prev Cardiol. https://doi.org/10.1093/eurjpc/zwaf083

Yokoi N, Hoshino M, Hidaka S, Yoshida E, Beppu M, Hoshikawa R et al (2013) A novel rat model of type 2 diabetes: the Zucker fatty diabetes mellitus ZFDM rat. J Diabetes Res 2013:103731. https://doi.org/10.1155/2013/103731

Youn J-Y, Zhou J, Cai H (2015) Bone Morphogenic protein 4 mediates NOX1-dependent eNOS uncoupling, endothelial dysfunction, and COX2 induction in type 2 diabetes mellitus. Mol Endocrinol 29(8):1123–1133. https://doi.org/10.1210/ME.2014-1313

Zaman AK, Fujii S, Goto D, Furumoto T, Mishima T, Nakai Y et al (2004) Salutary effects of attenuation of angiotensin II on coronary perivascular fibrosis associated with insulin resistance and obesity. J Mol Cell Cardiol 37(2):525–535. https://doi.org/10.1016/j.yjmcc.2004.05.006

Zaragoza C, Gomez-Guerrero C, Martin-Ventura LJ, Blanco-Colio L, Lavin B, Mallavia B et al (2011) Animal models of cardiovascular diseases. Biomed Res Int 2011(1):1–13. https://doi.org/10.1155/2011/497841

Zeeni N, Dagher-Hamalian C, Dimassi H, Faour WH (2015) Cafeteria diet-fed mice is a pertinent model of obesity-induced organ damage: a potential role of inflammation. Inflamm Res 64(7): 501–512. https://doi.org/10.1007/s00011-015-0831-z

Zeng X, Yang Y (2024) Molecular mechanisms underlying vascular remodeling in hypertension. Rev Cardiovasc Med 25(2):72. https://doi.org/10.31083/j.rcm2502072

Zeng M, Qiao Y, Wen Z, Liu J, Xiao E, Tan C et al (2017) The association between diffuse myocardial fibrosis on cardiac magnetic resonance T1 mapping and myocardial dysfunction in diabetic rabbits. Sci Rep 7(1):44937. https://doi.org/10.1038/srep44937

Zhang SH, Reddick RL, Piedrahita JA, Maeda N (1992) Spontaneous hypercholesterolemia and arterial lesions in mice lacking apolipoprotein E. Science 258(5081):468–471. https://doi.org/10.1126/science.1411543

Zhang X, Zhang R, Raab S, Zheng W, Wang J, Liu N et al (2011) Rhesus macaques develop metabolic syndrome with reversible vascular dysfunction responsive to pioglitazone. Circulation 124(1):77–86. https://doi.org/10.1161/circulationaha.110.990333

Zhang X, Li ZL, Eirin A, Ebrahimi B, Pawar AS, Zhu XY et al (2015) Cardiac metabolic alterations in hypertensive obese pigs. Hypertension 66(2):430–436. https://doi.org/10.1161/hypertensionaha.115.05478

Zhang G, Li M, Xu Y, Peng L, Yang C, Zhou Y, Zhang J (2016a) Antioxidation effect of simvastatin in aorta and hippocampus: A rabbit model fed high-cholesterol diet. Oxidative Med Cell Longev 2016:6929306. https://doi.org/10.1155/2016/6929306

Zhang Y, Wang J-H, Zhang Y-Y, Wang Y-Z, Wang J, Zhao Y et al (2016b) Deletion of interleukin-6 alleviated interstitial fibrosis in streptozotocin-induced diabetic cardiomyopathy of mice through affecting TGFβ1 and miR-29 pathways. Sci Rep 6(1):23010. https://doi.org/10.1038/srep23010

Zhang J, Qiu H, Huang J, Ding S, Huang B, Wu Q, Jiang Q (2018) Establishment of a diabetic myocardial hypertrophy model in Mus musculus castaneus mouse. Int J Exp Pathol 99(6):295–303. https://doi.org/10.1111/iep.12296

Zhang W, Li X, Ding H, Lu Y, Stilwell GE, Halvorsen YD, Welihinda A (2020) Metabolism and disposition of the SGLT2 inhibitor bexagliflozin in rats, monkeys and humans. Xenobiotica 50(5):559–569. https://doi.org/10.1080/00498254.2019.1654634

Zhao J, Cao T-T, Tian J, Chen H-h, Zhang C, Wei H-C et al (2016) Shengmai san ameliorates myocardial dysfunction and fibrosis in diabetic db/db mice. Evid Based Complement Alternat Med 2016(1):4621235. https://doi.org/10.1155/2016/4621235

Zhao H, Liu E, Zhang YQ (2023) Dog models of human atherosclerotic cardiovascular diseases. Mamm Genome 34(2):262–269. https://doi.org/10.1007/s00335-022-09965-w

Zheng H, Zhang C, Yang W, Wang Y, Lin Y, Yang P et al (2009) Fat and cholesterol diet induced lipid metabolic disorders and insulin resistance in rabbit. Exp Clin Endocrinol Diabetes 117(8):400–405. https://doi.org/10.1055/s-0028-1102918

Zheng S, Tan W, Li X, Li B, Gong B, Pyle WG et al (2021) Aged monkeys fed a high-fat/high-sugar diet recapitulate metabolic disorders and cardiac contractile dysfunction. J Cardiovasc Transl Res 14(5):799–815. https://doi.org/10.1007/s12265-021-10105-z

Zhou X, Ma L, Habibi J, Whaley-Connell A, Hayden MR, Tilmon RD et al (2010) Nebivolol improves diastolic dysfunction and myocardial remodeling through reductions in oxidative stress in the Zucker obese rat. Hypertension 55(4):880–888. https://doi.org/10.1161/hypertensionaha.109.145136

Zhou D, Lin S, Liu Z, Yuan J, Ren H, Tan H et al (2025) Metabolic syndrome, left ventricular diastolic dysfunction and heart failure with preserved ejective fraction. Front Endocrinol (Lausanne) 16:1544908. https://doi.org/10.3389/fendo.2025.1544908

Zhuhua Z, Zhiquan W, Zhen Y, Yixin N, Weiwei Z, Xiaoyong L et al (2015) A novel mice model of metabolic syndrome: the high-fat-high-fructose diet-fed ICR mice. Exp Anim 64(4):435–442. https://doi.org/10.1538/expanim.14-0086

Zinman B, Wanner C, Lachin JM, Fitchett D, Bluhmki E, Hantel S et al (2015) Empagliflozin, cardiovascular outcomes, and mortality in type 2 diabetes. N Engl J Med 373(22):2117–2128. https://doi.org/10.1056/NEJMoa1504720

Zucker LM, Zucker TF (1961) Fatty—new mutation in rat. J Hered 52(6):275. https://doi.org/10.1093/oxfordjournals.jhered.a107093

Sexual Dimorphism in the Development of Cardiometabolic Syndrome

Myrian Velasco, Alondra Albarado-Ibañez, Carlos Larqué, Pablo Pánico, Julián Torres-Jacome, and Marcia Hiriart

Contents

Authors Myrian Velasco and Alondra Albarado-Ibañez have equally contributed to this chapter.

M. Velasco · M. Hiriart (✉)
Department of Cognitive Neurosciences, Instituto de Fisiología Celular, Universidad Nacional Autónoma de México, México City, Mexico
e-mail: mhiriart@ifc.unam.mx

A. Albarado-Ibañez · J. Torres-Jacome
Laboratorio de Fisiopatología Cardiovascular. Centro de Investigación Fisicoquímica de Materiales, Instituto de Ciencias, Benemérita Universidad Autónoma de Puebla, Puebla, Mexico

C. Larqué
Laboratory of Embryology and Genetics, Departamento de Embriología y Genética, Facultad de Medicina, Universidad Nacional Autónoma de México, Mexico City, Mexico

P. Pánico
Department of Genomic Medicine and Environmental Toxicology, Instituto de Investigaciones Biomédicas, Universidad Nacional Autónoma de México, México City, Mexico

A. Rueda, M. Nieves-Cintrón (eds.), *Cardiovascular Alterations in Metabolic Diseases*, Handbook of Experimental Pharmacology 293,
https://doi.org/10.1007/164_2026_790

Abstract

Anatomical and physiological differences between sexes explain the sexual dimorphism in the development of diseases, such as obesity and metabolic syndrome. This syndrome is a condition that increases the risk of developing cardiovascular diseases, diabetes, and certain cancer types. Cardiovascular diseases remain the leading cause of mortality in both sexes worldwide. However, CVD mortality is higher in men than women, demonstrating that the differences between women and men might have an essential role in the development of CVD.

The CV system shows dimorphic variations, starting at early developmental stages. However, most studies on the CV system have been conducted predominantly in males. Understanding the differences in the CVD associated with sex is vital to improving the prevention, diagnosis, and treatment of these diseases. In this chapter, we highlight the differences found in the literature between sexes in physiological and pathological events within the cardiovascular system related to metabolic syndrome (MetS).

Keywords

Cardio · Cardiovascular aging · Heart rhythm · Metabolic syndrome · Sexual dimorphism · Sinoatrial node

1 The Cardiovascular System

The mammalian heart is formed by three layers of cells that form four cavities, which pump blood to the vessels and keep it moving throughout the body by the cardiomyocytes' contraction and relaxation cycles and by specialized cardiomyocytes that form the cardiac conduction system (Woodcock and Matkovich 2005). The function of the heart needs the coordinated activity of the pacemaker cells of the heart, formed by the sinoatrial node (SAN) located in the right atrium (Fig. 1), that generate pacemaker potentials that propagate into the atrium through the conduction system, the atrioventricular node (AVN), and finally excite the ventricles through the Purkinje fibers (St Pierre et al. 2022).

The anatomical and functional characteristics of the cardiovascular (CV) system differ between males and females. This fact is essential to understanding sexual differences in the presentation of cardiovascular diseases (CVD). Moreover, the metabolic syndrome, often observed, also shows sexual dimorphism and a close relationship between these two entities. In this review, we will emphasize both.

The heart changes and remodels throughout life. In newborns, the female heart is 5% larger than that of males. While hearts are comparable between sexes through their development, the heart in males grows faster at puberty. In adulthood, the

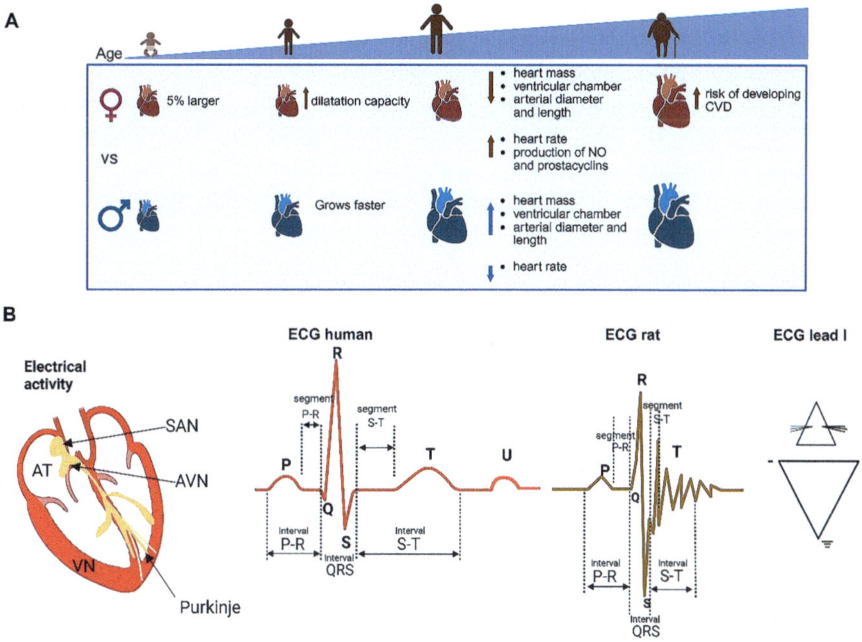

Fig. 1 Sexual dimorphism in the cardiovascular system and mammalian electrocardiogram. (**a**) Sexual differences in the human cardiovascular system. (**b**) The electrocardiogram (ECG) reflects the summation of the heart's electrical activity. Comparative analysis of human and rat ECGs recorded in the same configuration

female heart mass is nearly 25% lighter than the male heart. The heart mass keeps increasing with age, but it is always higher in males (St Pierre et al. 2022). Also, women have smaller ventricular chambers, arterial diameters, and lengths than men; there are also differences in stroke volume, and women exhibit a higher heart rate (Zaid et al. 2023).

Electrical activity is also different between the sexes. Women have a prolonged interval between ventricular depolarization and repolarization, represented by the QT interval in an electrocardiogram (ECG) (Smith et al. 2025b; Zaid et al. 2023). The longer depolarization-repolarization interval could explain the higher female prevalence of cardiac arrhythmias (Emerson et al. 2025). On the other hand, the diameter and length of the main arteries are also different, being smaller in females compared to males. The endothelium, which lines the lumen of the blood vessels, produces and releases both vasodilating and vasoconstricting factors, the most potent being nitric oxide (NO) and endothelin-1 (ET-1), respectively. The dilatation capacity is more significant in young women than in men. The decline in endothelial function begins at a younger age in men; however, after menopause, the rate of decline is higher in women (Kuczmarski et al. 2021).

Endothelial dysfunction is characterized by a reduced capacity for vasodilation, decreased nitric oxide (NO) production, and a proinflammatory and prothrombotic state within the endothelium. Estrogen and its receptors play a significant role in vascular health, particularly in women. Endothelial cells express estrogen receptors, which regulate ET-1 production and enhance the production of NO and prostacyclins, which enhance vasodilation. After menopause, estradiol production decreases, and type B receptors are reduced, increasing the risk of developing CVD in women (Kuczmarski et al. 2021). Aging is a primary risk factor for CVDs. It is interesting, considering that the heart of rats with metabolic syndrome shows premature signs of aging (Albarado-Ibañez et al. 2024).

2 Heart Rhythm and Electrocardiogram

SAN's automatic activity determines the heart rhythm (HR). Automaticity is the property of the pacemaker (core and subsidiary) that generates spontaneous action potentials. Although the SAN typically displays the highest intrinsic rate, there is a hierarchy of inherent rates of subsidiary pacemakers with automaticity. The SAN node fibers have faster intrinsic rates than the NAV junctional pacemakers, and the latter have more rapid rates than ventricular pacemakers (Albarado-Ibanez et al. 2013).

The ECG is a spatial and temporal recording of the heart's electrical activity, obtained from outside the body using surface electrodes placed on the skin (Zhang et al. 2025). For each ECG, different successive morphologies are recorded: the wave of atrial depolarization (P wave), the QRS complex, which represents ventricular depolarization, and the wave of ventricular repolarization (T wave). In some cases, physiological waves such as U waves may be recorded (see Fig. 1) (Antzelevitch and Di Diego 2022). These waves show different intervals representing the successive activation, depolarization, and repolarization of atria and ventricles (Naskar et al. 2024), which repeat one cardiac cycle after another.

Spontaneous sinus activity results from diastolic depolarization and is caused by a net inward current during the fourth phase of the action potential, which progressively brings the membrane potential to a threshold that allows the origin of the automaticity and consequently the spontaneous beating of the heart. The contraction-relaxation process of cardiac tissue is named the heartbeat and shows a cyclic pattern. The beats per minute produce the heart rate, a parameter that diagnoses some health problems (Torres-Jacome et al. 2022).

The normal resting heart rate, known as the human sinus rhythm, typically ranges from 60 to 90 beats per minute for both men and women. While there is limited information available about heart rate and rhythm, specifically in women, it is understood that hormones can lead to changes in these factors (Arroyo-Carmona et al. 2016). The HR is recorded in the ECG by evaluating the R-R intervals that occur within 6 s and multiplying by 10 (Dorsa et al. 2023). The electrical activity propagates to the atria and the AVN and reaches the ventricles, triggering their contraction from the apex to the base (Fig. 1). Any change in the origin and propagation of this electrical activity is denominated arrhythmia. When HR increases, it is called tachycardia, and a decrease in HR is called bradycardia.

Tachycardia is related to exercise, emotions, and the fight-or-flight phenomenon; bradycardia is related to sleep and rest (Albarado-Ibanez et al. 2019).

The autonomic nervous system (ANS) modulates the spontaneous activity of the SAN and the heart's conduction system (Albarado-Ibanez et al. 2013). The heart rate variability analysis is based on biological variations in sinus cycle length, generally attributed to the cardiac autonomic system. The SAN innervation is divided into the sympathetic (SNS) and parasympathetic (PNS) systems. They both have opposing effects on heart activity. The SNS innervating predominantly the ventricles increases the HR by norepinephrine, which stimulates the heart's adrenergic receptors (Albarado-Ibanez et al. 2019; Arroyo-Carmona et al. 2016). The PNS has an inhibitory effect on the rate of spontaneous activity through acetylcholine acting on muscarinic receptors (Torres-Jacome et al. 2022).

Some hypothalamic nuclei, like dorsomedial (Carrillo-Franco et al. 2024) and paraventricular, are connected to other brain areas involved in cardiovascular function, generating complex neuroendocrine and autonomic regulation patterns and controlling the homeostasis between sympathetic and parasympathetic cardiovascular systems. Poincaré plots and the standard deviation of the heart rhythm are good methods to study the central nervous system modulation. Although the genesis of these mechanisms is of central importance, the interactions of the afferents from the peripheral reflex arc, such as the baroreflex, are still in discussion (Arroyo-Carmona et al. 2024).

The heart rate variability (HRV) analysis assesses cardiac function in patients with several pathologic conditions; however, gender has not been included as a variable in these studies. It is known that women before the menopause have a minor proportion of lethal arrhythmias compared to men. One accepted hypothesis is that female hormones protect cardiac function and myocardial injuries (Albarado-Ibanez et al. 2019; Barajas-Martinez et al. 2021).

HRV analysis is based on subtle variations in sinus cycle length and has been used to assess cardiac autonomic status by two methods. The time-domain method identifies the R-R interval sequences and then applies statistical techniques to express the variance. The HRV suggests an ability to differentiate the cardiac rhythm according to sex. Sex steroid hormones interact with their receptors, affecting postsynaptic target cell responses and influencing presynaptic adrenergic function. Cardiomyocytes are not only a target for sex steroid hormones, but they also synthesize other steroids and metabolize these hormones. They express nuclear steroid hormone receptors that modulate gene expression and non-nuclear receptors that exert nongenomic effects (Barajas-Martinez et al. 2021).

A study by Albarado-Ibanez and collaborators analyzed the changes in HRV and cardiac function considering sex and heart rate. The patients in the study exhibited alterations in HRV in SD1 and SD2 related to being overweight. On the other hand, obese patients exhibited alterations in heart rhythm, such as bradycardia and HRV; the results did not show a significant difference between males (78 ± 16 bpm) and females (80 ± 14 bpm). However, HRV in women showed significant variability in both SD1 (0.053) and SD2 (0.28) compared to men (0.017 and 0.06, respectively). This data suggests that women have a more significant regulation of HRV by the autonomic nervous system than men (Albarado-Ibanez et al. 2013; Arroyo-Carmona et al. 2024).

3 Heart-Liver Axis

The relationship between the heart and the liver is evident in pathological conditions, but there are fewer observations concerning the physiological connection of the cardio-hepatic axis. The liver is highly responsive to changes in blood flow and hemodynamics, and these organs have a close circulatory connection. Also, the hemodynamic changes driven by cardiac pathology will affect liver function (Hollenberg and Waldman 2016). Moreover, specific cytokines secreted by each organ can directly influence the normal functioning of the other (Cheung et al. 2025).

Metabolic dysfunction-associated fatty liver disease (MASLD) is a global health concern, especially related to metabolic syndrome. The relationship between MASLD, atrial fibrillation, and cardiac failure may initially be related to mild metabolic inflammation (Cheung et al. 2025). Moreover, the ectopic fat accumulation observed in MetS probably releases adipokines that activate the immune system and increase inflammation, which can also produce myocardial inflammation (Hollenberg and Waldman 2016).

The cardio-hepatic syndrome refers to liver injuries observed in patients with cardiac fibrosis due to uncompensated heart failure and hemodynamic imbalance. Various pathologies of the right heart increase cardiac filling pressures, leading to low cardiac output and venous congestion, which in turn increases the pressure in hepatic sinusoids. The increase in retrograde pressure increases liver enzymes and may cause hepatocyte necrosis (Hollenberg and Waldman 2016).

On the other hand, some patients show splanchnic and arterial vasodilatation, and the increased flux leads to portal hypertension and altered bile circulation that leads to cholestasis. The hyperdynamic state increases heart rate and cardiac output. Also, the cardiomyocytes have bile acid receptors, which have a cardiotoxic effect (Voiosu et al. 2017).

The most common cause of death in metabolic dysfunction-associated steatosis liver disease (MASLD; see below) is CVD in both sexes. There is considerable overlap in signs present in MetS and both pathologies, including obesity, hypertension, insulin resistance, and hyperlipidemia. Even though the MASLD prevalence is higher in men, women have a higher risk of death than men when data are stratified by age. It is interesting that in middle-aged groups, women with MASLD lose their sex-protective advantage and may show a 10-year early aging (Ren and Zheng 2023).

The sex-dimorphic details of the heart-liver axis must be further studied because there is little literature about it.

4 Sexual Dimorphism in Metabolic Syndrome

Metabolic syndrome (MetS) is a cluster of signs that increases the risk of developing type 2 diabetes mellitus and cardiovascular diseases. MetS includes central obesity (with a circumference of 88 cm in women and 90 cm in men, or a body mass index (BMI) ≥30), hypertension (≥140/90 mmHg), dyslipidemia (such as hypertriglyceridemia with levels ≥150 mg/dl and low high-density lipoprotein levels ≤40 mg/dl in women and ≤35 mg/dl in men), impaired fasting glucose (greater than 100 mg/dl) or glucose intolerance (plasma glucose between 140 and 199 mg/dl 2 h after glucose load administration in an oral glucose tolerance test (OGTT). Finally, insulin resistance, considered the most critical sign of metabolic syndrome, is also present. For clinical diagnosis of MetS, at least three of these signs must be present, including insulin resistance or fasting glucose abnormalities (Hiriart et al. 2014; Samson and Garber 2014).

The etiology of MetS is multifactorial, comprising both environmental (diet and sedentary lifestyle) and genetic factors. According to the National Health and Nutrition Examination Survey (NHANES), the prevalence of MetS in the US was 34 (Mozumdar and Liguori 2011). The prevalence of metabolic syndrome varies around the world, by several factors such as diet and lifestyle, education, age, and sex, NHANES reported that the prevalence of MetS was significantly higher in women than men (35.6% vs 30.3%), and there are differences in all the signs of MetS between women and men (Aguilar et al. 2015; Rochlani et al. 2015).

5 Sexual Dimorphism in White Adipose Tissue

Sexual dimorphism, in all organisms, includes anatomical, physiological, and metabolic differences between females and males. In humans, these differences impact the distribution and function of white adipose tissue (Valencak et al. 2017). Women tend to store fat subcutaneously in the glute-femoral region (gynoid phenotype). At the same time, men accumulate more visceral fat (android phenotype), which is linked to higher metabolic risk. This fat distribution is influenced by sex hormones such as estrogens, which promote subcutaneous fat storage and modulate leptin actions in the central nervous system. At the same time, androgens reduce subcuta neous fat in men (Karastergiou and Fried 2017; Karastergiou et al. 2012).

Studies in small animals and humans show that losing estrogens or androgens alters fat distribution. Additionally, sex-specific differences in gene expression, adipocyte size, enzyme activity (such as LPL), and adrenergic receptor distribution across fat depots affect lipolysis. Variations are observed in fatty acid oxidation, leptin, adiponectin, VLDL, and energy expenditure, with the latter being lower in women due to reduced lean mass and body weight (Lee et al. 2013; Lovejoy et al. 2009).

Increased calorie intake combined with low physical activity has contributed to the global rise in obesity (Gonzalez-Muniesa et al. 2017). Although obesity affects both sexes, its prevalence is higher in women, who also tend to have greater total body fat (Meyer et al. 2011). This sexual dimorphism is linked to differences in fat quantity and distribution and the capability of fat depots to store and release fatty acids (Tchkonia et al. 2013). Under physiological conditions, adipocytes and immune cells such as eosinophils, ILC2s, NKT, T regulatory cells, and M2 macrophages maintain WAT homeostasis, which supports an anti-inflammatory Th2 response (Wensveen et al. 2015).

In obesity, excess caloric intake leads to adipocyte hypertrophy, hypoxia, activation of Hif-1a, and a shift toward a proinflammatory M1 macrophage profile. This promotes chronic low-grade local and systemic inflammation (Castoldi et al. 2015). In animal models, these inflammatory changes are more pronounced in males than females (Singer et al. 2015), highlighting sex-based differences in obesity-related inflammation.

6 Sex Differences in Lipid Metabolism, Dyslipidemia, Blood Pressure, and Hypertension

Sex differences in lipid metabolism and blood pressure regulation have clinically relevant implications. Premenopausal women exhibit lower cardiovascular risk, partially attributed to the protective effects of estrogens. After menopause, the decline in estrogen levels increases the risk of cardiovascular disease and dyslipidemia (Benjamin et al. 2017; Palmisano et al. 2018; Wilmot et al. 2015).

6.1 Lipid Metabolism and Dyslipidemia

Estrogens influence lipid metabolism through the receptors ERα, ERβ, and GPER, which are expressed in the liver, adipose tissue, intestine, and central nervous system. These receptors regulate the distribution of free fatty acids and lipoproteins, including VLDL, LDL, and HDL. In women, hepatic production of triglyceride-rich VLDL is lower during obesity, partially due to greater fatty acid clearance by muscle and lower intramuscular triglyceride accumulation, preserving insulin sensitivity (Palmisano et al. 2018).

Moreover, estrogens enhance reverse cholesterol transport, facilitating the excretion of hepatic cholesterol through bile. Estradiol carried on HDL potentiates cholesterol efflux capacity from macrophages, potentially contributing to the lower incidence of atherosclerosis in women. However, the specific roles of each estrogen receptor in humans remain unclear (Wang et al. 2004).

Estrogens also regulate intracellular pathways through non-genomic mechanisms, activating signaling cascades such as ERK1/2 and PI3K. GPER, a G-protein-coupled estrogen receptor, contributes to LDL regulation and vascular protection (Palmisano et al. 2018). In adipocytes, estrogens promote subcutaneous fat storage by increasing sensitivity to insulin and adiponectin, as well as enhancing white adipocyte differentiation. After menopause, fat redistribution toward the visceral compartment is associated with a decline in ovarian hormones (Santosa and Jensen 2012). Sex differences also exist in free fatty acid uptake, which is more active in females, independently of lipoprotein lipase.

Additionally, studies using the Four Core Genotype (FCG) mouse model demonstrate that sex chromosomes influence lipid metabolism and obesity (Burgoyne and Arnold 2016). Mice with two X chromosomes show greater adiposity and weight gain even without gonadal hormones, suggesting that X-linked genes, X chromosome inactivation scope, and microRNA expression can modulate metabolism independently of sex hormones (Zore et al. 2018).

6.2 Blood Pressure and Hypertension

Premenopausal women have a lower prevalence of hypertension, which rises significantly after menopause. Blood pressure (BP) increases with age in a sex-specific manner: in women, this rise is steeper after the age of 60, eventually surpassing that of men (Colafella and Denton 2018).

Sex hormones and chromosomes regulate key vascular and renal mechanisms, including endothelial function, sodium reabsorption, and the renin-angiotensin-aldosterone system (RAAS) activation. In females, estrogens induce vasodilation and modulate the expression of RAAS components, downregulating AT1R and upregulating AT2R. They also reduce the production of endothelin-1 and its vasoconstrictive receptors, contributing to natriuretic and antihypertensive effects (Colafella and Denton 2018; Mirabito et al. 2014).

Aging and cellular senescence, driven by oxidative stress and mitochondrial dysfunction, also play a role. In rats, chronic RAAS activation contributes to age-related loss of renal function, particularly in males (Colafella and Denton 2018). In postmenopausal women, increased adiposity has been associated with greater telomere shortening, a marker of vascular senescence (Walker et al. 2016).

Finally, sex chromosomes influence the pressor response to angiotensin II and the development of atherosclerosis (Ji et al. 2010). Genes such as Sry (located on the Y chromosome) increase the synthesis of sympathetic neurotransmitters, which may be related to the pathogenesis of hypertension. In contrast, the double dosage of genes like ACE2 and ATR2 (located on the X chromosome) may confer cardiovascular protection in females (Hilliard et al. 2013).

6.3 Insulin Resistance

Since its description by Reaven, insulin resistance has been considered a central factor in the pathophysiology of MetS and a hallmark of type 2 diabetes (Reaven 1988). Several mechanisms have been proposed for its development, with obesity, often driven by high-calorie diets, being a key trigger (Alejandro et al. 2015). Excessive nutrient intake leads to hyperinsulinemia, which promotes insulin resistance in tissues, partly through inflammatory adipokines such as TNF-α and IL-6. In adipose tissue, insulin resistance enhances lipolysis, elevating plasma-free fatty acids and toxic lipids that impair insulin signaling. At the molecular level, insulin receptor expression and signal transduction are reduced. The soluble insulin receptor (SIR), which increases with hyperinsulinemia, may further contribute to insulin resistance by limiting insulin availability (Hiriart et al. 2014).

The unregulated inhibition of the insulin signaling pathway mainly occurs at the proximal phase, targeting critical nodes such as insulin receptor substrate 1 (IRS1) and Akt. IRS1 is phosphorylated at inhibitory serine/threonine residues by kinases such as c-Jun N-terminal Kinase (JNK1), IkB kinase (IKKB), and suppressors of cytokine signaling (SOCS). These kinases are activated by proinflammatory cytokine signaling pathways, including TNFα, IL-6, and IL-1β, and by nutrients such as free fatty acids (FFAs), which can activate JNK1 and IKKB. This illustrates how obesity impairs insulin signaling and leads to metabolic disturbances (Rochlani et al. 2017).

In obesity, the ribosomal kinase S6K1, which plays a role in the protein synthesis pathway, may become overstimulated, phosphorylating IRS1 at serine 1101 (Ser1101), leading to IRS1 degradation. This disrupts signal transmission between the insulin receptor and IRS1, impairing the pathway. Akt kinase is a critical node in the insulin signaling cascade. Studies have shown that accumulating ceramides and diacylglycerols (DAG) can impair Akt function by activating PKCZ, which alters Akt localization at the membrane. Moreover, protein phosphatases such as PP2A (protein phosphatase 2A) and PHLPPL (Pleckstrin homology domain leucine-rich repeat protein phosphatase-like) can dephosphorylate Akt, reducing activity (Haeusler et al. 2018).

6.4 Sex Dimorphism in Conditions Associated with MetS and CVD

Metabolic dysfunction-associated steatosis liver disease (MASLD) is the most prevalent chronic liver disease, characterized by excessive lipid accumulation in hepatocytes. This condition is strongly associated with metabolic syndrome and contributes to the development of CVD due to the liver's influence on systemic insulin resistance, dyslipidemia, inflammation, and gut dysbiosis (Padureanu et al. 2025).

MASLD is more prevalent in men and postmenopausal women than in premenopausal women (Cherubini et al. 2024). In males, androgen signaling prevents the development of MASLD due to the effects of the androgen receptor (AR) signaling on the formation of lipid droplets, inflammation, and hepatocyte apoptosis (Cherubini et al. 2024). Conversely, androgen signaling in females exacerbates lipid accumulation in obese premenopausal women and in patients with polycystic ovary syndrome (Cherubini et al. 2024). Nevertheless, androgen signaling promotes the progression of MASLD towards liver fibrosis and hepatocellular carcinoma in both males and females (Nagral et al. 2022).

Contrarily, estrogen signaling prevents the development and progression of MASLD in both males and females (Nagral et al. 2022). The protective effects of estrogens include the promotion of hepatocyte regeneration, insulin sensitivity, and free fatty acid oxidation, while they inhibit triglyceride synthesis and inflammation (Cherubini et al. 2024). Notably, the decrease in estrogen production during menopause is related to the increase in MASLD prevalence in postmenopausal women (Nagral et al. 2022), and decreased hepatic levels of estrogen receptor α (ERα) enhance lipid accumulation and induce atherosclerosis and cardiovascular alterations (Cherubini et al. 2024). Thus, the pathophysiology of MASLD is heavily influenced by sex hormones, driving metabolic alterations that can promote the development of CVD in a sex-specific manner.

Metabolic syndrome also promotes the development of sarcopenic obesity, a condition characterized by the coexistence of low skeletal muscle mass and function and a high body fat percentage (Donini et al. 2022). This condition increases the risk of developing T2DM, CVD, frailty syndrome, and premature death (Donini et al. 2022). Due to the cross-communication between WAT, skeletal muscle, and bone, sarcopenic obesity can result in osteoporosis, reduced mobility, loss of independence, and worsening metabolic alterations due to increased sedentarism (Rubio-Ruiz et al. 2019).

There are disparities in the diagnostic criteria of sarcopenic obesity, but it is generally recognized that men lose more muscle mass during aging than women (McMillin et al. 2022). However, by applying the current diagnostic criteria for sarcopenic obesity, the prevalence is higher in women (Danielewicz et al. 2024), and the prevalence of frailty syndrome increases after menopause in women (Conforto et al. 2024).

In women, estrogen deficits promote low-grade systemic inflammation, impair mitochondrial function, and increase oxidative stress, all known factors contributing to loss of myofibrillar proteins and reduced force production (McMillin et al. 2022; Rubio-Ruiz et al. 2019). Moreover, female rats with diet-induced obesity develop more muscle steatosis compared with males (Smith et al. 2025a).

Contrarily, testosterone promotes protein anabolism and satellite cell differentiation in skeletal muscle, contributing to the higher muscle mass observed in males (Rubio-Ruiz et al. 2019). Moreover, testosterone levels stimulate insulin-like growth factor-1 (IGF-1) secretion in muscle, which acts as a myokine that promotes protein synthesis in the muscle. The decreased testosterone concentrations observed in men during aging promote the loss of muscle mass due to reduced protein synthesis and increased proteolytic activity in skeletal muscle (Rubio-Ruiz et al. 2019) (Fig. 2).

7 Premature Cardiovascular Aging

Women and men have differences in structure, function, and electrical activity of the heart; the latter is clinically evaluated by ECG, which has characteristic differences between women and men throughout life (childhood, adulthood, and old age). ECG in healthy newborns (third to fourth day of life) has shown that heart rates are higher in females than in males. In addition, the QT interval and the cycle length were shorter in females than in males. The mean QTc was not different between females and males (Stramba-Badiale et al. 1995).

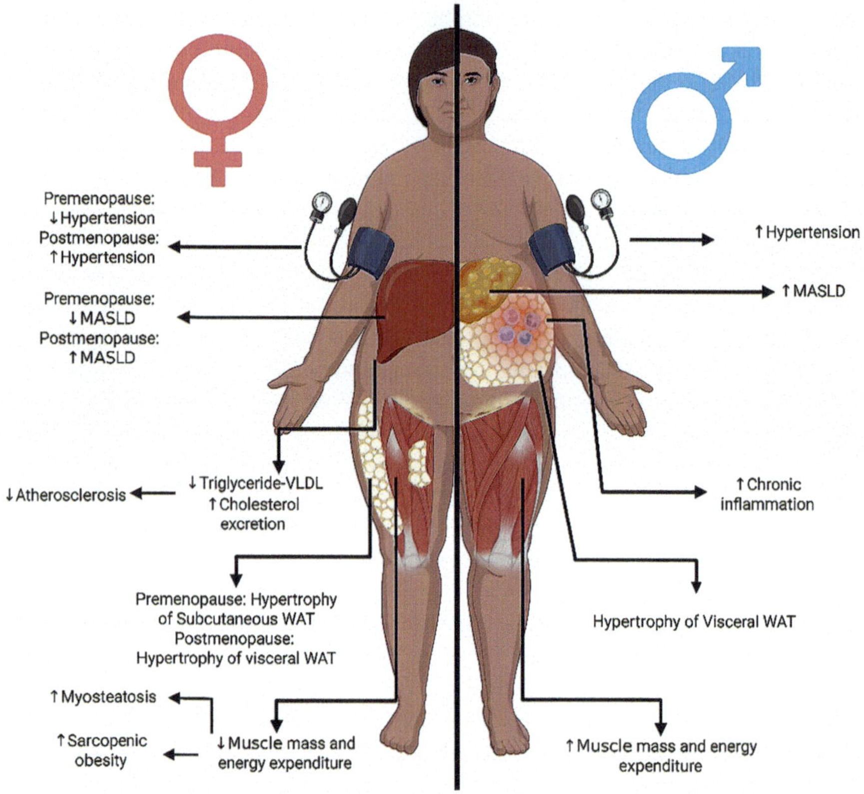

Fig. 2 Sexual dimorphism in metabolic syndrome

In infants, the heart is typically vertically oriented and physiologically dominated by the right ventricle, leading to right axis deviation and a QRS complex shifted to the right. Biphasic T waves are commonly seen in the right precordial leads (V1 to V3–V4), reflecting normal age-related repolarization patterns. This characteristic morphology may be present until adolescence, particularly in females. Additionally, boys and girls under 15 years of age have similar heart rates and QTc intervals. Some adolescents show an R wave with high voltage in precordial leads I (60 mm) without left ventricular enlargement. Sometimes, there is an evident increase in the heart rate with inspiration (Albarado-Ibañez et al. 2024).

In adulthood, the QTc interval decreases by approximately 20 ms in men, while in women it remains unchanged. As a result, women tend to have longer QTc intervals than men, regardless of the correction method used. In men, the QTc interval gradually increases with age, and this age-related change is more pronounced in men than in women. In older individuals, the ECG exhibits the following age-related changes. A slower HR and longer PR interval (normal up to 0.22 s), an AP shifted to the right, are associated with pulmonary emphysema, characterized by an S wave in lead V6 and a QRS complex shifted to the left. There is poor R-wave progression from V1 to V3 due to septal fibrosis. Unspecific alterations of repolarization (slightly depressed ST segment and/or flattened T wave). A U wave is frequently present, particularly in the intermediate precordial leads (Tang et al. 2018).

The aging process is associated with a decline in heart rate in humans in both genders, primarily due to a reduction in intrinsic factors that regulate heart rate. This age-related phenomenon is associated with a decrease in the excitability and function of individual pacemaker cells in the sinoatrial node. In contrast, the occurrence of sudden arrhythmias originates within the pacemaker, but these arrhythmias could be due to electrical activity in the ventricles. Any change in HRV is a predictor of mortality from cardiovascular disease and is associated with cardiac disease morbidity. Factors contributing to changes in HRV include hypertension, obesity, family history, and stressful work environments. The decrease in HR related to aging is inevitable. This process is related to an increased accumulation of lipids in non-adipose tissues, insulin resistance, and hardening of the extracellular matrix, as well as the inflammatory process and electrical changes observed in left ventricular hypertrophy, heart failure, and atrial fibrillation (Albarado-Ibanez et al. 2013).

Recent studies have shown that metabolic diseases like obesity produce early aging (Albarado-Ibañez et al. 2024). Most of the early evidence on the CV benefits of weight reduction was gleaned from observational studies in which weight loss was a secondary endpoint. However, many of the adverse consequences of obesity are mediated through resultant risk factors acting in the pathophysiologic pathway of atherosclerotic vascular disease.

Weight reduction has been shown to improve most risk factors, including glucose tolerance, insulin sensitivity, blood pressure, and dyslipidemia. These conditions produced alterations in cardiac rhythm and arrhythmias in humans. A trilogy of heart diseases manifests during aging: left ventricular hypertrophy, heart failure, and atrial fibrillation (Lakatta and Levy 2003). These alterations increase dramatically with MetS. Heart failure and left ventricular hypertrophy are associated with hypertension and obesity (Lauer et al. 1999).

However, atrial fibrillation is present in 4% of healthy volunteers over 60 years of age, excluding clinical coronary artery disease, without identifiable cause. The association between aging and heart failure is most likely the result of decades of inadequate treatment of underlying risk factors rather than aging alone, even lethal arrhythmias (Abidov et al. 2004).

We recently described that exposing young adult male Wistar rats to high sucrose drinking water for 2 and 6 months is enough to induce MetS. These MetS models show differences in the severity of obesity and lipid plasma levels, hyperinsulinemia, glucose tolerance, and MASLD. Moreover, these models exhibit morphological changes and altered electrical activity in the pacemaker. At 2 months, we observed supraventricular arrhythmia, while at 6 months, animals with MetS predominantly showed QT-long arrhythmia (Fig. 3). These changes in electrical SAN are associated with MetS and cause cardiovascular frailty and premature aging of the heart (Albarado-Ibanez et al. 2013, 2024; Torres-Jacome et al. 2022).

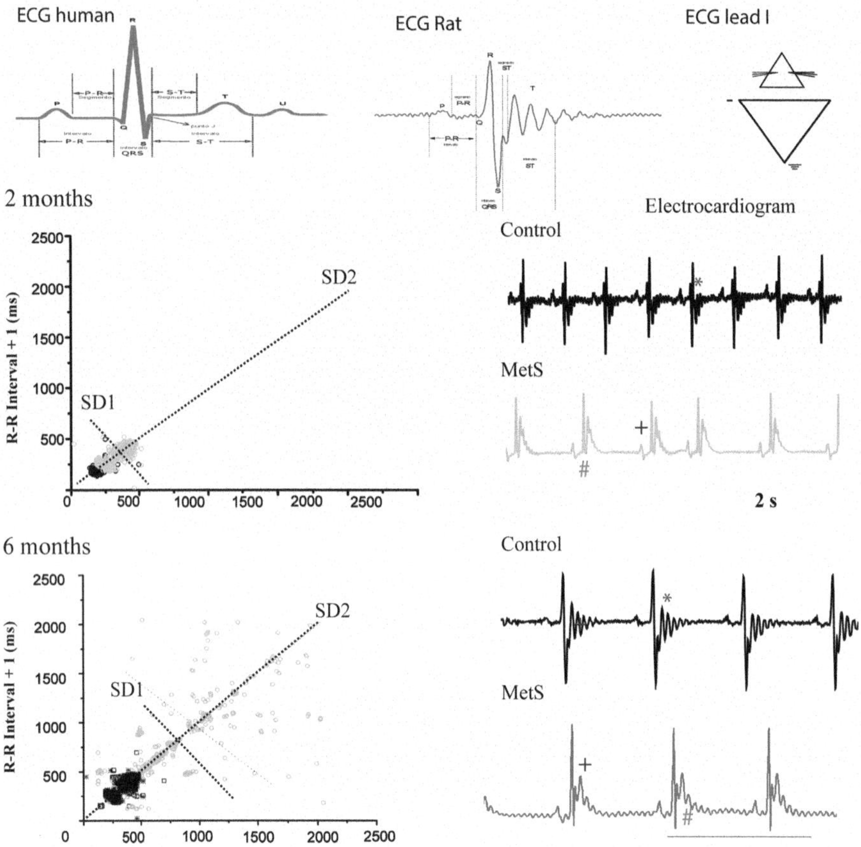

Fig. 3 Metabolic syndrome produces premature ageing. Decrease heart rate, * T wave elevation, + increase PR Interval, P wave elevation, # inhibition T wave

8 Perspectives

Changes in the way we eat and exercise are crucial to prevent the cardiovascular risks associated with MetS. In addition, differences in gene expression between men and women, resulting from sex chromosomes and sex hormones, are mediated by epigenetic control.

The regulation affects sex differences observed during different stages of development and may contribute to the marked sex differences present in CVD. Sexual dimorphism exists in metabolism and the cardiovascular system and needs to be further investigated to improve understanding and treatments. These may differ, not only in the dosing but also in the type of approach.

A better understanding of MSLAD is also needed to develop better treatments that will target the liver with medicines that can prevent, in time, the development of cirrhosis and heart damage.

Finally, developing ways to prevent CV damage during each developmental stage is essential.

References

Abidov A, Hachamovitch R, Rozanski A, Hayes SW, Santos MM, Sciammarella MG et al (2004) Prognostic implications of atrial fibrillation in patients undergoing myocardial perfusion single-photon emission computed tomography. J Am Coll Cardiol 44(5):1062–1070. https://doi.org/10.1016/j.jacc.2004.05.076

Aguilar M, Bhuket T, Torres S, Liu B, Wong RJ (2015) Prevalence of the metabolic syndrome in the United States, 2003–2012. JAMA 313(19):1973–1974. https://doi.org/10.1001/jama.2015.4260

Albarado-Ibanez A, Avelino-Cruz JE, Velasco M, Torres-Jacome J, Hiriart M (2013) Metabolic syndrome remodels electrical activity of the sinoatrial node and produces arrhythmias in rats. PLoS One 8(11):e76534. https://doi.org/10.1371/journal.pone.0076534

Albarado-Ibanez A, Arroyo-Carmona RE, Sanchez-Hernandez R, Ramos-Ortiz G, Frank A, Garcia-Gudino D, Torres-Jacome J (2019) The role of the autonomic nervous system on cardiac rhythm during the evolution of diabetes mellitus using heart rate variability as a biomarker. J Diabetes Res 2019:5157024. https://doi.org/10.1155/2019/5157024

Albarado-Ibañez A, Torres -Jacome J, Hiriart M (2024) Chronic metabolic syndrome develops a frailty of cardiac rhythm similar to aging in rats. Med Res Arch 12(10):1–10. https://doi.org/10.18103/mra.v12i10.5939

Alejandro EU, Gregg B, Blandino-Rosano M, Cras-Meneur C, Bernal-Mizrachi E (2015) Natural history of beta-cell adaptation and failure in type 2 diabetes. Mol Asp Med 42:19–41. https://doi.org/10.1016/j.mam.2014.12.002

Antzelevitch C, Di Diego JM (2022) J wave syndromes: what's new? Trends Cardiovasc Med 32(6):350–363. https://doi.org/10.1016/j.tcm.2021.07.001

Arroyo-Carmona RE, Lopez-Serrano AL, Albarado-Ibanez A, Mendoza-Lucero FM, Medel-Cajica D, Lopez-Mayorga RM, Torres-Jacome J (2016) Heart rate variability as early biomarker for the evaluation of diabetes mellitus progress. J Diabetes Res 2016:8483537. https://doi.org/10.1155/2016/8483537

Arroyo-Carmona RE, Mitre-Velasco Y, Martinez-Laguna Y, Torres-Jacome J, Albarado-Ibanez A (2024) A maternal diet high in carbohydrates causes bradyarrhythmias and changes in heart rate variability in the offspring sex-dependent in mice. Lab Anim Res 40(1):34. https://doi.org/10.1186/s12826 024 00222 6

Barajas-Martinez A, Ibarra-Coronado E, Fossion R, Toledo-Roy JC, Martinez-Garces V, Lopez-Rivera JA et al (2021) Sex differences in the physiological network of healthy Young subjects. Front Physiol 12:678507. https://doi.org/10.3389/fphys.2021.678507

Benjamin EJ, Blaha MJ, Chiuve SE, Cushman M, Das SR, Deo R et al (2017) Heart disease and stroke Statistics-2017 update: A report from the American Heart Association. Circulation 135(10):e146–e603. https://doi.org/10.1161/CIR.0000000000000485

Burgoyne PS, Arnold AP (2016) A primer on the use of mouse models for identifying direct sex chromosome effects that cause sex differences in non-gonadal tissues. Biol Sex Differ 7:68. https://doi.org/10.1186/s13293-016-0115-5

Carrillo-Franco L, Gonzalez-Garcia M, Morales-Luque C, Dawid-Milner MS, Lopez-Gonzalez MV (2024) Hypothalamic regulation of cardiorespiratory functions: insights into the dorsomedial and perifornical pathways. Biology (Basel) 13(11). https://doi.org/10.3390/biology13110933

Castoldi A, Naffah de Souza C, Camara NO, Moraes-Vieira PM (2015) The macrophage switch in obesity development. Front Immunol 6:637. https://doi.org/10.3389/fimmu.2015.00637

Cherubini A, Della Torre S, Pelusi S, Valenti L (2024) Sexual dimorphism of metabolic dysfunction-associated steatotic liver disease. Trends Mol Med 30(12):1126–1136. https://doi.org/10.1016/j.molmed.2024.05.013

Cheung J, Cheung BM, Yiu KH, Tse HF, Chan YH (2025) Role of metabolic dysfunction-associated fatty liver disease in atrial fibrillation and heart failure: molecular and clinical aspects. Front Cardiovasc Med 12:1573841. https://doi.org/10.3389/fcvm.2025.1573841

Colafella KMM, Denton KM (2018) Sex-specific differences in hypertension and associated cardiovascular disease. Nat Rev Nephrol 14(3):185–201. https://doi.org/10.1038/nrneph.2017.189

Conforto R, Rizzo V, Russo R, Mazza E, Maurotti S, Pujia C et al (2024) Advances in body composition and gender differences in susceptibility to frailty syndrome: role of osteosarcopenic obesity. Metabolism 161:156052. https://doi.org/10.1016/j.metabol.2024.156052

Danielewicz AL, Marra A, Tringali G, Micheli R, Abbruzzese L, Fanari P et al (2024) Analysis of sarcopenic obesity prevalence and diagnostic agreement according to the 2022 ESPEN and EASO Consensus in hospitalized older adults with severe obesity. Front Endocrinol (Lausanne) 15:1366229. https://doi.org/10.3389/fendo.2024.1366229

Donini LM, Busetto L, Bischoff SC, Cederholm T, Ballesteros-Pomar MD, Batsis JA et al (2022) Definition and diagnostic criteria for Sarcopenic obesity: ESPEN and EASO consensus statement. Obes Facts 15(3):321–335. https://doi.org/10.1159/000521241

Dorsa EPM, Banta A, Post A, Razavi M, Aazhang B (2023) A novel method for 12-lead ECG reconstruction. Conf Rec Asilomar Conf Signals Syst Comput 2023:1054–1058. https://doi.org/10.1109/ieeeconf59524.2023.10476822

Emerson JI, Shi W, Paredes-Larios J, Walker WG, Hutton JE, Cristea IM et al (2025) X-chromosome-linked miRNAs regulate sex differences in cardiac physiology. Circ Res 136(3): 258–275. https://doi.org/10.1161/CIRCRESAHA.124.325447

Gonzalez-Muniesa P, Martinez-Gonzalez MA, Hu FB, Despres JP, Matsuzawa Y, Loos RJF et al (2017) Obesity. Nat Rev Dis Primers 3:17034. https://doi.org/10.1038/nrdp.2017.34

Haeusler RA, McGraw TE, Accili D (2018) Biochemical and cellular properties of insulin receptor signalling. Nat Rev Mol Cell Biol 19(1):31–44. https://doi.org/10.1038/nrm.2017.89

Hilliard LM, Sampson AK, Brown RD, Denton KM (2013) The "his and hers" of the renin-angiotensin system. Curr Hypertens Rep 15(1):71–79. https://doi.org/10.1007/s11906-012-0319-y

Hiriart M, Sanchez-Soto C, Diaz-Garcia CM, Castanares DT, Avitia M, Velasco M et al (2014) Hyperinsulinemia is associated with increased soluble insulin receptors release from hepatocytes. Front Endocrinol (Lausanne) 5:95. https://doi.org/10.3389/fendo.2014.00095

Hollenberg SM, Waldman B (2016) The circulatory system in liver disease. Crit Care Clin 32(3): 331–342. https://doi.org/10.1016/j.ccc.2016.02.004

Ji H, Zheng W, Wu X, Liu J, Ecelbarger CM, Watkins R et al (2010) Sex chromosome effects unmasked in angiotensin II-induced hypertension. Hypertension 55(5):1275–1282. https://doi.org/10.1161/HYPERTENSIONAHA.109.144949

Karastergiou K, Fried SK (2017) Cellular mechanisms driving sex differences in adipose tissue biology and body shape in humans and mouse models. Adv Exp Med Biol 1043:29–51. https://doi.org/10.1007/978-3-319-70178-3_3

Karastergiou K, Smith SR, Greenberg AS, Fried SK (2012) Sex differences in human adipose tissues – the biology of pear shape. Biol Sex Differ 3(1):13. https://doi.org/10.1186/2042-6410-3-13

Kuczmarski AV, Welti LM, Moreau KL, Wenner MM (2021) ET-1 as a sex-specific mechanism impacting age-related changes in vascular function. Front Aging 2:727416. https://doi.org/10.3389/fragi.2021.727416

Lakatta EG, Levy D (2003) Arterial and cardiac aging: major shareholders in cardiovascular disease enterprises: part I: aging arteries: a "set up" for vascular disease. Circulation 107(1):139–146. https://doi.org/10.1161/01.cir.0000048892.83521.58

Lauer MS, Larson MG, Evans JC, Levy D (1999) Association of left ventricular dilatation and hypertrophy with chronotropic incompetence in the Framingham Heart Study. Am Heart J 137(5):903–909. https://doi.org/10.1016/s0002-8703(99)70415-1

Lee MJ, Wu Y, Fried SK (2013) Adipose tissue heterogeneity: implication of depot differences in adipose tissue for obesity complications. Mol Asp Med 34(1):1–11. https://doi.org/10.1016/j.mam.2012.10.001

Lovejoy JC, Sainsbury A, Stock Conference Working, G (2009) Sex differences in obesity and the regulation of energy homeostasis. Obes Rev 10(2):154–167. https://doi.org/10.1111/j.1467-789X.2008.00529.x

McMillin SL, Minchew EC, Lowe DA, Spangenburg EE (2022) Skeletal muscle wasting: the estrogen side of sexual dimorphism. Am J Physiol Cell Physiol 322(1):C24–C37. https://doi.org/10.1152/ajpcell.00333.2021

Meyer MR, Clegg DJ, Prossnitz ER, Barton M (2011) Obesity, insulin resistance and diabetes: sex differences and role of oestrogen receptors. Acta Physiol (Oxf) 203(1):259–269. https://doi.org/10.1111/j.1748-1716.2010.02237.x

Mirabito KM, Hilliard LM, Kett MM, Brown RD, Booth SC, Widdop RE et al (2014) Sex- and age-related differences in the chronic pressure-natriuresis relationship: role of the angiotensin type 2 receptor. Am J Physiol Renal Physiol 307(8):F901–F907. https://doi.org/10.1152/ajprenal.00288.2014

Mozumdar A, Liguori G (2011) Persistent increase of prevalence of metabolic syndrome among U.S. adults: NHANES III to NHANES 1999-2006. Diabetes Care 34(1):216–219. https://doi.org/10.2337/dc10-0879

Nagral A, Bangar M, Menezes S, Bhatia S, Butt N, Ghosh J et al (2022) Gender differences in nonalcoholic fatty liver disease. Euroasian J Hepatogastroenterol 12(Suppl 1):S19–S25. https://doi.org/10.5005/jp-journals-10018-1370

Naskar K, Mukherjee S, Ghosh S, Adhikari S (2024) Coupled 3D (J >/= 0) time-dependent wave packet calculation for the F + H(2) reaction on accurate Ab initio multi-state diabatic potential energy surfaces. J Phys Chem A 128(8):1438–1456. https://doi.org/10.1021/acs.jpca.3c05590

Padureanu V, Fortofoiu MC, Pirscoveanu M, Padureanu R, Radulescu D, Donoiu I, Pirscoveanu DFV (2025) Cardiovascular manifestations of patients with non-alcoholic fatty liver disease. Metabolites 15(3). https://doi.org/10.3390/metabo15030149

Palmisano BT, Zhu L, Eckel RH, Stafford JM (2018) Sex differences in lipid and lipoprotein metabolism. Mol Metab 15:45–55. https://doi.org/10.1016/j.molmet.2018.05.008

Reaven GM (1988) Banting lecture 1988. Role of insulin resistance in human disease. Diabetes 37(12):1595–1607. Retrieved from http://www.ncbi.nlm.nih.gov/pubmed/3056758

Ren R, Zheng Y (2023) Sex differences in cardiovascular and all-cause mortality in nonalcoholic fatty liver disease in the US population. Nutr Metab Cardiovasc Dis 33(7):1349–1357. https://doi.org/10.1016/j.numecd.2023.03.003

Rochlani Y, Pothineni NV, Mehta JL (2015) Metabolic syndrome: does it differ between women and men? Cardiovasc Drugs Ther 29(4):329–338. https://doi.org/10.1007/s10557-015-6593-6

Rochlani Y, Pothineni NV, Kovelamudi S, Mehta JL (2017) Metabolic syndrome: pathophysiology, management, and modulation by natural compounds. Ther Adv Cardiovasc Dis 11(8):215–225. https://doi.org/10.1177/1753944717711379

Rubio-Ruiz ME, Guarner-Lans V, Perez-Torres I, Soto ME (2019) Mechanisms underlying metabolic syndrome-related sarcopenia and possible therapeutic measures. Int J Mol Sci 20(3). https://doi.org/10.3390/ijms20030647

Samson SL, Garber AJ (2014) Metabolic syndrome. Endocrinol Metab Clin N Am 43(1):1–23. https://doi.org/10.1016/j.ecl.2013.09.009

Santosa S, Jensen MD (2012) Effects of male hypogonadism on regional adipose tissue fatty acid storage and lipogenic proteins. PLoS One 7(2):e31473. https://doi.org/10.1371/journal.pone.0031473

Singer K, Maley N, Mergian T, DelProposto J, Cho KW, Zamarron BF et al (2015) Differences in hematopoietic stem cells contribute to sexually dimorphic inflammatory responses to high fat diet-induced obesity. J Biol Chem 290(21):13250–13262. https://doi.org/10.1074/jbc.M114.634568

Smith HE, Abughazaleh N, Seerattan RA, Syed F, Young D, Dufour A et al (2025a) Sex-specific response of intramuscular fat to diet-induced obesity in rats. Sci Rep 15(1):2147. https://doi.org/10.1038/s41598-024-85084-7

Smith CER, Ni H, Grandi E (2025b) Sex differences in electrophysiology and calcium handling in atrial health and fibrillation. Annu Rev Physiol 87(1):1–24. https://doi.org/10.1146/annurev-physiol-022724-104938

St Pierre SR, Peirlinck M, Kuhl E (2022) Sex matters: a comprehensive comparison of female and male hearts. Front Physiol 13:831179. https://doi.org/10.3389/fphys.2022.831179

Stramba-Badiale M, Spagnolo D, Bosi G, Schwartz PJ (1995) Are gender differences in QTc present at birth? MISNES Investigators. Multicenter Italian Study on Neonatal electrocardiography and sudden infant death syndrome. Am J Cardiol 75(17):1277–1278. Retrieved from http://www.ncbi.nlm.nih.gov/pubmed/7778558

Tang WH, Ho WH, Chen YJ (2018) Retrieving hidden atrial repolarization waves from standard surface ECGs. Biomed Eng Online 17(Suppl 2):146. https://doi.org/10.1186/s12938-018-0576-3

Tchkonia T, Thomou T, Zhu Y, Karagiannides I, Pothoulakis C, Jensen MD, Kirkland JL (2013) Mechanisms and metabolic implications of regional differences among fat depots. Cell Metab 17(5):644–656. https://doi.org/10.1016/j.cmet.2013.03.008

Torres-Jacome J, Ortiz-Fuentes BS, Bernabe-Sanchez D, Lopez-Silva B, Velasco M, Ita-Amador ML, Albarado-Ibanez A (2022) Ventricular dysfunction in obese and nonobese rats with metabolic syndrome. J Diabetes Res 2022:9321445. https://doi.org/10.1155/2022/9321445

Valencak TG, Osterrieder A, Schulz TJ (2017) Sex matters: the effects of biological sex on adipose tissue biology and energy metabolism. Redox Biol 12:806–813. https://doi.org/10.1016/j.redox.2017.04.012

Voiosu A, Wiese S, Voiosu T, Bendtsen F, Moller S (2017) Bile acids and cardiovascular function in cirrhosis. Liver Int 37(10):1420–1430. https://doi.org/10.1111/liv.13394

Walker AE, Morgan RG, Ives SJ, Cawthon RM, Andtbacka RH, Noyes D et al (2016) Age-related arterial telomere uncapping and senescence is greater in women compared with men. Exp Gerontol 73:65–71. https://doi.org/10.1016/j.exger.2015.11.009

Wang HH, Afdhal NH, Wang DQH (2004) Estrogen receptor alpha, but not beta, plays a major role in 17beta-estradiol-induced murine cholesterol gallstones. Gastroenterology 127(1):239–249. Retrieved from https://www.ncbi.nlm.nih.gov/pubmed/15236189

Wensveen FM, Valentic S, Sestan M, Turk Wensveen T, Polic B (2015) The "Big Bang" in obese fat: events initiating obesity-induced adipose tissue inflammation. Eur J Immunol 45(9):2446–2456. https://doi.org/10.1002/eji.201545502

Wilmot KA, O'Flaherty M, Capewell S, Ford ES, Vaccarino V (2015) Coronary heart disease mortality declines in the United States from 1979 through 2011: evidence for stagnation in young adults, especially women. Circulation 132(11):997–1002. https://doi.org/10.1161/CIRCULATIONAHA.115.015293

Woodcock EA, Matkovich SJ (2005) Cardiomyocytes structure, function and associated pathologies. Int J Biochem Cell Biol 37(9):1746–1751. https://doi.org/10.1016/j.biocel.2005.04.011

Zaid M, Sala L, Despins L, Heise D, Popescu M, Skubic M et al (2023) Cardiovascular sex-differences: insights via physiology-based modeling and potential for noninvasive sensing via ballistocardiography. Front Cardiovasc Med 10:1215958. https://doi.org/10.3389/fcvm.2023.1215958

Zhang ZH, Barajas-Martinez H, Duan HY, Fan GH, Jiang H, Antzelevitch C et al (2025) Characterization of novel arrhythmogenic patterns arising secondary to heterogeneous expression and activation of Nav1.8. Front Cardiovasc Med 12:1546803. https://doi.org/10.3389/fcvm.2025.1546803
Zore T, Palafox M, Reue K (2018) Sex differences in obesity, lipid metabolism, and inflammation-A role for the sex chromosomes? Mol Metab 15:35–44. https://doi.org/10.1016/j.molmet.2018.04.003

Cardiac Cell Remodeling in Obesity and Diabetes

Avelino-Cruz José Everardo, Yang-Bennett Daniela Sarahi, and Galindo-Ramírez Fabián

Contents

A.-C. José Everardo (✉)
Laboratory of Molecular Cardiology, Institute of Physiology, Benemérita Universidad Autónoma de Puebla, Puebla, Mexico
e-mail: jose.avelino@correo.buap.mx

Y.-B. Daniela Sarahi
Laboratory of Molecular Cardiology, Institute of Physiology, Benemérita Universidad Autónoma de Puebla, Puebla, Mexico

Division of Cardiovascular Medicine, Department of Internal Medicine, Abboud Cardiovascular Research Center, University of Iowa, Iowa City, IA, USA
e-mail: danielasarahi-yangbennett@uiowa.edu

G.-R. Fabián
Laboratory of Cancer and intercellular communication, Institute of Physiology, Benemérita Universidad Autónoma de Puebla, Puebla, Mexico
e-mail: fabian.galindo@correo.buap.mx

A. Rueda, M. Nieves-Cintrón (eds.), *Cardiovascular Alterations in Metabolic Diseases*, Handbook of Experimental Pharmacology 293,
https://doi.org/10.1007/164_2026_789

Abstract

The contractile activity of the heart depends on the coordinated activation of cardiac muscle cells, as well as the activation of each region within these cells. The conversion of an electrical signal into a mechanical process is known as excitation-contraction coupling; this process depends on the accurate organization and functional coupling between the different participating structures. The T-tubules and the sarcoplasmic reticulum constitute the dyads, a functional structure where the activity of voltage-gated calcium channels is coupled with the type 2 ryanodine receptor to generate calcium-induced calcium release. This phenomenon increases the intracellular calcium concentration, allowing cell contraction. The relaxation process occurs at the same time as calcium extrusion or recapture into the sarcoplasmic reticulum. The formation of the T tubules, the organization of the dyad, and the distribution of the proteins that regulate the entry, reuptake, and extrusion of calcium involve different structural proteins whose expression, localization, and function can be affected in pathological processes such as heart failure. In this chapter, we give an overview of the proteins involved in cardiac cell ultrastructural organization and an insight into changes and possible causes of these changes found in diabetes, obesity, and heart failure models.

Keywords

BIN1 · Cardiomyocyte ultrastructure · Heart failure · Junctophilin 2 · Metabolic remodeling

1 Introduction

In this chapter, we examine the intricate relationship between metabolic disorders, specifically obesity and diabetes, and their impact on cardiac function. As the global prevalence of these conditions continues to rise, elucidating their effects on cardiovascular health has become increasingly critical.

We discuss how obesity and diabetes induce profound metabolic alterations that detrimentally affect cardiac cells, with particular emphasis on oxidative stress as a pivotal mediator between lipid accumulation, inflammation, and cardiac dysfunction, which typically manifests as myocardial fibrosis, hypertrophy, and, ultimately, heart failure.

Further, we explore the cellular mechanisms underlying cardiac performance, with a focus on excitation–contraction coupling, a process that is frequently disrupted under pathological conditions. Notably, the structural disorganization of the transverse tubule (T-tubule) system in such states impairs the coordinated function of key calcium-handling proteins, including the ryanodine receptor type 2 (RyR2), L-type calcium channel (LTCC), sodium–calcium exchanger (NCX), sarcoplasmic/endoplasmic reticulum calcium ATPase (SERCA), and caveolin-3

(Cav-3). These disruptions compromise calcium homeostasis in cardiomyocytes, leading to impaired relaxation and contractility.

In summary, this chapter provides a comprehensive overview of the mechanisms through which obesity and diabetes contribute to pathological cardiac remodeling and dysfunction, ultimately promoting heart failure. The insights presented herein are essential for guiding the development of targeted therapeutic strategies to reduce cardiovascular risk associated with these metabolic conditions.

2 Obesity and Diabetes

Diabetes encompasses a group of metabolic disorders characterized by hyperglycemia, resulting from defects in insulin secretion or in its functional mechanism (Magliano and Boyko 2021). The leading cause of death among diabetic patients is cardiovascular disease (Wong and Sattar 2023).

Obesity is a chronic disease characterized by the consumption of more energy than is expended, resulting in progressive weight gain. This condition is viewed as a low-intensity inflammatory process that correlates with other pathologies, including cardiac diseases, systemic arterial hypertension, type 2 diabetes, and dyslipidemias, among others (Vasconcelos et al. 2016).

Excess caloric intake is stored in adipose tissue, the main energy storage in the body. White adipose tissue (WAT), besides being an active endocrine tissue, can secrete free fatty acids and adipokines. On the other hand, brown adipose tissue (BAT) is enriched with mitochondria, which express the uncoupling protein I (UCP1), and is associated with the thermogenesis process (Tam et al. 2012; Vasconcelos et al. 2016). Visceral/abdominal and pericardial fat tissue accumulation correlates with a higher incidence of death and cardiovascular diseases (Powell-Wiley et al. 2021; Lopez-Jimenez et al. 2022).

Both obesity and diabetes involve an inflammatory process characterized by alterations in the secretion of adipokines and cytokines, including adiponectin, resistin, tumor necrosis factor alpha (TNF-α), interleukins 1 and 6 (IL-1 and IL-6), angiotensinogen and angiotensin II (Ang II), leptin, and ghrelin, as well as plasminogen activator inhibitor type I (PAI-I) (Leon 2015; Vasconcelos et al. 2016). Changes in these factors perpetuate the inflammatory process and link these conditions to cardiovascular diseases. Furthermore, they contribute to lipid accumulation, endothelial dysfunction, an increase in plasma fatty acids, glucose production in the liver, and the accumulation of triglycerides in the muscles (Leon 2015).

By 2021, the prevalence of diabetes worldwide was 10.5% (Magliano and Boyko 2021). According to the World Health Organization (WHO), the global incidence of obesity and overweight was 15.3% and 42.8%, respectively (WHO).

3 General Effects on the Heart

In the heart, adipose tissue is stored in the outer and inner layers of the pericardium. It accumulates over the right ventricle and the atria, around the coronary arteries, and at the level of the pulmonary vein (Lavie et al. 2017; Goette and Lendeckel 2021). In addition to its mechanical role in cardiac function, the accumulation of fat tissue is associated with increased proinflammatory cytokine secretion, such as TNF (Ng et al. 2021). This increase exacerbates insulin resistance and elevates the production of Ang II and endothelin, leading to vasoconstriction and inflammation (Lavie et al. 2017; Goette and Lendeckel 2021). Functionally, the accumulation of adipose tissue could disrupt the physiological conduction pathways in the heart, promoting re-entry circuits and fibrosis by mobilizing certain types of progenitor cells, cardiac dilation, alterations in intracellular calcium homeostasis, extracellular remodeling, and reduction in sarcomere shortening, thereby favoring contractile dysfunction (Ward 2014; Lavie et al. 2017; Ng et al. 2021; Goette and Lendeckel 2021; Kruszewska et al. 2022).

It is important to consider that the cardiac remodeling process happens gradually at a structural, functional, and metabolic level, which makes it difficult to identify which event occurs first. In this sense, different animal models have been used to determine the causes and alterations in cardiac remodeling.

Electrophysiological alterations, including electrocardiographic changes and alterations in atrial and ventricular action potential morphology, have been identified in animal models of obesity and hyperglycemia. These changes are seen in the sodium (I_{Na}) and potassium ionic currents (I_{Kur}, I_{to}, I_{Kr}, I_{Ks}, and I_{K1}) during electrical remodeling (Albarado-Ibañez et al. 2013; Aromolaran and Boutjdir 2017; Bernardi et al. 2021).

At a metabolic level, a common factor involved in different cardiovascular pathologies is oxidative stress, specifically an increase in reactive oxygen species (ROS) and nitrogen species (RNS) formation (Murfitt et al. 2015). Both obesity and diabetes share the same effect in ROS/RNS increment, as well as mitochondrial metabolism dysregulation and its impact on intracellular calcium handling and contractile dysfunction at a cellular level (Fig. 1) (Goette and Lendeckel 2021).

When using animal models to study alterations in obesity or diabetes, it is essential to consider the pathology induction method since this determines the speed of cardiac remodeling and the results obtained (Table 1). However, clinical data in humans are clear in establishing that as independent factors, glycemic control, weight loss, as well as nutritional status, determine the appearance, severity, and frequency of cardiovascular diseases (Menezes et al. 2013; Bernardi et al. 2021; Ng et al. 2021; Chien et al. 2021).

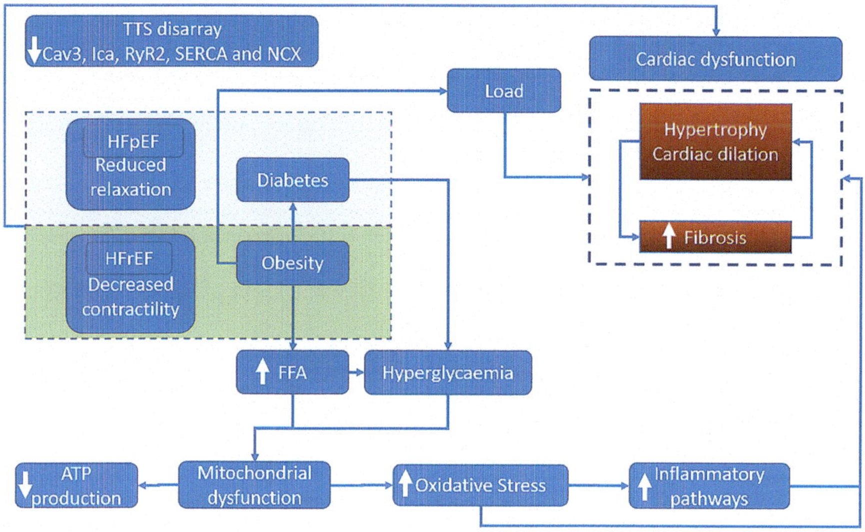

Fig. 1 Relationship between diabetes, obesity, and cardiac dysfunction
Both obesity and diabetes are well-established risk factors for the development of heart failure. Experimental models of obesity have shown that cardiomyocytes exhibit reduced contractile capacity, a characteristic primarily associated with heart failure with reduced ejection fraction (HFrEF). Conversely, in diabetes, impairments in cardiomyocyte relaxation have been observed, linking this condition to heart failure with preserved ejection fraction (HFpEF). Although the temporal progression of these pathological mechanisms remains incompletely understood, elevated levels of free fatty acids (FFAs) and hyperglycemia have been identified as critical contributors to mitochondrial dysfunction, a common feature in both obesity and diabetes. Mitochondrial dysfunction leads to reduced ATP synthesis, increased oxidative stress, and the activation of pro-inflammatory pathways, all of which contribute to myocardial fibrosis, cardiac hypertrophy, and ventricular dilation—key features of cardiac dysfunction. In obesity, the increased body mass further elevates cardiac afterload, a burden compounded by vascular abnormalities such as endothelial dysfunction, thereby exacerbating myocardial impairment. At the cellular level, disturbances in energy metabolism and mechanical overload are accompanied by dysregulation of key proteins involved in intracellular calcium homeostasis, including the sodium-calcium exchanger (NCX), the sarco/endoplasmic reticulum calcium ATPase (SERCA), and the ryanodine receptor type 2 (RyR2). Structural disruptions in the transverse T-tubule system and alterations in the expression of caveolin-3 (Cav3), critical components for action potential propagation and efficient excitation-contraction coupling in cardiomyocytes, have also been reported

4 Metabolic Alterations

Under physiological conditions, energy production in the heart is carried out via beta-oxidation. In the mitochondria, the oxidation of fatty acids is the main route of generating Acetyl Co-A (60–90%), while the remaining 10–40% is derived from glucose oxidation, lactate, and ketones (Wisneski et al. 1985; Stanley et al. 2005).

In obesity and diabetes, a vicious cycle is established. This cycle involves changing the metabolic substrate of the heart to obtain energy by increasing fatty

Table 1 Summary of alterations in T-tubule organization and protein expression involved in calcium regulation during contraction

Effect	Ob	DM1	DM2	Reference
BIN1				
Downregulation disrupts calcium handling			*	Li et al. (2023)
T tubule system				
Decreased density	*		*	Stølen et al. (2009)
T tubule disarray and enlargement			*	McGrath et al. (2009)
T tubule disarray and decreased density	*			Kemi et al. (2011)
Increased density			*	Frisk et al. (2021)
T tubule disarray		*		Romanelli et al. (2024)
Calcium channel				
Decrease calcium current and current inactivation		*		Chattou et al. (1999)
Decrease expression at membrane		*		Lu et al. (2007)
Decrease calcium current		*		Bracken et al. (2006)
Decrease current and inactivation	*		*	Howarth et al. (2011)
Decrease on functional channels	*		*	Pereira et al. (2006)
No changes reported			*	Al Kury et al. (2018)
		*		Lacombe et al. (2007)
Junctophilin-2				
Regulates calcium handling and apoptosis in lipotoxicity	*		*	Ji (2019)
Its mutation leads to lipid regulation			*	Lahiri et al. (2024)
Nexilin				
No changes reported in literature				
Sarcomere				
Length modifications preserve systolic function		*	*	Isola et al. (2021)
Diastolic dysfunction without systolic impairment			*	Flagg et al. (2009)
Altered left ventricular structure	*			De Feria et al. (2021)
Costamere				
Increases stiffness		*		Romanelli et al. (2024)
Ryanodine receptor type 2				
Decrease protein expression			*	Reuter et al. (2008), Lee et al. (2013)
Increased phosphorylation	*		*	Reuter et al. (2008), Okatan et al. (2016)
Increased RyR2 oxidation			*	Oda et al. (2015), Joseph et al. (2016)
Increased RyR2 phosphorylation at ser 2,809	*			Dincer et al. (2006)
Decreased mRNA		*		Teshima et al. (2000)

(continued)

Table 1 (continued)

Effect	Ob	DM1	DM2	Reference
Decreased protein expression		*		Yu et al. (1994)
Decreased activity		*		Choi et al. (2002), Yaras et al. (2005)
Altered sensitivity to calcium due to receptor oxidation		*		Bidasee et al. (2003), Gilca et al. (2017)
Increase RyR2 phosphorylation		*		Shao et al. (2009)
Increased sensitivity to calcium		*		Tian et al. (2011)
Sarco/endoplasmic reticulum calcium ATPase				
Decrease SERCA activity	*			Okatan et al. (2016), Ponce-Balbuena et al. (2024)
Decreased function, enhanced CaMKII-mediated phosphorylation of PLB	*		*	Stølen et al. (2009)
Decreased activity without protein expression changes	*		*	Wold et al. (2005)
Decreased expression	*		*	Young et al. (2002)
Upregulated expression	*		*	Fredersdorf et al. (2012)
Decrease in mRNA levels		*		Teshima et al. (2000)
Decreases sensitivity to calcium		*		Kim et al. (2001)
Increase in non-phosphorylated PLB		*		Kim et al. (2001), Choi et al. (2002)
Decreased SERCA expression		*		Choi et al. (2002), Bidasee et al. (2004) and Lee et al. (2013)
Sodium calcium exchanger				
Decreased activity			*	Golfman et al. (1998)
Increase activity	*		*	Stølen et al. (2009)
Increase NCX gene expression			*	Ashrafi et al. (2017)
Reduced NCX current and inactivation		*		Chattou et al. (1999), Sheikh et al. (2012) and Al Kury et al. (2021)
Decreased mRNA and protein		*		Hattori et al. (2000), Lee et al. (2013)

Ob Obesity, *DM1* Diabetes mellitus type I, *DM2* Diabetes mellitus type 2

acid oxidation instead of glucose, up until it completely depends on it, generating ROS and oxidative stress (Murfitt et al. 2015; Ng et al. 2021). At the same time, a rise in peroxisome proliferator-activated receptor alpha (PPAR alpha) expression is established, consolidating the fatty acid oxidation pathway. The accumulation of fatty acids generates phosphorylation of Insulin Receptor Substrate I (IRS-I), inhibiting its activation and leading to insulin resistance (Murfitt et al. 2015).

An increase in fatty acid intake and its accumulation in the heart has been seen in patients with obesity and diabetes (McGavock et al. 2007). This, in addition to insulin resistance, causes an increase in lipolysis, exceeding the mitochondria's beta oxidative capacity, leading to lipotoxicity, generating intermediates such as ceramide and diacylglycerol (DAG), which, when accumulated, cause apoptosis and, eventually, replacement fibrosis and contractile dysfunction (Listenberger et al. 2001; Peterson et al. 2004).

In this process, oxidative stress could be the link between fatty accumulation, free fatty acid increase, activation of different metabolic pathways, inflammation, and effects on the heart such as hypertrophy and fibrosis (Listenberger et al. 2001; Murfitt et al. 2015). See Fig. 1.

5 Excitation-Contraction Coupling

Excitation-contraction coupling (ECC) plays a fundamental role in cardiac function. It largely depends on the ultrastructural organization of the cell, in addition to a sequence of events that lead to the electrical signal transduction into a mechanical one (Eisner et al. 2017). T-tubules allow action potential propagation in cardiac cells and trigger calcium-induced calcium release (CICR) by coupling with the sarcoplasmic reticulum (SR) through the activation of the type 2 ryanodine receptor (RyR2). Junctophilin 2 (JP2) is a protein that allows the sarcoplasmic reticulum and the T-tubule system (TTS) to form the cardiac dyad, while Bridging Integrator-1 (BIN1) enables the formation of T-tubules, as well as different functional domains with other proteins that are involved in calcium handling (Hong and Shaw 2017).

5.1 T-Tubules

T-tubules play a significant role in the ECC process and serve as a functional and structural anchoring platform for different proteins. Recently, up to 78 new proteins were identified that could be potentially expressed in the T-tubule (Cheah et al. 2019).

T-tubules are invaginations of the cardiomyocyte membrane that are regularly distributed every 1.8–2.2 μm in distance. When they are perpendicular to the surface and the long axis of the cell, they are called transverse T-tubules and represent approximately 60% of the total TTS. The remaining 40% corresponds to the axial T-tubules, which are extensions of the same system that run through the cell parallel to the myofilaments and interconnect the transverse components (Brette and Orchard 2003; Hong and Shaw 2017). Approximately 60% of the transverse T-tubules are located 0.5 μm from the Z line of the sarcomere (Soeller and Cannell 1999) and surround the contractile myofilaments, forming a radial tubular structure that will establish a connection with the flattened ends of the SR to shape the dyad (Hayashi et al. 2009; Pinali et al. 2013; Hong and Shaw 2017). Furthermore, the T-tubules are relatively fixed, both inside the cell in the costamer and in the extracellular part with the extracellular matrix (ECM), interacting with both structures through the vinculin-talin-integrin protein complexes, as well as with dystrophin (Dp71) (Fabbrizio et al. 1994; Kawada et al. 2003; Martin et al. 2022).

T-tubules vary in size between 20 and 450 nm, depending on the species. They are 6.7 μm long in each branch, occupy 0.8–3.6% of the cardiomyocyte total volume, and, on average, 30% of the cell's capacitance. That means a third of the cell surface corresponds to the TTS (Soeller and Cannell 1999; Pinali et al. 2013; Hong and Shaw 2017).

The development of TTS begins in the fetal stage for large species or at birth for small species. In both cases, T-tubule generation coincides with the expression of JP2 and BIN1. The loss, decrease, or change in JP2 expression site correlates with T-tubule loss (Zhang et al. 2014; Prins et al. 2016; Jones et al. 2018). The same happens with BIN 1 expression, whose levels go along with the number of T-tubules and their folding (Hong et al. 2014; Caldwell et al. 2014). In fact, circulating BIN1 levels in the blood have been proposed as an indicator of cardiovascular risk since this protein is continually replaced, and in some cardiac pathologies such as heart failure, the turnover rate or its expression decreases, and therefore its circulating levels (Hong et al. 2012; Li et al. 2021b).

The expression of the TTS is variable. In small species with a high heart rate, the TTS is extensive, but in cardiomyocytes from larger species, the density of this tubule network decreases (Song et al. 2005; Jones et al. 2018). Similarly, in atrial cardiomyocytes compared to ventricular ones, a less organized network of T-tubules with a predominance of longitudinal tubules has been reported, especially in small cells (Smyrnias et al. 2010; Gadeberg et al. 2016; Arora et al. 2017).

Another critical factor in T-tubule development and maintenance is related to mechanical stress on the membrane surface, which could trigger T-tubule degradation, folding, and formation (Frisk et al. 2016). Furthermore, increased cardiac muscle tension could lead to fibrosis and ECM remodeling. Crossman et al. (2017) demonstrated the presence of collagen and filopodia of cardiac fibroblasts inside the T-tubules of cardiomyocytes with ventricular failure (Crossman et al. 2017). It has also been reported that the most significant loss of T-tubules coincides with regions closer to an infarcted area, where membrane tension increases, and in fibrotic areas during heart failure (Frisk et al. 2016; Seidel et al. 2017). These data suggest that the expression regulation of the TTS depends partially on local mechanical signals transmitted through the ECM and cytoskeleton.

We must see T-tubules as a dynamic structure in size and shape and with different microdomains that regulate cardiac contractile activity throughout life, both in physiological and pathological conditions (Hong et al. 2014; Uchida and Lopatin 2018). The integrity of the TTS is essential for an accurate synchronization of calcium release and contraction and for optimal action potential propagation on its surface (Louch 2004; Song et al. 2006; Sacconi et al. 2012). Microdomain development and TTS interaction with the SR depend on the proteins BIN1, JP2, ankyrin b, caveolin 3, and nexilin, among others (Hong and Shaw 2017; Poulet et al. 2021).

5.2 Sarcoplasmic Reticulum

The SR is a network consisting of tubules and sacs surrounding the contractile myofilaments and present widening in the vicinity of the T-tubules. Calsequestrin, a calcium-chelating protein, is expressed in its lumen. This protein allows a high calcium concentration inside the SR and helps to regulate this organelle's size and calcium release (Terentyev et al. 2003). RyR2 is a channel expressed in the SR membrane that allows stored calcium to be released to the cytosol during CICR. In contrast, the sarco/endoplasmic reticulum calcium ATPase (SERCA) pumps the calcium back into the SR. Changes in SERCA and calsequestrin expression produce changes in the SR volume and in the TTS organization and expression as a compensatory mechanism for the SR loss of function (Denegri et al. 2012; Swift et al. 2012). Another common finding is the relocation of calcium-releasing unit proteins, specifically RyR2 and SERCA. Furthermore, the SR is positioned by JP2, meaning that changes in its expression could also lead to spatial organization modifications within the sarcomere by decreasing contact with the T-tubule or diminishing the area of RyR2 expression within the dyad, increasing orphan RyR2 (Louch 2004; Song et al. 2006; Louch et al. 2006).

5.3 Dyad

The macrostructural organization of the dyads and the specific arrangement of calcium channels and RyR2 within each dyad are crucial for ECC to occur. Likewise, its remodeling during development, pathological processes, or fine regulation under physiological conditions is essential for cardiac function (Sun et al. 1995; Jones et al. 2018).

A point to highlight is that CICR depends on the TTS and the SR and that T-tubule integrity depends on a delicate balance between the load to which the heart is subjected, the degree of development or cell differentiation, the pathophysiological state of the heart, and the energy availability to maintain calcium gradients (Frisk et al. 2016; Watson et al. 2016).

The cardiac dyad is formed by the structural and functional interaction between the T-tubule and the terminal cisternae of the SR membranes, and it is precisely in that space where the electrical activity is transduced into mechanical activity by the expression of calcium regulatory proteins and their spatial arrangement. This allows a rapid increase in intracellular calcium concentration and the binding to troponin, which will start the contractile process (Hayashi et al. 2009; Trafford et al. 2013; Eisner et al. 2017). In each dyad, a group of type L calcium channels (LTCC), also known as voltage-gated calcium channels 1.2 (Cav1.2), are found in the T-tubule membrane in juxtaposition with a group of RyR2 in the SR (Scriven et al. 2013). The membranes of both structures will be anchored by JP2, interacting with both Cav1.2 and RyR2 (Jones et al. 2018; Poulet et al. 2021; Dibb et al. 2022).

Type L calcium channels (LTCC) are expressed in the T-tubule within the dyad. Its location within the dyad is due to several factors. On one hand, there is a preferential channel expression in the T-tubule concerning the membrane surface. LTCCs are expressed in regions enriched with caveolin 3 (Cav-3), where protein kinase A (PKA) is also anchored. PKA is an enzyme that phosphorylates the channel and increases its activity (Kamp and Hell 2000; Bryant et al. 2018). Also, its localization is directed by BIN1 expression, which creates a microdomain in the T-tubule, where the positive end of the microtubules is anchored, allowing calcium channel transport from the endoplasmic reticulum to the T-tubule (Hong and Shaw 2017). Another important fact is the union of the calcium channel with RyR2 through JP2 and that the opening probability of the LTCC increases when they are grouped and joined through their carboxyl-terminal ends (Dixon et al. 2015). In failing cardiomyocytes, there is an LTCC relocation from the T-tubule to the membrane surface, which causes a decrease in calcium current in the T-tubules and, consequently, a reduction in CICR (Bryant et al. 2015; Sanchez-Alonso et al. 2016).

RyR2 is predominantly expressed in the terminal cisterna of the SR. Its localization is partly maintained by interactions with JP2 and the functional domain formed with BIN1 (Munro et al. 2016; Hong and Shaw 2017; Hou et al. 2021). Initially, it was thought that RyR2s were grouped regularly in dyads. However, it has been shown that it is organized in groups of approximately 45 receptors, although about a third of the groups contain up to 15 RyR2 tetramers (Hayashi et al. 2009; Jayasinghe et al. 2018). Each group is separated by about 150 nm (Macquaide et al. 2015). Within each group, the receptors are organized dispersedly and in small groups that can adopt a side-by-side conformation or, when phosphorylated, adopt a checkerboard crystalline conformation (Cabra et al. 2016; Jones et al. 2018). This spatial organization would establish calcium spark formation and, eventually, their possible propagation. Therefore, the loss of this organization can cause a slowdown in the calcium sparks kinetics (Louch et al. 2013; Kolstad et al. 2018). Under conditions that promote their activity, RyR2 are found at the periphery of the clusters and can move within the dyad, either laterally or towards the surface or the interior, to the extent of changing their position by up to 1 μm in just 12 min; that means that they can travel half of a sarcomere (Hiess et al. 2018; Dries et al. 2018). This is important since RyR2 localization and activity can change in pathological processes (Louch et al. 2013; Kolstad et al. 2018).

6 Structural Proteins of the Dyad

BIN1, or Amphiphysin 2, belongs to the large Bin-Amphiphysin-Rvs proteins (BAR) family. These proteins cause plasma membrane deformation and participate in other processes, such as membrane trafficking, remodeling, and cytoskeletal reorganization (Prokic et al. 2014; Gruber and Balbach 2015).

There are ten isoforms of this protein, all of which are encoded by a single gene with 20 different exons (Hong and Shaw 2017). Of the six isoforms that are expressed in the heart, BIN1 + 13 + 17 contains an NH3 domain conserved in all isoforms; exon 17 is ubiquitously expressed, and a proline-rich domain is encoded by exon 13 (Wechsler-Reya et al. 1997; Li et al. 2021a). The amino end interacts with membrane phospholipids to create the curvatures that will arise in the T-tubules (Gruber and Balbach 2015).

The BIN1 +13+17 protein has different functions at the cardiac level. On one side, it participates in T-tubule formation and maintenance (Hong et al. 2014; Picas et al. 2014; Gruber and Balbach 2015). It creates functional domains in the dyad for LTCCs and RyR2 interaction and other intracellular calcium regulatory proteins (Gorelik et al. 2013; Hong et al. 2014; Fu et al. 2016). It serves as an anchoring point for the positive end of the microtubules that transport LTCCs from the Golgi to the T-tubules, accumulating up to 80% of the total channels in that area (Hong et al. 2010, 2012; Westhoff and Dixon 2021). It also recruits phosphorylated RyR2 to the SR terminal cisterna and facilitates its organization in juxtaposition with LTCCs in the T-tubule (Dibb et al. 2022). It affects the capture of cytosolic calcium by grouping SERCA A2 along the SR membrane (Li et al. 2021a). When expressed in a high concentration at the T-tubules, it creates microfolds and slows ionic diffusion regions in the lumen of the tubule, allowing for the maintenance of electrical stability of the cell (Hong et al. 2014). It has been shown that BIN1 downregulation disrupts calcium handling and affects glucose uptake, contributing to diabetic cardiomyopathy (Li et al. 2023).

Within the T-tubules, in addition to the microdomains and folds formed by BIN1, *Cav-3* can form small invaginations of the plasma membrane called caveolae by binding mainly to sphingomyelin and cholesterol (Hong and Shaw 2017). These areas will also serve to recruit proteins such as β2 adrenergic receptors, ion channels like HCN4, Kv1.5, Nav1.5, Cav1.2, and the sodium-calcium exchanger (NCX) (Bosman et al. 2013; Wright et al. 2014).

Ankyrin B and *ankyrin G* are two proteins with structural functions that participate in membrane biogenesis, transport of proteins involved in calcium homeostasis, and cardiomyocyte electrical activity (Cunha and Mohler 2006). *Ankyrin B* has four functional domains: the membrane binding domain (MBD), the death domain (DD), the spectrin binding domain (SBD), and the carboxy-terminal domain (CTD). Through the interaction of the MBD domain, ankyrin B can form a protein complex that brings together the NCX, the sodium-potassium pump, and the inositol 1,4,5-trisphosphate (IP3) receptor in cardiac activity (Mohler et al. 2005; Hashemi et al. 2009). Changes in ankyrin B expression are followed by alterations in intracellular calcium regulation, a decrease in $Cav_{1.2}$ calcium current expression, and the proteins above (Hashemi et al. 2009). Similarly, ankyrin G regulates not only the trafficking and correct expression of the cardiac sodium channel, $Nav_{1.5,}$ but also its biophysical properties (Cunha and Mohler 2006).

The membranes of the T-tubule and the sarcoplasmic reticulum are kept together at a constant distance, thanks to *JP2*. This protein anchors to the SR membrane at its amino terminus and interacts with the T-tubule membrane through the 8 Membrane on Receptor Nexus (MORN) domains present at its carboxyl end (Scriven et al. 2013; Poulet et al. 2021). The distance between both structures is 12–15 nm, partly due to the protein's flexibility when binding to IP3 (Bennett et al. 2013). Maintaining the dyadic cleft is crucial for an accurate ECC since functional coupling requires the formation of the microdomain between both membranes and, especially, for the formation of the couplon (Takeshima 2000; Scriven et al. 2013).

JP2 also binds to RyR2 and LTCC (Poulet et al. 2021; Gross et al. 2021). Furthermore, the amino-terminal end of the protein, in the presence of high calcium concentrations, is cleaved by calpain and can translocate to the nucleus and bind to DNA, triggering the transcription of different genes that prevent the development of hypertrophy and heart failure (Guo et al. 2018). Likewise, the carboxy-terminal end can translocate to the nucleus and have the opposite effect (Lahiri et al. 2020). Mutations in this protein lead to lipid regulation issues, potentially contributing to hypertrophic cardiomyopathy (Lahiri et al. 2024). Additionally, it has been reported that this protein protects cardiac myocytes from lipotoxicity-induced damage by regulating calcium handling and apoptosis (Ji 2019).

Striated muscle preferentially expressed protein kinase (SPEG) is a serine/threonine kinase of the myosin light chain and has been found to immunoprecipitate with RyR2 and JP2, indicating a possible interaction between the three proteins. It decreases the intradyadic calcium concentration by phosphorylating RyR2 at serine 2367, reducing its probability of intracellular opening and increasing calcium reuptake by SERCA by phosphorylating it at threonine 484 (London 2017; Quick et al. 2017; Dibb et al. 2022). The decrease in SPEG expression causes a reduction in ejection fraction, contractile dysfunction, ventricular dilation, and atrial fibrosis. At a cellular level, it causes a junctional membrane complex disarrangement, disorganization, and loss of T-tubules. These changes are associated with decreased calcium transient amplitude and calcium storage within the SR, with no SERCA activity changes (Quick et al. 2017).

Nexillin is an actin-binding protein found in the Z-line junctional membrane complex, as it binds to other proteins of the cardiac dyad, such as RyR2 and JP2. In addition, it is an essential protein for TTS development, generation, and maintenance (Liu et al. 2019). The absence of nexillin in cardiac cells results in a transverse tubule loss, a deficiency of RyR2 and SERCA and prolonged relaxation along with decreased shortening, which correlates with a lower calcium transient amplitude and a decrease in calcium clearance rate (Liu et al. 2019), making nexillin one of the proteins necessary to maintain TTS and junctional membrane complex arrangement (Spinozzi et al. 2020; Wang et al. 2020). The global KO of nexilin, as well as the inducible one, develops premature death and dilated cardiomyopathy, which is evidenced by an increase in ventricular diameter and thinning of the wall, as well as an increase in the expression of collagen type Ia1 and 3a1 (Spinozzi et al. 2020).

7 Cellular Remodeling

Obesity is a risk factor for developing diabetes, and both independently increase the likelihood of suffering from heart failure. The failing heart loses its ability to function effectively as a pump. Clinically, heart failure can be categorized as heart failure with reduced ejection fraction (HFrEF), the most common type, which typically occurs in individuals with obesity, or as heart failure with preserved ejection fraction (HFpEF), which is more commonly seen in people with diabetes (Frisk et al. 2021; Hulot and Livrozet 2021). Eventually, both will compromise cardiac output and alter cardiac structure, causing hypertrophy and cardiac dilation (Fig. 1).

HFrEF has been associated with a disorder of the T-tubule system, while HFpEF has been related to an increase in T-tubule density, showing a widening and increase in the number of these structures (Guo et al. 2013; Frisk et al. 2021). See Table 1.

The ECC requires a high spatial organization of the components that intervene in each phase of the process, such as action potential propagation, CICR, and calcium reuptake into the SR. For this, the cardiac dyad and the couplon organization are of utmost importance (Scriven et al. 2013; Trafford et al. 2013; Kolstad et al. 2018). In this sense, the TTS organization is crucial to maintain stable functional domains and guarantee the correct transduction of the electrical signal into mechanical ones (Stølen et al. 2009; Ibrahim et al. 2011). Small alterations in its density, shape, or distribution can have serious functional consequences.

In different experimental models of diabetes, with or without obesity, as well as in those of heart failure, various degrees of alterations occur in cardiomyocytes. However, most coincide with a contractile capacity reduction, a decrease in the amplitude of calcium transients, and a slower calcium clearance rate (Al Kury 2020; Jaquenod De Giusti et al. 2022). It has been reported that changes in sarcomere length and increased cross-bridge density in diabetic hearts are a compensatory mechanism (Isola et al. 2021), as well as impaired diastolic function in lipid metabolism disorders due to myofilament calcium sensitivity changes (Flagg et al. 2009). Furthermore, diabetes induces changes in costameric proteins, increasing stiffness in cardiac myocytes (Romanelli et al. 2024). These functional alterations occur along with changes in protein expression that regulate intracellular calcium and, therefore, contraction. Although it is difficult to distinguish changes in T-tubules between pathological models, there are some studies where TTS remodeling is specifically identified in diabetes and metabolic syndrome (McGrath et al. 2009; Stølen et al. 2009; Ibrahim and Terracciano 2013; Frisk et al. 2021; Hulot and Livrozet 2021; Romanelli et al. 2024). See Table 1.

It is essential to consider that the cardiomyocyte structural remodeling occurs gradually and concomitantly with metabolic changes and in the expression of ion channels or calcium regulatory proteins (Peterson et al. 2004; Al Kury 2020; Jaquenod De Giusti et al. 2022). Murfitt et al. (2015) propose mitochondrial dysfunction and oxidative stress increment as a common point in alterations caused by hyperglycemia and the increase in circulating fatty acids in diabetes and obesity (Murfitt et al. 2015). The rise of oxidative stress can lead to the activation of apoptosis, fibrosis, and hypertrophy-promoting pathways, as well as the activation of inflammatory pathways, which act as a positive feedback loop for the pathological process (Murfitt et al. 2015; Ng et al. 2021).

In a review of the different diabetes models, Russell et al. (2017) emphasize the remodeling of plasma membrane components such as cholesterol, fatty acids, and phosphoinositides that would result in compensatory changes in the expression of Cav-3 and IP3 kinase (Russell et al. 2017). The membrane domains, comprised of caveolin and phosphoinositides, are crucial for the anchoring of JP2 and BIN1 and for all the functions that depend on these proteins to be carried out, as well as for insulin signaling in cardiomyocytes (Bennett et al. 2013; Picas et al. 2014; Murfitt et al. 2015).

Energetically, maintaining the CICR in the cardiac dyad is expensive, and in the metabolic remodeling that cardiomyocytes undergo in obesity and diabetes, there is a reduction in cellular ATP reserves (Leon 2015; Watson et al. 2016; Ng et al. 2021). Let us also consider that in both diabetes and obesity, changes in cardiac wall tension have been proven due to fibrosis, hypertrophy, or dilation, which represents a direct effect on the load experienced by the cardiomyocyte and affects the disorganization of the TTS (Frisk et al. 2016; Watson et al. 2016).

8 Conclusions

Obesity and diabetes are two syndromes that increase the risk of suffering from cardiovascular diseases, and both cause alterations in cardiac activity, reducing the efficiency of the heart as a pump. The changes underlying these deficiencies include remodeling at the metabolic level, with complete dependence on beta-oxidation of fatty acids as an energy source, and the promotion of pro-inflammatory, pro-fibrotic, and hypertrophic signaling pathways. At a structural level, the changes include derangement in the T-tubule system, in the dyad, and in the expression and localization of structural and calcium regulation proteins, leading to alterations in calcium regulation and a decrease in contractile capacity of cardiomyocytes and heart failure.

References

Al Kury LT (2020) Calcium homeostasis in ventricular myocytes of diabetic cardiomyopathy. J Diabetes Res 2020:1–12. https://doi.org/10.1155/2020/1942086

Al Kury L, Sydorenko V, Smail MMA et al (2018) Voltage dependence of the Ca^{2+} transient in endocardial and epicardial myocytes from the left ventricle of Goto–Kakizaki type 2 diabetic rats. Mol Cell Biochem 446:25–33. https://doi.org/10.1007/s11010-018-3269-0

Al Kury LT, Sydorenko V, Smail MM et al (2021) Calcium signaling in endocardial and epicardial ventricular myocytes from streptozotocin-induced diabetic rats. J Diabetes Investig 12:493–500. https://doi.org/10.1111/jdi.13451

Albarado-Ibañez A, Avelino-Cruz JE, Velasco M et al (2013) Metabolic syndrome remodels electrical activity of the sinoatrial node and produces arrhythmias in rats. PLoS One 8: e76534. https://doi.org/10.1371/journal.pone.0076534

Aromolaran AS, Boutjdir M (2017) Cardiac Ion Channel regulation in obesity and the metabolic syndrome: relevance to long QT syndrome and atrial fibrillation. Front Physiol 8:431. https://doi.org/10.3389/fphys.2017.00431

Arora R, Aistrup GL, Supple S et al (2017) Regional distribution of T-tubule density in left and right atria in dogs. Heart Rhythm 14:273–281. https://doi.org/10.1016/j.hrthm.2016.09.022

Ashrafi R, Modi P, Oo AY et al (2017) Arrhythmogenic gene remodelling in elderly patients with type 2 diabetes with aortic stenosis and normal left ventricular ejection fraction. Exp Physiol 102:1424–1434. https://doi.org/10.1113/EP086412

Bennett HJ, Davenport JB, Collins RF et al (2013) Human junctophilin-2 undergoes a structural rearrangement upon binding PtdIns(3,4,5) *P* 3 and the S101R mutation identified in hypertrophic cardiomyopathy obviates this response. Biochem J 456:205–217. https://doi.org/10.1042/BJ20130591

Bernardi J, Aromolaran KA, Zhu H, Aromolaran AS (2021) Circadian mechanisms: cardiac Ion Channel remodeling and arrhythmias. Front Physiol 11:611860. https://doi.org/10.3389/fphys.2020.611860

Bidasee KR, Nallani K, Yu Y et al (2003) Chronic diabetes increases advanced glycation end products on cardiac ryanodine receptors/calcium-release channels. Diabetes 52:1825–1836. https://doi.org/10.2337/diabetes.52.7.1825

Bidasee KR, Zhang Y, Shao CH et al (2004) Diabetes increases formation of advanced glycation end products on Sarco(endo)plasmic reticulum Ca^{2+}-ATPase. Diabetes 53:463–473. https://doi.org/10.2337/diabetes.53.2.463

Bosman A, Sartiani L, Spinelli V et al (2013) Molecular and functional evidence of HCN4 and Caveolin-3 interaction during Cardiomyocyte differentiation from human embryonic stem cells. Stem Cells Dev 22:1717–1727. https://doi.org/10.1089/scd.2012.0247

Bracken N, Howarth FC, Singh J (2006) Effects of streptozotocin-induced diabetes on contraction and calcium transport in rat ventricular cardiomyocytes. In: Diabetes mellitus and its complications, pp 208–222. https://doi.org/10.1196/annals.1372.018

Brette F, Orchard C (2003) T-tubule function in mammalian cardiac myocytes. Circ Res 92:1182–1192. https://doi.org/10.1161/01.RES.0000074908.17214.FD

Bryant SM, Kong CHT, Watson J et al (2015) Altered distribution of ICa impairs Ca release at the t-tubules of ventricular myocytes from failing hearts. J Mol Cell Cardiol 86:23–31. https://doi.org/10.1016/j.yjmcc.2015.06.012

Bryant SM, Kong CHT, Watson JJ et al (2018) Caveolin-3 KO disrupts t-tubule structure and decreases t-tubular I_{Ca} density in mouse ventricular myocytes. Am J Phys Heart Circ Phys 315: H1101–H1111. https://doi.org/10.1152/ajpheart.00209.2018

Cabra V, Murayama T, Samsó M (2016) Ultrastructural analysis of self-associated RyR2s. Biophys J 110:2651–2662. https://doi.org/10.1016/j.bpj.2016.05.013

Caldwell JL, Smith CER, Taylor RF et al (2014) Dependence of cardiac transverse tubules on the BAR domain protein Amphiphysin II (BIN-1). Circ Res 115:986–996. https://doi.org/10.1161/CIRCRESAHA.116.303448

Chattou, Diacono, Feuvray (1999) Decrease in sodium–calcium exchange and calcium currents in diabetic rat ventricular myocytes. Acta Physiol Scand 166:137–144. https://doi.org/10.1046/j.1365-201x.1999.00547.x

Cheah JX, Nieuwenhuis TO, Halushka MK (2019) An expanded proteome of cardiac t-tubules. Cardiovasc Pathol 42:15–20. https://doi.org/10.1016/j.carpath.2019.05.001

Chien S-C, Chandramouli C, Lo C-I et al (2021) Associations of obesity and malnutrition with cardiac remodeling and cardiovascular outcomes in Asian adults: a cohort study. PLoS Med 18: e1003661. https://doi.org/10.1371/journal.pmed.1003661

Choi KM, Zhong Y, Hoit BD et al (2002) Defective intracellular Ca^{2+} signaling contributes to cardiomyopathy in type 1 diabetic rats. Am J Phys Heart Circ Phys 283:H1398–H1408. https://doi.org/10.1152/ajpheart.00313.2002

Crossman DJ, Shen X, Jüllig M et al (2017) Increased collagen within the transverse tubules in human heart failure. Cardiovasc Res 113:879–891. https://doi.org/10.1093/cvr/cvx055

Cunha S, Mohler P (2006) Cardiac ankyrins: essential components for development and maintenance of excitable membrane domains in heart. Cardiovasc Res 71:22–29. https://doi.org/10.1016/j.cardiores.2006.03.018

De Feria AE, Kott AE, Becker JR (2021) Sarcomere mutation negative hypertrophic cardiomyopathy is associated with ageing and obesity. Open Heart 8:e001560. https://doi.org/10.1136/openhrt-2020-001560

Denegri M, Avelino-Cruz JE, Boncompagni S et al (2012) Viral gene transfer rescues Arrhythmogenic phenotype and ultrastructural abnormalities in adult Calsequestrin-null mice with inherited arrhythmias. Circ Res 110:663–668. https://doi.org/10.1161/CIRCRESAHA.111.263939

Dibb KM, Louch WE, Trafford AW (2022) Cardiac transverse tubules in physiology and heart failure. Annu Rev Physiol 84:229–255. https://doi.org/10.1146/annurev-physiol-061121-040148

Dincer UD, Araiza A, Knudson JD et al (2006) Dysfunction of cardiac ryanodine receptors in the metabolic syndrome. J Mol Cell Cardiol 41:108–114. https://doi.org/10.1016/j.yjmcc.2006.04.018

Dixon RE, Moreno CM, Yuan C et al (2015) Graded Ca^{2+}/calmodulin-dependent coupling of voltage-gated CaV1.2 channels. eLife 4:e05608. https://doi.org/10.7554/eLife.05608

Dries E, Santiago DJ, Gilbert G et al (2018) Hyperactive ryanodine receptors in human heart failure and ischaemic cardiomyopathy reside outside of couplons. Cardiovasc Res 114:1512–1524. https://doi.org/10.1093/cvr/cvy088

Eisner DA, Caldwell JL, Kistamás K, Trafford AW (2017) Calcium and excitation-contraction coupling in the heart. Circ Res 121:181–195. https://doi.org/10.1161/CIRCRESAHA.117.310230

Fabbrizio E, Nudel U, Hugon G et al (1994) Characterization and localization of a 77 kDa protein related to the dystrophin gene family. Biochem J 299:359–365. https://doi.org/10.1042/bj2990359

Flagg TP, Cazorla O, Remedi MS et al (2009) Ca^{2+} -independent alterations in diastolic sarcomere length and relaxation kinetics in a mouse model of Lipotoxic diabetic cardiomyopathy. Circ Res 104:95–103. https://doi.org/10.1161/CIRCRESAHA.108.186809

Fredersdorf S, Thumann C, Zimmermann WH et al (2012) Increased myocardial SERCA expression in early type 2 diabetes mellitus is insulin dependent: in vivo and in vitro data. Cardiovasc Diabetol 11:57. https://doi.org/10.1186/1475-2840-11-57

Frisk M, Ruud M, Espe EKS et al (2016) Elevated ventricular wall stress disrupts cardiomyocyte t-tubule structure and calcium homeostasis. Cardiovasc Res 112:443–451. https://doi.org/10.1093/cvr/cvw111

Frisk M, Le C, Shen X et al (2021) Etiology-dependent impairment of diastolic cardiomyocyte calcium homeostasis in heart failure with preserved ejection fraction. J Am Coll Cardiol 77:405–419. https://doi.org/10.1016/j.jacc.2020.11.044

Fu Y, Shaw SA, Naami R et al (2016) Isoproterenol promotes rapid ryanodine receptor movement to bridging integrator 1 (BIN1)–organized dyads. Circulation 133:388–397. https://doi.org/10.1161/CIRCULATIONAHA.115.018535

Gadeberg HC, Bond RC, Kong CHT et al (2016) Heterogeneity of T-tubules in pig hearts. PLoS One 11:e0156862. https://doi.org/10.1371/journal.pone.0156862

Gilca G-E, Stefanescu G, Badulescu O et al (2017) Diabetic cardiomyopathy: current approach and potential diagnostic and therapeutic targets. J Diabetes Res 2017:1–7. https://doi.org/10.1155/2017/1310265

Goette A, Lendeckel U (2021) Atrial cardiomyopathy: pathophysiology and clinical consequences. Cells 10:2605. https://doi.org/10.3390/cells10102605

Golfman L, Dixon IM, Takeda N et al (1998) Cardiac sarcolemmal Na(+)-Ca^{2+} exchange and Na (+)-K+ ATPase activities and gene expression in alloxan-induced diabetes in rats. Mol Cell Biochem 188:91–101

Gorelik J, Wright PT, Lyon AR, Harding SE (2013) Spatial control of the βAR system in heart failure: the transverse tubule and beyond. Cardiovasc Res 98:216–224. https://doi.org/10.1093/cvr/cvt005

Gross P, Johnson J, Romero CM et al (2021) Interaction of the joining region in Junctophilin-2 with the L-type Ca^{2+} channel is pivotal for cardiac dyad assembly and intracellular Ca^{2+} dynamics. Circ Res 128:92–114. https://doi.org/10.1161/CIRCRESAHA.119.315715

Gruber T, Balbach J (2015) Protein folding mechanism of the dimeric AmphiphysinII/Bin1 N-BAR domain. PLoS One 10:e0136922. https://doi.org/10.1371/journal.pone.0136922

Guo A, Zhang C, Wei S et al (2013) Emerging mechanisms of T-tubule remodelling in heart failure. Cardiovasc Res 98:204–215. https://doi.org/10.1093/cvr/cvt020

Guo A, Wang Y, Chen B et al (2018) E-C coupling structural protein junctophilin-2 encodes a stress-adaptive transcription regulator. Science 362:eaan3303. https://doi.org/10.1126/science.aan3303

Hashemi SM, Hund TJ, Mohler PJ (2009) Cardiac ankyrins in health and disease. J Mol Cell Cardiol 47:203–209. https://doi.org/10.1016/j.yjmcc.2009.04.010

Hattori Y, Matsuda N, Kimura J et al (2000) Diminished function and expression of the cardiac Na^+-Ca^{2+} exchanger in diabetic rats: implication in Ca^{2+} overload. J Physiol 527:85–94. https://doi.org/10.1111/j.1469-7793.2000.00085.x

Hayashi T, Martone ME, Yu Z et al (2009) Three-dimensional electron microscopy reveals new details of membrane systems for Ca^{2+} signaling in the heart. J Cell Sci 122:1005–1013. https://doi.org/10.1242/jcs.028175

Hiess F, Detampel P, Nolla-Colomer C et al (2018) Dynamic and irregular distribution of RyR2 clusters in the periphery of live ventricular myocytes. Biophys J 114:343–354. https://doi.org/10.1016/j.bpj.2017.11.026

Hong T, Shaw RM (2017) Cardiac T-tubule microanatomy and function. Physiol Rev 97:227–252. https://doi.org/10.1152/physrev.00037.2015

Hong T-T, Smyth JW, Gao D et al (2010) BIN1 localizes the L-type Calcium Channel to cardiac T-tubules. PLoS Biol 8:e1000312. https://doi.org/10.1371/journal.pbio.1000312

Hong T-T, Smyth JW, Chu KY et al (2012) BIN1 is reduced and Cav1.2 trafficking is impaired in human failing cardiomyocytes. Heart Rhythm 9:812–820. https://doi.org/10.1016/j.hrthm.2011.11.055

Hong T, Yang H, Zhang S-S et al (2014) Cardiac BIN1 folds T-tubule membrane, controlling ion flux and limiting arrhythmia. Nat Med 20:624–632. https://doi.org/10.1038/nm.3543

Hou Y, Bai J, Shen X et al (2021) Nanoscale organisation of ryanodine receptors and Junctophilin-2 in the failing human heart. Front Physiol 12:724372. https://doi.org/10.3389/fphys.2021.724372

Howarth FC, Qureshi MA, Hassan Z et al (2011) Changing pattern of gene expression is associated with ventricular myocyte dysfunction and altered mechanisms of Ca^{2+} signalling in young type 2 Zucker diabetic fatty rat heart: cardiac dysfunction in Zucker diabetic fatty rats. Exp Physiol 96:325–337. https://doi.org/10.1113/expphysiol.2010.055574

Hulot J-S, Livrozet M (2021) HFpEF: should we consider diabetic patients separately? J Am Coll Cardiol 77:420–422. https://doi.org/10.1016/j.jacc.2020.11.051

Ibrahim M, Terracciano CM (2013) Reversibility of T-tubule remodelling in heart failure: mechanical load as a dynamic regulator of the T-tubules. Cardiovasc Res 98:225–232. https://doi.org/10.1093/cvr/cvt016

Ibrahim M, Gorelik J, Yacoub MH, Terracciano CM (2011) The structure and function of cardiac t-tubules in health and disease. Proc R Soc B 278:2714–2723. https://doi.org/10.1098/rspb.2011.0624

Isola R, Broccia F, Casti A et al (2021) STZ-diabetic rat heart maintains developed tension amplitude by increasing sarcomere length and crossbridge density. Exp Physiol 106:1572–1586. https://doi.org/10.1113/EP089000

Jaquenod De Giusti C, Palomeque J, Mattiazzi A (2022) Ca^{2+} mishandling and mitochondrial dysfunction: a converging road to prediabetic and diabetic cardiomyopathy. Pflugers Arch – Eur J Physiol 474:33–61. https://doi.org/10.1007/s00424-021-02650-y

Jayasinghe I, Clowsley AH, Lin R et al (2018) True molecular scale visualization of variable clustering properties of ryanodine receptors. Cell Rep 22:557–567. https://doi.org/10.1016/j.celrep.2017.12.045

Ji X (2019) Junctophilin-2 protects Cardiomyocytes against palmitate-induced injury. Master of Science, The University of Western Ontario

Jones PP, MacQuaide N, Louch WE (2018) Dyadic plasticity in cardiomyocytes. Front Physiol 9:1773. https://doi.org/10.3389/fphys.2018.01773

Joseph LC, Subramanyam P, Radlicz C et al (2016) Mitochondrial oxidative stress during cardiac lipid overload causes intracellular calcium leak and arrhythmia. Heart Rhythm 13:1699–1706. https://doi.org/10.1016/j.hrthm.2016.05.002

Kamp TJ, Hell JW (2000) Regulation of cardiac L-type calcium channels by protein kinase a and protein kinase C. Circ Res 87:1095–1102. https://doi.org/10.1161/01.RES.87.12.1095

Kawada T, Hemmi C, Fukuda S et al (2003) Sarcolemmal fragility secondary to the degradation of dystrophin in dilated cardiomyopathy, as estimated by electron microscopy. Exp Clin Cardiol 8: 67

Kemi OJ, Hoydal MA, MacQuaide N et al (2011) The effect of exercise training on transverse tubules in normal, remodeled, and reverse remodeled hearts. J Cell Physiol 226:2235–2243. https://doi.org/10.1002/jcp.22559

Kim HW, Cho YS, Lee HR et al (2001) Diabetic alterations in cardiac sarcoplasmic reticulum Ca^{2+}-ATPase and phospholamban protein expression. Life Sci. https://doi.org/10.1016/s0024-3205(01)01483-7

Kolstad TR, Van Den Brink J, MacQuaide N et al (2018) Ryanodine receptor dispersion disrupts Ca^{2+} release in failing cardiac myocytes. eLife 7:e39427. https://doi.org/10.7554/eLife.39427

Kruszewska J, Cudnoch-Jedrzejewska A, Czarzasta K (2022) Remodeling and fibrosis of the cardiac muscle in the course of obesity—pathogenesis and involvement of the extracellular matrix. IJMS 23:4195. https://doi.org/10.3390/ijms23084195

Lacombe VA, Viatchenko-Karpinski S, Terentyev D et al (2007) Mechanisms of impaired calcium handling underlying subclinical diastolic dysfunction in diabetes. Am J Phys Regul Integr Comp Phys 293:R1787–R1797. https://doi.org/10.1152/ajpregu.00059.2007

Lahiri SK, Quick AP, Samson-Couterie B et al (2020) Nuclear localization of a novel calpain-2 mediated junctophilin-2 C-terminal cleavage peptide promotes cardiomyocyte remodeling. Basic Res Cardiol 115:49. https://doi.org/10.1007/s00395-020-0807-1

Lahiri SK, Jin F, Zhou Y et al (2024) Altered myocardial lipid regulation in junctophilin-2–associated familial cardiomyopathies. Life Sci Alliance 7:e202302330. https://doi.org/10.26508/lsa.202302330

Lavie CJ, Pandey A, Lau DH et al (2017) Obesity and atrial fibrillation prevalence, pathogenesis, and prognosis. J Am Coll Cardiol 70:2022–2035. https://doi.org/10.1016/j.jacc.2017.09.002

Lee T-I, Chen Y-C, Kao Y-H et al (2013) Rosiglitazone induces arrhythmogenesis in diabetic hypertensive rats with calcium handling alteration. Int J Cardiol 165:299–307. https://doi.org/10.1016/j.ijcard.2011.08.072

Leon BM (2015) Diabetes and cardiovascular disease: epidemiology, biological mechanisms, treatment recommendations and future research. WJD 6:1246. https://doi.org/10.4239/wjd.v6.i13.1246

Li J, Richmond B, Hong T (2021a) Cardiac T-tubule cBIN1-microdomain, a diagnostic marker and therapeutic target of heart failure. IJMS 22:2299. https://doi.org/10.3390/ijms22052299

Li T, Li G, Guo X et al (2021b) The influence of diabetes and prediabetes on left heart remodeling: a population-based study. J Diabetes Complicat 35:107771. https://doi.org/10.1016/j.jdiacomp.2020.107771

Li J, Richmond B, Cluntun AA et al (2023) Cardiac gene therapy treats diabetic cardiomyopathy and lowers blood glucose. JCI Insight 8:e166713. https://doi.org/10.1172/jci.insight.166713

Listenberger LL, Ory DS, Schaffer JE (2001) Palmitate-induced apoptosis can occur through a ceramide-independent pathway. J Biol Chem 276:14890–14895. https://doi.org/10.1074/jbc.M010286200

Liu C, Spinozzi S, Chen J-Y et al (2019) Nexilin is a new component of junctional membrane complexes required for cardiac T-tubule formation. Circulation 140:55–66. https://doi.org/10.1161/CIRCULATIONAHA.119.039751

London B (2017) Defining the complexity of the junctional membrane complex. Circ Res 120:11–12. https://doi.org/10.1161/CIRCRESAHA.116.310214

Lopez-Jimenez F, Almahmeed W, Bays H et al (2022) Obesity and cardiovascular disease: mechanistic insights and management strategies. A joint position paper by the world heart federation and world obesity federation. Eur J Prev Cardiol 29:2218–2237. https://doi.org/10.1093/eurjpc/zwac187

Louch W (2004) Reduced synchrony of Ca^{2+} release with loss of T-tubules—a comparison to Ca^{2+} release in human failing cardiomyocytes. Cardiovasc Res 62:63–73. https://doi.org/10.1016/j.cardiores.2003.12.031

Louch WE, Mørk HK, Sexton J et al (2006) T-tubule disorganization and reduced synchrony of Ca^{2+} release in murine cardiomyocytes following myocardial infarction. J Physiol 574:519–533. https://doi.org/10.1113/jphysiol.2006.107227

Louch WE, Hake J, Mørk HK et al (2013) Slow Ca^{2+} sparks de-synchronize Ca^{2+} release in failing cardiomyocytes: evidence for altered configuration of Ca^{2+} release units? J Mol Cell Cardiol 58:41–52. https://doi.org/10.1016/j.yjmcc.2013.01.014

Lu Z, Jiang Y-P, Xu X-H et al (2007) Decreased L- type Ca^{2+} current in cardiac myocytes of type 1 diabetic Akita mice due to reduced phosphatidylinositol 3-kinase signaling. Diabetes 56:2780–2789. https://doi.org/10.2337/db06-1629

Macquaide N, Tuan H-TM, Hotta J et al (2015) Ryanodine receptor cluster fragmentation and redistribution in persistent atrial fibrillation enhance calcium release. Cardiovasc Res 108:387–398. https://doi.org/10.1093/cvr/cvv231

Magliano D, Boyko EJ (2021) IDF diabetes atlas, 10th edn. International Diabetes Federation, Brussels

Martin AA, Thompson BR, Hahn D et al (2022) Cardiac sarcomere signaling in health and disease. Int J Mol Sci 23:16223. https://doi.org/10.3390/ijms232416223

McGavock JM, Lingvay I, Zib I et al (2007) Cardiac steatosis in diabetes mellitus: a 1H-magnetic resonance spectroscopy study. Circulation 116:1170–1175. https://doi.org/10.1161/CIRCULATIONAHA.106.645614

McGrath KF, Yuki A, Manaka Y et al (2009) Morphological characteristics of cardiac calcium release units in animals with metabolic and circulatory disorders. J Muscle Res Cell Motil 30:225–231. https://doi.org/10.1007/s10974-009-9191-z

Menezes AR, Lavie CJ, DiNicolantonio JJ et al (2013) Atrial fibrillation in the 21st century: a current understanding of risk factors and primary prevention strategies. Mayo Clin Proc 88:394–409. https://doi.org/10.1016/j.mayocp.2013.01.022

Mohler PJ, Davis JQ, Bennett V (2005) Ankyrin-B coordinates the Na/K ATPase, Na/ca exchanger, and InsP3 receptor in a cardiac T-tubule/SR microdomain. PLoS Biol 3:e423. https://doi.org/10.1371/journal.pbio.0030423

Munro ML, Jayasinghe I, Wang Q et al (2016) Junctophilin-2 in the nanoscale organisation and functional signalling of ryanodine receptor clusters in cardiomyocytes. J Cell Sci 129:4388–4398. https://doi.org/10.1242/jcs.196873

Murfitt L, Whiteley G, Iqbal MM, Kitmitto A (2015) Targeting caveolin-3 for the treatment of diabetic cardiomyopathy. Pharmacol Ther 151:50–71. https://doi.org/10.1016/j.pharmthera.2015.03.002

Ng ACT, Delgado V, Borlaug BA, Bax JJ (2021) Diabesity: the combined burden of obesity and diabetes on heart disease and the role of imaging. Nat Rev Cardiol 18:291–304. https://doi.org/10.1038/s41569-020-00465-5

Oda T, Yang Y, Uchinoumi H et al (2015) Oxidation of ryanodine receptor (RyR) and calmodulin enhance Ca release and pathologically alter, RyR structure and calmodulin affinity. J Mol Cell Cardiol 85:240–248. https://doi.org/10.1016/j.yjmcc.2015.06.009

Okatan EN, Durak AT, Turan B (2016) Electrophysiological basis of metabolic-syndrome-induced cardiac dysfunction. Can J Physiol Pharmacol 94:1064–1073. https://doi.org/10.1139/cjpp-2015-0531

Pereira L, Matthes J, Schuster I et al (2006) Mechanisms of [Ca2+]i transient decrease in cardiomyopathy of *db/db* Type 2 diabetic mice. Diabetes 55:608–615. https://doi.org/10.2337/diabetes.55.03.06.db05-1284

Peterson LR, Herrero P, Schechtman KB et al (2004) Effect of obesity and insulin resistance on myocardial substrate metabolism and efficiency in Young women. Circulation 109:2191–2196. https://doi.org/10.1161/01.CIR.0000127959.28627.F8
Picas L, Viaud J, Schauer K et al (2014) BIN1/M-Amphiphysin2 induces clustering of phosphoinositides to recruit its downstream partner dynamin. Nat Commun 5:5647. https://doi.org/10.1038/ncomms6647
Pinali C, Bennett H, Davenport JB et al (2013) Three-dimensional reconstruction of cardiac sarcoplasmic reticulum reveals a continuous network linking transverse-tubules: this organization is perturbed in heart failure. Circ Res 113:1219–1230. https://doi.org/10.1161/CIRCRESAHA.113.301348
Ponce-Balbuena D, Tyrrell DJ, Cruz-Cortés C et al (2024) Paradoxical SERCA dysregulation contributes to atrial fibrillation in a model of diet-induced obesity. bioRxiv. https://doi.org/10.1101/2024.08.02.606385
Poulet C, Sanchez-Alonso J, Swiatlowska P et al (2021) Junctophilin-2 tethers T-tubules and recruits functional L-type calcium channels to lipid rafts in adult cardiomyocytes. Cardiovasc Res 117:149–161. https://doi.org/10.1093/cvr/cvaa033
Powell-Wiley TM, Poirier P, Burke LE et al (2021) Obesity and cardiovascular disease: a scientific statement from the American Heart Association. Circulation 143. https://doi.org/10.1161/CIR.0000000000000973
Prins KW, Asp ML, Zhang H et al (2016) Microtubule-mediated Misregulation of Junctophilin-2 underlies T-tubule disruptions and calcium mishandling in mdx mice. JACC: Basic Transl Sci 1:122–130. https://doi.org/10.1016/j.jacbts.2016.02.002
Prokic I, Cowling BS, Laporte J (2014) Amphiphysin 2 (BIN1) in physiology and diseases. J Mol Med 92:453–463. https://doi.org/10.1007/s00109-014-1138-1
Quick AP, Wang Q, Philippen LE et al (2017) SPEG (striated muscle preferentially expressed protein kinase) is essential for cardiac function by regulating junctional membrane complex activity. Circ Res 120:110–119. https://doi.org/10.1161/CIRCRESAHA.116.309977
Reuter H, Grönke S, Adam C et al (2008) Sarcoplasmic Ca^{2+} release is prolonged in nonfailing myocardium of diabetic patients. Mol Cell Biochem 308:141–149. https://doi.org/10.1007/s11010-007-9622-3
Romanelli G, Villarreal L, Espasandín C, Benech JC (2024) Diabetes induces differences in costameric proteins and increases cardiomyocyte stiffness. Am J Physiol Cell Physiol. https://doi.org/10.1152/ajpcell.00273.2024
Russell J, Du Toit EF, Peart JN et al (2017) Myocyte membrane and microdomain modifications in diabetes: determinants of ischemic tolerance and cardioprotection. Cardiovasc Diabetol 16:155. https://doi.org/10.1186/s12933-017-0638-z
Sacconi L, Ferrantini C, Lotti J et al (2012) Action potential propagation in transverse-axial tubular system is impaired in heart failure. Proc Natl Acad Sci USA 109:5815–5819. https://doi.org/10.1073/pnas.1120188109
Sanchez-Alonso JL, Bhargava A, O'Hara T et al (2016) Microdomain-specific modulation of L-type calcium channels leads to triggered ventricular arrhythmia in heart failure. Circ Res 119:944–955. https://doi.org/10.1161/CIRCRESAHA.116.308698
Scriven DRL, Asghari P, Moore EDW (2013) Microarchitecture of the dyad. Cardiovasc Res 98:169–176. https://doi.org/10.1093/cvr/cvt025
Seidel T, Sankarankutty AC, Sachse FB (2017) Remodeling of the transverse tubular system after myocardial infarction in rabbit correlates with local fibrosis: a potential role of biomechanics. Prog Biophys Mol Biol 130:302–314. https://doi.org/10.1016/j.pbiomolbio.2017.07.006
Shao C-H, Wehrens XHT, Wyatt TA et al (2009) Exercise training during diabetes attenuates cardiac ryanodine receptor dysregulation. J Appl Physiol 106:1280–1292. https://doi.org/10.1152/japplphysiol.91280.2008
Sheikh AQ, Hurley JR, Huang W et al (2012) Diabetes alters intracellular calcium transients in cardiac endothelial cells. PLoS One 7:e36840. https://doi.org/10.1371/journal.pone.0036840

Smyrnias I, Mair W, Harzheim D et al (2010) Comparison of the T-tubule system in adult rat ventricular and atrial myocytes, and its role in excitation–contraction coupling and inotropic stimulation. Cell Calcium 47:210–223. https://doi.org/10.1016/j.ceca.2009.10.001

Soeller C, Cannell MB (1999) Examination of the transverse tubular system in living cardiac rat myocytes by 2-photon microscopy and digital image–processing techniques. Circ Res 84:266–275. https://doi.org/10.1161/01.RES.84.3.266

Song L, Guatimosim S, Gómez-Viquez L et al (2005) Calcium biology of the transverse tubules in heart. Ann N Y Acad Sci 1047:99–111. https://doi.org/10.1196/annals.1341.009

Song L-S, Sobie EA, McCulle S et al (2006) Orphaned ryanodine receptors in the failing heart. Proc Natl Acad Sci USA 103:4305–4310. https://doi.org/10.1073/pnas.0509324103

Spinozzi S, Liu C, Chen Z et al (2020) Nexilin is necessary for maintaining the transverse-axial tubular system in adult Cardiomyocytes. Circ: Heart Failure 13:e006935. https://doi.org/10.1161/CIRCHEARTFAILURE.120.006935

Stanley WC, Recchia FA, Lopaschuk GD (2005) Myocardial substrate metabolism in the Normal and failing heart. Physiol Rev 85:1093–1129. https://doi.org/10.1152/physrev.00006.2004

Stølen TO, Høydal MA, Kemi OJ et al (2009) Interval training normalizes Cardiomyocyte function, diastolic Ca^{2+} control, and SR Ca^{2+} release synchronicity in a mouse model of diabetic cardiomyopathy. Circ Res 105:527–536. https://doi.org/10.1161/CIRCRESAHA.109.199810

Sun XH, Protasi F, Takahashi M et al (1995) Molecular architecture of membranes involved in excitation-contraction coupling of cardiac muscle. J Cell Biol 129:659–671. https://doi.org/10.1083/jcb.129.3.659

Swift F, Franzini-Armstrong C, Øyehaug L et al (2012) Extreme sarcoplasmic reticulum volume loss and compensatory T-tubule remodeling after *Serca2* knockout. Proc Natl Acad Sci USA 109:3997–4001. https://doi.org/10.1073/pnas.1120172109

Takeshima H (2000) JunctophilinsA novel family of junctional membrane complex proteins. Mol Cell 6:11–22. https://doi.org/10.1016/S1097-2765(00)00003-4

Tam CS, Lecoultre V, Ravussin E (2012) Brown adipose tissue: mechanisms and potential therapeutic targets. Circulation 125:2782–2791. https://doi.org/10.1161/CIRCULATIONAHA.111.042929

Terentyev D, Viatchenko-Karpinski S, Györke I et al (2003) Calsequestrin determines the functional size and stability of cardiac intracellular calcium stores: mechanism for hereditary arrhythmia. Proc Natl Acad Sci USA 100:11759–11764. https://doi.org/10.1073/pnas.1932318100

Teshima Y, Takahashi N, Saikawa T et al (2000) Diminished expression of sarcoplasmic reticulum Ca(2+)-ATPase and ryanodine sensitive Ca(2+)Channel mRNA in Streptozotocin-induced diabetic rat heart. J Mol Cell Cardiol 32:655–664. https://doi.org/10.1006/jmcc.2000.1107

Tian C, Hong Shao C, Moore CJ et al (2011) Gain of function of cardiac ryanodine receptor in a rat model of type 1 diabetes. Cardiovasc Res 91:300–309. https://doi.org/10.1093/cvr/cvr076

Trafford AW, Clarke JD, Richards MA et al (2013) Calcium signalling microdomains and the t-tubular system in atrial mycoytes: potential roles in cardiac disease and arrhythmias. Cardiovasc Res 98:192–203. https://doi.org/10.1093/cvr/cvt018

Uchida K, Lopatin AN (2018) Diffusional and electrical properties of T-tubules are governed by their constrictions and dilations. Biophys J 114:437–449. https://doi.org/10.1016/j.bpj.2017.11.3742

Vasconcelos LHC, Souza ILL, Pinheiro LS, Silva BA (2016) Ion channels in obesity: pathophysiology and potential therapeutic targets. Front Pharmacol 7. https://doi.org/10.3389/fphar.2016.00058

Wang J, Hall DD, Song L-S (2020) Nexilin is a new player for shaping T-tubules in cardiomyocytes. Circulation: Heart Failure 13:e007196. https://doi.org/10.1161/CIRCHEARTFAILURE.120.007196

Ward M-L (2014) Mechanisms underlying the impaired contractility of diabetic cardiomyopathy. WJC 6:577. https://doi.org/10.4330/wjc.v6.i7.577

Watson SA, Perbellini F, Terracciano CM (2016) Cardiac t-tubules: where structural plasticity meets functional adaptation. Cardiovasc Res 112:423–425. https://doi.org/10.1093/cvr/cvw198
Wechsler-Reya R, Sakamuro D, Zhang J et al (1997) Structural analysis of the human BIN1 gene. J Biol Chem 272:31453–31458. https://doi.org/10.1074/jbc.272.50.31453
Westhoff M, Dixon RE (2021) Mechanisms and regulation of cardiac CaV1.2 trafficking. IJMS 22: 5927. https://doi.org/10.3390/ijms22115927
Wisneski JA, Gertz EW, Neese RA et al (1985) Metabolic fate of extracted glucose in normal human myocardium. J Clin Invest 76:1819–1827. https://doi.org/10.1172/JCI112174
Wold L, Dutta K, Mason M et al (2005) Impaired SERCA function contributes to cardiomyocyte dysfunction in insulin resistant rats. J Mol Cell Cardiol 39:297–307. https://doi.org/10.1016/j.yjmcc.2005.03.014
Wong ND, Sattar N (2023) Cardiovascular risk in diabetes mellitus: epidemiology, assessment and prevention. Nat Rev Cardiol 20:685–695. https://doi.org/10.1038/s41569-023-00877-z
Wright PT, Nikolaev VO, O'Hara T et al (2014) Caveolin-3 regulates compartmentation of cardiomyocyte beta2-adrenergic receptor-mediated cAMP signaling. J Mol Cell Cardiol 67: 38–48. https://doi.org/10.1016/j.yjmcc.2013.12.003
Yaras N, Ugur M, Ozdemir S et al (2005) Effects of diabetes on ryanodine receptor ca Release Channel (RyR2) and Ca^{2+} homeostasis in rat heart. Diabetes 54:3082–3088. https://doi.org/10.2337/diabetes.54.11.3082
Young ME, Guthrie PH, Razeghi P et al (2002) Impaired long-chain fatty acid oxidation and contractile dysfunction in the obese Zucker rat heart. Diabetes 51:2587–2595. https://doi.org/10.2337/diabetes.51.8.2587
Yu Z, Tibbits GF, McNeill JH (1994) Cellular functions of diabetic cardiomyocytes: contractility, rapid-cooling contracture, and ryanodine binding. Am J Phys Heart Circ Phys 266:H2082–H2089. https://doi.org/10.1152/ajpheart.1994.266.5.H2082
Zhang C, Chen B, Guo A et al (2014) Microtubule-mediated defects in Junctophilin-2 trafficking contribute to myocyte transverse-tubule remodeling and Ca^{2+} handling dysfunction in heart failure. Circulation 129:1742–1750. https://doi.org/10.1161/CIRCULATIONAHA.113.008452

Calcium Signaling Dysregulation in Diabetic Cardiomyopathy: Roles of STIM and Orai Channels

Tarik Smani, Beltzane Dominguez-Liste, Marta de Jesús Gutiérrez-Barranco, Carlos Aspron-Martin, Celia Cordero-Sánchez, Eva M. Calderón-Sánchez, Juan Antonio Rosado, and Abdelkrim Hmadcha

Contents

Authors Beltzane Dominguez-Liste, Marta de Jesús Gutiérrez-Barranco, Carlos Aspron-Martin and Celia Cordero-Sánchez have equally contributed to this chapter.

T. Smani (✉) · B. Dominguez-Liste · M. de Jesús Gutiérrez-Barranco · C. Aspron-Martin · C. Cordero-Sánchez
Group of Cardiovascular Pathophysiology, Institute of Biomedicine of Seville, University Hospital of Virgen del Rocio/University of Seville/CSIC, Seville, Spain

Department of Medical Physiology and Biophysics, Faculty of Medicine, University of Seville, Seville, Spain
e-mail: tasmani@us.es

E. M. Calderón-Sánchez
Group of Cardiovascular Pathophysiology, Institute of Biomedicine of Seville, University Hospital of Virgen del Rocio/University of Seville/CSIC, Seville, Spain

J. A. Rosado
Department of Physiology, Cell Physiology Research Group, University of Extremadura, Cáceres, Spain

A. Hmadcha
Biosanitary Research Institute (IIB-VIU), Valencian International University (VIU), Valencia, Spain

A. Rueda, M. Nieves-Cintrón (eds.), *Cardiovascular Alterations in Metabolic Diseases*, Handbook of Experimental Pharmacology 293,
https://doi.org/10.1007/164_2026_797

Abstract

Diabetes mellitus is a major metabolic disorder that significantly increases the risk of cardiovascular disease. Altered calcium (Ca^{2+}) homeostasis, particularly through store-operated calcium entry (SOCE), has emerged as a critical pathway linking diabetes with cardiac dysfunction. Evidence indicates that SOCE is dysregulated in diabetes, but findings remain controversial. Some studies report reduced SOCE due to downregulation or impaired coupling of STIM1 and Orai1, leading to altered Ca^{2+} homeostasis and cardiac dysfunction. Others demonstrate enhanced SOCE linked to Orai and STIM isoforms upregulation, contributing to mitochondrial dysfunction, maladaptive hypertrophy, and metabolic remodeling in diabetic cardiomyopathy. Recent work also highlighted an unexpected role of STIM1 in fatty acid metabolism, linking Ca^{2+} signaling with energy substrate preference in the diabetic heart. This chapter synthesizes current evidence on the molecular mechanisms of STIM and Orai proteins in the regulation of SOCE under diabetic conditions, highlighting their roles in heart dysfunction.

Keywords

Diabetic Cardiomyopathy · Fatty acid metabolism · Orai isoforms · STIM · Store-operated calcium entry

1 Overview of Diabetes and Its Cardiovascular Impact

Diabetes mellitus (DM) is a metabolic disorder characterized by chronic hyperglycemia resulting from defects in insulin secretion, its action, or both. Sustained long-term hyperglycemia leads to progressive damage in multiple organs, particularly the heart and blood vessels (American Diabetes Association 2011). The World Health Organization classifies DM into two main types: type 1 (T1DM), caused by autoimmune destruction of pancreatic β-cells, and type 2 (T2DM), mainly associated with insulin resistance and impaired insulin secretion (Darenskaya et al. 2021). T1DM is more common in children and adolescents and usually develops rapidly. In contrast, T2DM is generally diagnosed in adulthood and progresses slowly, typically accompanying obesity, sedentary lifestyle, and associated with genetic predisposition (Maahs et al. 2010; Młynarska et al. 2025).

The relationship between DM and cardiovascular diseases was first identified in 1972 through a postmortem analysis of 27 patients (Rubler et al. 1972). Since then, substantial investigations have been dedicated to elucidating the mechanisms that connect these two major pathologies (Jia et al. 2018). In fact, among diabetic complications, cardiovascular diseases are the most prevalent, including ischemic heart disease, stroke, limb ischemia, and heart failure (Avagimyan et al. 2024). A particularly concerning condition is diabetic cardiomyopathy (DCM) characterized by cardiac dysfunction and heart failure occurring independently of coronary artery disease, hypertension, or valvular heart disease (Tarquini et al. 2011; Zhao et al. 2022). DCM also affects cardiac endothelial cells, marked by impaired Ca^{2+} signaling, reduced nitric oxide bioavailability, and heightened oxidative and inflammatory stress, promoting coronary microvascular dysfunction and myocardial stiffening, key pathophysiological mechanisms that link diabetes to the development of heart failure with preserved ejection fraction (HFpEF) (Zhao et al. 2022). Actually, DCM results from a complex interplay of molecular, cellular, and metabolic mechanisms that contribute to structural and functional alterations in the myocardium, leading to adverse cardiac remodeling. Key mechanisms include chronic metabolic disturbances caused by hyperglycemia and insulin resistance, oxidative stress contributing to endothelial dysfunction, atherosclerosis, and direct myocardial injury in patients with diabetes (Teo and Rafiq 2021; He et al. 2025). Additionally, under diabetes myocardial lipotoxicity, chronic inflammation, mitochondrial dysfunction, and endoplasmic reticulum (ER) stress, marked by protein misfolding and disrupted Ca^{2+} homeostasis, all contribute to impaired cardiac function (Dong et al. 2017; Chen et al. 2025; Congur et al. 2025; Luong et al. 2025). Among these, Ca^{2+} dysregulation has emerged as a pivotal mechanism, affecting both contractility and arrhythmogenesis. In fact, intracellular Ca^{2+} handling, a key determinant of excitation-contraction coupling in cardiomyocytes, is affected in DCM (Ren et al. 1997; Romero-García et al. 2020). Ca^{2+} ion is especially important in muscle cells (Fabiato 1985), where membrane components of the sarcolemma and the ER, and a lesser extent, the mitochondria, are involved in maintaining Ca^{2+} homeostasis (Bers 2002). ER mainly functions as Ca^{2+} storage necessary for contractile functions (Terrell et al. 2023). More recently, growing evidence implicates the dysregulation of store-operated calcium entry (SOCE) in the adverse cardiac remodeling (Eder 2017; Avila-Medina et al. 2020; Sabourin et al. 2022). However, only few reports associate DCM with SOCE signaling pathway, which is often underappreciated in cardiac Ca^{2+} homeostasis.

This chapter aims to provide a comprehensive overview of the role of SOCE and related proteins in cardiovascular behavior within the context of diabetes. Understanding the molecular and cellular mechanisms linking diabetes with cardiovascular diseases is essential for developing more effective therapeutic strategies.

2 Intracellular Ca^{2+} Mishandling in Diabetic Heart

In the heart, Ca^{2+} homeostasis plays distinct but interconnected roles in cardiac myocytes, coronary smooth muscle, and endothelial cells. In cardiac myocytes, Ca^{2+} is tightly regulated through excitation–contraction coupling mechanism. In coronary smooth muscle cells, Ca^{2+} influx mainly through voltage-gated activates calmodulin–myosin light chain kinase signaling, leading to contraction and regulation of vascular tone; Ca^{2+} efflux and sequestration ensure relaxation. In endothelial cells, Ca^{2+} signaling is crucial for nitric oxide production, promoting smooth muscle relaxation, and regulate barrier function and angiogenic signaling. Together, these cell-specific Ca^{2+} dynamics coordinate cardiac contraction, vascular tone, and blood flow regulation, which are affected under cardiovascular disease. Here, we will focus on the impact of diabetes on cardiomyocytes.

2.1 Critical Players of Ca^{2+} Homeostasis in Heart Cells

In cardiomyocytes, excitation–contraction coupling relies on Ca^{2+} influx through L-type Ca^{2+} voltage-gated channels in the sarcolemma, resulting in Ca^{2+} influx and a subsequent increase in intracellular Ca^{2+} concentration ($[Ca^{2+}]_i$). This rise in $[Ca^{2+}]_i$ triggers the release of additional Ca^{2+} from the sarcoplasmic reticulum (SR) via ryanodine-sensitive receptors (RyRs), through a process known as Ca^{2+}-induced Ca^{2+} release (CICR) (Fabiato 1985). Cardiac relaxation begins when most cytosolic Ca^{2+} is actively sequestered into the SR by the sarcoplasmic/endoplasmic Ca^{2+}-ATPase pump (SERCA), while another fraction is extruded from the cell via the Na^+/Ca^{2+} exchanger (NCX) under physiological conditions (Bers 2002). In adult ventricular cardiomyocytes, SR Ca^{2+} refilling is mediated predominantly by Ca^{2+} influx through L-type voltage-gated Ca^{2+} channels during membrane depolarization, followed by SERCA-dependent uptake into the SR. Unlike other muscle cell, store-operated Ca^{2+} entry (SOCE) does not contribute significantly to physiological SR Ca^{2+} refilling under normal pacing conditions. Although SOCE can be activated following severe SR Ca^{2+} depletion or in neonatal and pathological cardiac states, its contribution in mature ventricular myocytes appears minimal due to low STIM1/Orai1 activity and the dominance of excitation–contraction coupling–linked Ca^{2+} influx. However, increasing evidence suggested the participation of store-operated Ca^{2+} and TRPC channels in agonist-induced Ca^{2+} influx, particularly during cardiac development or under stress conditions, such as ischemia/reperfusion (I/R) and pressure overload caused by transverse aortic constriction (TAC) (Bartoli et al. 2020; Falcón et al. 2024); although, the participation of SOCE in DCM remains unclear.

2.2 Store-Operated Ca^{2+} Signaling

SOCE is a widespread mechanism that maintains intracellular Ca^{2+} homeostasis which was first described by Putney in 1986 (Putney 1986). SOCE plays key roles in gene transcription, cell proliferation, immune responses, and memory, among others (Emrich et al. 2021). SOCE is initiated when ER Ca^{2+} levels decrease, triggering conformational changes in STIM1, Ca^{2+} sensor located in the ER membrane (Fig. 1). Ca^{2+} dissociation induces STIM1 unfolding and the consequent conformational change leads to STIM1 dimerization and accumulation into puncta at the ER/plasma membrane junctions. Previous studies have shown that STIM1 accumulation is regulated by its interaction with EB1, a microtubule-plus-end binding protein that transiently traps STIM1 molecules and modulates their mobility (Chang et al. 2018; Ahmad et al. 2022). Additional works have shown that proteins such as EMC1, as

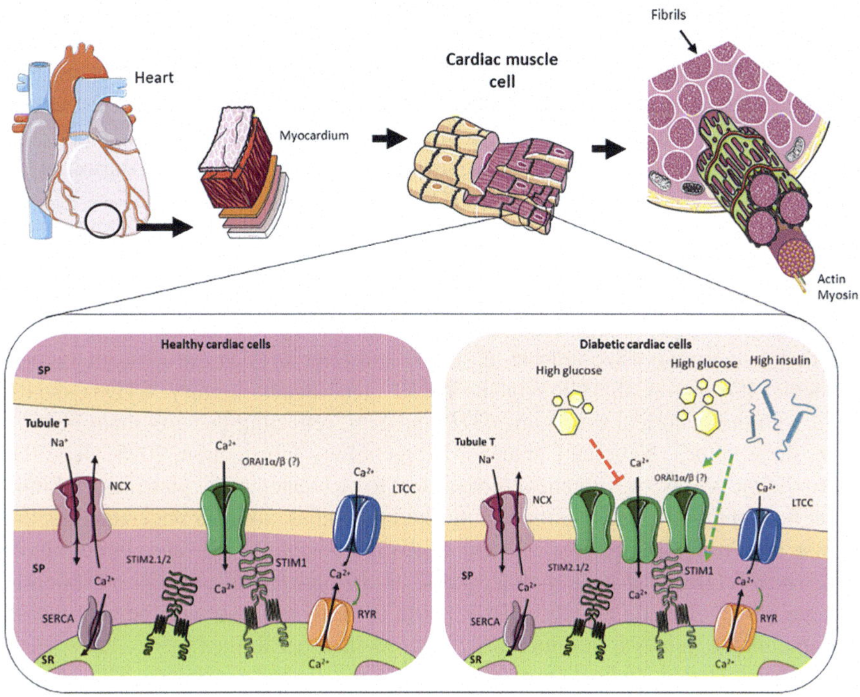

Fig. 1 Schematic representation of store-operated calcium entry in cardiac muscle in physical conditions and in diabetic cardiomyopathy. In healthy cardiomyocyte, the store-operated calcium entry (SOCE) is initiated upon store depletion by the interaction of STIM1 with Orai1, allowing Ca^{2+} influx. Under diabetes, the expression of Orai1 seems sensitive to hyperglycemia. Green arrows indicate activation. Red arrows indicate inhibition. Abbreviation: L-Type Calcium Channels (LTCC); Na+/Ca2+ exchanger (NCX); Ryanodine receptors (RYR); Sarcoplasmic/endoplasmic Ca^{2+}-ATPase pump (SERCA); Sarcoplasmic Reticulum (SR); Sarcoplasm (SP); STIM: Stromal Interaction Molecule. (Figure created through Smart Servier Medical Art)

well as actin cytoskeleton organization, contribute to the formation and stabilization of STIM1 puncta (Wang et al. 2018; Yu et al. 2019). Once clustered, STIM1 recruits Orai1 channels to these junctions and activates them leading to the opening of Ca^{2+} release-activated Ca^{2+} (CRAC) channels, and the subsequent influx of extracellular Ca^{2+}. Despite the broad relevance of SOCE, its presence in cardiomyocytes has been initially overlooked and its contribution to normal cardiac physiology remains under debate (Collins et al. 2013; Bootman and Rietdorf 2017). However, there is consensus that SOCE becomes upregulated in cardiomyocytes through increased ion channel expression during the reactivated fetal gene program, or via enhanced channel activity in chronic cardiac disease as reviewed elsewhere (Eder and Molkentin 2011; Luo et al. 2012).

Strong evidence supports the presence of SOCE, especially in neonatal cardiomyocytes whose stimulation with SERCA inhibitor, thapsigargin, or agonists activating G protein–coupled receptors, evokes persistent Ca^{2+} influx that is insensitive to LTCC or NCX inhibition, but sensitive to blockers of SOCE (Kojima et al. 2012; Bartoli and Sabourin 2017; Domínguez-Rodríguez et al. 2018; Falcón et al. 2024; Narayanasamy et al. 2024). The interaction between STIM proteins and Orai channels is necessary for SOCE-mediated Ca^{2+} influx (Fig. 1), which contributes not only to contractile function in heart but also to gene expression and cellular adaptation during cardiac development and remodeling (Bartoli et al. 2020; Durak et al. 2022; Falcón et al. 2024).

2.2.1 STIM Proteins

STIM1 was initially identified under different names in two independent studies: first as GOK, a type I transmembrane protein associated with rhabdomyosarcomas and rhabdoid tumors (Sabbioni et al. 1999) and later as SIM (stromal interacting molecule) (Oritani et al. 1996). In the NCBI Gene database entry, STIM1 is still listed with the historical synonyms *GOK* and *SIM*, reflecting its early identification under these names (National Center for Biotecnology Information, 2025, Gene ID: 6786). In both cases, the protein was described to be located at the plasma membrane rather than in the ER. These early findings laid the foundations for understanding the diverse roles of STIM proteins, including their long-standing relevance in immunology, where STIM1 and its homolog STIM2 are recognized as essential sensors that activate SOCE (Nelson and Roe 2018). Both proteins are known to be single-pass transmembrane sensors predominantly located in the ER membrane, with small fractions detected in acidic compartments and at the plasma membrane. This historical background is consistent with more recent studies, which highlighted the involvement of STIM proteins in cancer growth (Narayanasamy et al. 2024).

STIM1 (aa 1–685) and STIM2 (aa 1–721) share a conserved domain architecture. Their N-terminal luminal region contains a highly conserved EF-SAM domain composed of two EF-hands and an adjacent sterile α-motif (SAM) (Collins and Meyer 2011; Fahrner et al. 2020; Grabmayr et al. 2021). The canonical EF-hand directly binds Ca^{2+}, with half-maximal dissociation occurring at ~200 μM for STIM1 and ~ 400 μM for STIM2, whereas the non-canonical EF-hand, which does not bind Ca^{2+}, stabilizes the Ca^{2+}-bound state of the EF-SAM module. The SAM domain further reinforces the EF-SAM packing by enlarging the hydrophobic pocket and enhancing the overall structural stability (Stathopulos et al. 2006; Zheng et al. 2011; Kamath and Matreyek 2025). Depletion of luminal Ca^{2+} leads to the destabilization of the quaternary conformation of STIM, triggering a conformational rearrangement that leads to the EF-SAM unfolding and subsequent dimerization (Stathopulos et al. 2006;). The cytosolic C-terminus contains three coiled-coil domains (CC1–CC3), collectively known as the Orai-activating small fragment (OASF), CRAC-activating domain (CAD), or STIM-Orai-activating region (SOAR). These domains drive STIM1 oligomerization (Convington et al. 2010), targeting of STIM to the ER-PM junctions, and the activation of Orai channel (Baba et al. 2006; Huang et al. 2006; Liou et al. 2007).

In the heart, STIM1 is the predominant isoform, regulating Ca^{2+} homeostasis and contributing to pathological hypertrophy under stress conditions, such as TAC or I/R (Sabourin et al. 2018; Wu et al. 2025). Indeed, STIM1 is upregulated during hypertrophic remodeling in animal model subjected to aortic banding (Hulot et al. 2011; Troupes et al. 2017). Its activity promotes Ca^{2+} influx that stimulates downstream pathways, including Ca^{2+}/calmodulin-dependent protein kinase II (CaMKII), thereby driving hypertrophic gene expression (Collins et al. 2019). Moreover, cardiomyocyte-specific deletion of STIM1 in mice impaired Ca^{2+} handling, disrupted mitochondrial function, and induced dilated cardiomyopathy, underscoring its essential role in cardiac metabolism and structural integrity (Collins et al. 2019). STIM1 also modulates electrical activity as cardiomyocyte-specific knockdown of STIM1 enhanced arrhythmogenesis and altered action potential dynamics in mice (Cacheux et al. 2019). By contrast, transgenic mice overexpressing STIM1 developed cardiac hypertrophy and heart failure and were predisposed to increased cardiac disease after TAC (Correll et al. 2015).

STIM2 has been less extensively studied in the heart, but it may play a complementary role as it responds to smaller decreases in ER Ca^{2+} compared with STIM1 (Collins et al. 2022). Like STIM1, STIM2 expression increases in pressure overload–induced left ventricular hypertrophy and dysfunction in mice (Bartoli et al. 2020). STIM2 is also upregulated after I/R injury in the H9C2 cardiomyoblast cell line, where it contributed to mitochondrial Ca^{2+} overload and apoptosis (Tu et al. 2020). Furthermore, splice variants STIM2.1 and STIM2.2 are expressed in cardiac myocytes and exert opposing effects on Orai1-mediated SOCE in neonatal rat ventricular myocytes (Luo et al. 2024). More recently, duplication of the STIM2 gene has been associated with severe congenital heart disease in a young patient (Liang et al. 2017).

2.2.2 Orai Proteins

The Orai family comprises three tetraspanning plasma membrane proteins, Orai1, Orai2, and Orai3, with both termini facing the cytosol. Orai1, the principal channel underlying SOCE, was first identified in 2006 as the gene responsible for severe combined immunodeficiency and was initially considered the sole CRAC channel subunit alongside STIM1 (Feske et al. 2006). Activated CRAC channels conduct highly selective Ca^{2+} currents with a reversal potential of +60 mV and exhibit two Ca^{2+}-dependent inactivation (CDI) mechanisms: fast CDI (milliseconds, local Ca^{2+}) and slow CDI (seconds, global Ca^{2+} rise) (Prakriya et al. 2006).

In 2012, the structure of *Drosophila* Orai was crystallized, revealing CRAC channels as hexameric complexes in which the first transmembrane domains form the ion pore (Hou et al. 2012). Although tetrameric and pentameric stoichiometries of human Orai channels have been proposed, it is now generally accepted that Orai1 proteins form a hexamer (Penna et al. 2008; Maruyama et al. 2009; Demuro et al. 2011).

Two additional members of the Orai family, Orai2 and Orai3, were identified (Lis et al. 2007; DeHaven et al. 2007). The three isoforms are capable of forming functional channels with STIM1, but they exhibit distinct biophysical and pharmacological properties. Orai1-mediated currents are the largest, whereas Orai2 and Orai3 exhibit more pronounced fast CDI. Thus, the relative expression of each isoform shapes CRAC channel architecture and Ca^{2+} signaling. Recent evidence indicates that native CRAC channels are heteromers of Orai1, Orai2, and/or Orai3 (Vaeth et al. 2017; Tsvilovskyy et al. 2018; Eckstein et al. 2019). The presence of Orai2 and Orai3 in these channels ensures that the magnitude of Ca^{2+} influx is proportional to the strength of agonist stimulation (Yoast et al. 2020a, b). However, several studies have shown that Orai2 and Orai3 can attenuate or alter current amplitudes of SOCE, indicating a physiological regulation of Ca2+ entry in specific cell types (Emrich et al. 2021).

Orai1 exists in two isoforms generated by alternative translation initiation (Jardin et al. 2022). The full-length human variant, Orai1α, contains 301 amino acids, while the short form, Orai1β, arises from alternative initiation at methionine 64 or 71, thereby lacking the N-terminal 63 or 70 residues present in Orai1α (Fukushima et al. 2012; Willoughby et al. 2012). Both isoforms mediate CRAC currents, but Orai1α harbors additional regulatory motifs. Its N-terminus includes phosphorylation sites (Ser27, Ser30 by PKC; Ser34 by PKA), an adenylyl cyclase 8 (AC8) interaction domain linking Ca^{2+} and cAMP signaling, a PIP_2-binding motif, an AKAP79-binding site, and a caveolin-binding domain (Kar et al. 2021; Kawasaki et al. 2010; Calloway et al. 2011; Willoughby et al. 2012). These features render Orai1α more sensitive to phosphorylation-dependent inhibition compared with Orai1β. Recent evidence shows that Orai1α and Orai1β mostly form separate CRAC channels, although a small subset of heteromeric channels containing both variants has been observed (Lopez et al. 2025).

While Orai1 is expressed ubiquitously during development, including in embryonic and adult cardiomyocytes, its importance in adult cardiac function appears more conditional. In whole heart tissue, all three Orai isoforms are detectable, but their expression is sensitive to pathological stress such as pressure overload–induced hypertrophy, heart failure, or I/R (Saliba et al. 2015; Bartoli et al. 2020; Falcón et al. 2024). Functional studies demonstrated that cardiomyocyte-specific expression of non-conducting Orai1 mutant preserved normal Ca^{2+} handling in mice subjected to TAC (Bartoli et al. 2020). Similarly, Orai1 downregulation by AAV9 targeting AC8 prevented I/R-induced cardiac dysfunction and diastolic Ca^{2+} increase in rats (Falcón et al. 2024). More recently, cardiomyocyte-specific deletion of Orai3 was shown to cause dilated cardiomyopathy and heart failure in mice (Gammons et al. 2021), underscoring the pivotal role of Orai1 and Orai3 in maintaining myocardial integrity. Evidence for a specific role of Orai2 in heart remains sparse. Orai2 is expressed in the heart, but its cardiac-specific functions are not yet well characterized (Domínguez-Rodríguez et al. 2018).

3 Role of SOCE in Diabetes-Associated Cardiovascular Diseases

While alterations in SOCE and Orai/STIM signaling are well documented in hypertrophy and I/R injury, their direct contribution to DCM remains less clear and underexplored. Early studies concluded that diabetes and hyperglycemia mainly inhibit SOCE in smooth muscle, macrophages, endothelial cells, as well as in cardiomyocytes (Chaudhari and Ma 2016). For instance, rat aortic smooth muscle treated with 25 mM glucose exhibited significant decrease in SOCE response (Rivera et al. 1995). In coronary endothelial cells from diabetic mice ER Ca^{2+} levels seem reduced associated with significantly decrease in STIM1 protein levels compared with nondiabetic controls (Estrada et al. 2012). Subsequent overexpression of STIM1 restored ER Ca^{2+} levels and improved endothelium-dependent relaxation of diabetic coronary arteries (Estrada et al. 2012). Interestingly, platelets from patients with T2DM exhibited decreased SOCE and attenuated association between STIM1 and Orai1 (Jardín et al. 2011). In accordance with these findings, the exposition of cardiomyocytes to short-term hyperglycemia significantly decreased SOCE induced by angiotensin II and thapsigargin and significantly inhibited the Ca^{2+}-dependent hypertrophic response as well as the Ca^{2+}-sensitive nuclear translocation of nuclear factor of activated T-cells (NFAT) (Pang et al. 2002). More recently, in diabetic rat, hearts evoked by streptozotocin (STZ), STIM1, and Orai1 expressions were found to be lower than in controls, although this downregulation could not be directly associated with the myocardial damage observed (Liu and Wu 2023). These findings do not clarify whether SOCE inhibition is beneficial or detrimental for the heart under these circumstances since SOCE prevention of pro-hypertrophic signaling may be determinant for heart adaptative remodeling in the early stage of diabetes.

Conversely, other studies reported that hyperglycemia enhanced SOCE in cardiomyocytes through the upregulation of Orai and STIM isoforms. In fact, neonatal rat ventricular myocytes exposed to hyperglycemia exhibited increased SOCE and CRAC current. Likewise, in adult cardiomyocytes from STZ-induced diabetic rat, upregulation of Orai1, Orai2, and STIM1 was observed (Wang et al. 2017). Similarly, increased expression of Orai1 and Orai3 has been reported in hearts of STZ-induced diabetic rats, although SOCE currents paradoxically decreased (Gökçe et al. 2022). This discrepancy was attributed to impaired STIM interaction with Orai, a phenomenon also observed in T2DM platelets (Jardín et al. 2011). In Zucker diabetic fatty rats, a recent study provided further insight into the contribution of Orai1 to cardiac hypertrophy by using Orai1 silencing with RNA interference in neonatal rat ventricular myocytes which reduced cardiac hypertrophy and improved mitochondrial function by decreasing Drp1, calcineurin, and ERK1/2 activities (Wu et al. 2021). In models of metabolic syndrome, which exhibited significantly higher fasting blood glucose and insulin levels compared with controls, STIM1 and Orai1 upregulation was associated with increased Ca^{2+} spark frequency due to RyR leak and altered contractile dynamics (Durak et al. 2022).

Taken together, these findings agree that Orai and STIM isoforms play an important role in glucose homeostasis changes and diabetes, mainly through their involvement in SOCE and key pathways. Despite the evidence that Orai and STIM contribute to SOCE decrease in diabetic cardiomyopathy, these proteins are not limited to regulating SOCE. They can also modulate additional Ca^{2+}-dependent targets involved in this pathology such as Drp1, calcineurin, and ERK1/2 pathways which contribute to cardiac hypertrophy in diabetes. Further studies are still needed to clarify whether discrepancies in the expression and function of Orai and STIM isoforms arise from differences in animal and cellular models used and to determine their precise role in cardiac dysfunction under diabetic conditions.

4 STIM1 Role in Fatty Acid Metabolism in Diabetic Cardiomyopathy

Glucose and long-chain fatty acids (FA) are the major cardiac metabolic substrates under physiological conditions. However, in DCM, a shift in substrate preference toward FA is observed, leading to lipotoxicity and cardiac dysfunction (Glatz et al. 2020; Lopaschuk et al. 2021). STIM1, as a multifunctional protein integrating Ca^{2+} signaling with structural, electrical, and metabolic responses, has emerged as a key regulator of cardiac energy preferences both in cardiac hypertrophy and in DCM (Liu et al. 2023). In diabetic cardiomyocytes from obese Zucker rats (Fig. 2), FA uptake is primarily mediated by CD36, whose translocation to the sarcolemma is

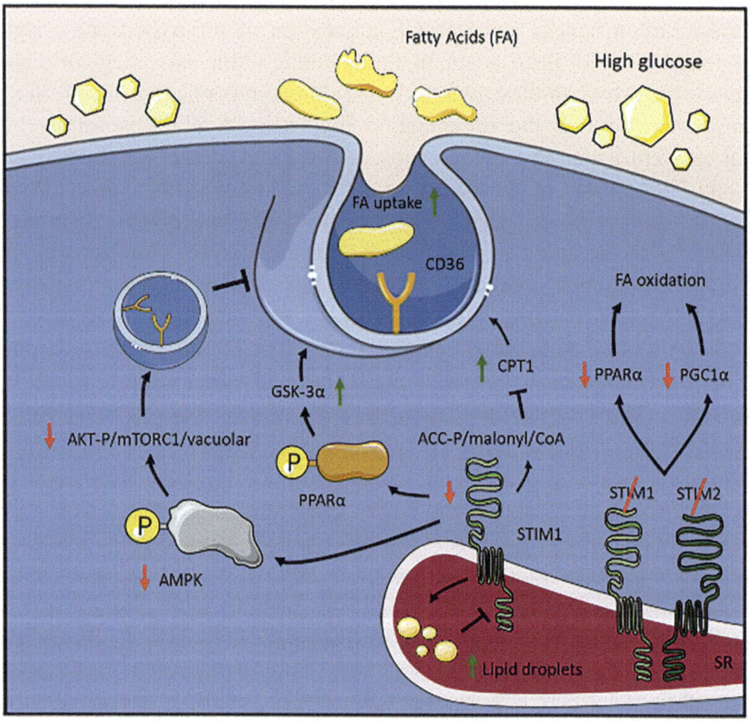

Fig. 2 Role of STIM1 in the metabolism of diabetic cardiomyopathy. The cartoon shows the role of STIM1 in different signaling pathways associated with fatty acid metabolism, such as AKT/mTORC1/vacuolar, GSK-3α, and ACC/malonyl/CoA. Green arrows indicate activation. Red arrows indicate inhibition. CPT1 Carnitine-palmitoyl transferase 1; GSK-3α Glycogen Synthase kinase-3α; FA Fatty Acids; SR Sarcoplasmic Reticulum; STIM Stromal Interaction Molecule. (Figure created through Smart Servier Medical Art)

enhanced (Coort et al. 2004). While AMPK phosphorylation typically regulated this process, STIM1 knockout (KO) hearts show reduced AMPK activity, suggesting that STIM1 may influence CD36 relocation via the AKT/mTORC1/vacuolar H^+-ATPase signaling axis (Wang et al. 2021). Reduced STIM1 expression also decreased AKT phosphorylation, impairing vacuolar H^+-ATPase assembly and promoting CD36 translocation, thereby increasing FA uptake (Collins et al. 2019).

Additionally, STIM1 apparently interacts with glycogen synthase kinase-3α (GSK-3α), enhancing FA uptake and their storage via PPARα phosphorylation. Consistently, hearts from diabetic patients exhibited increased GSK-3α activity together with reduced STIM1 expression, suggesting a regulatory link (Nakamura et al. 2019). STIM1 also modulates FA oxidation by regulating the expression and activity of carnitine-palmitoyl transferase 1 (CPT1), a key enzyme in mitochondrial FA transport (Collins et al. 2019). In STIM1 KO hearts, CPT1 levels and activity are elevated, indicating that STIM1 normally suppresses FA oxidation (Collins et al. 2019). This suppression may occur through the ACC/malonyl/CoA pathway, where STIM1-dependent phosphorylation of ACC reduced CPT1 activity (Collins et al. 2019).

Although STIM1 alone does not affect the expression of transcriptional regulators of FA oxidation, PPARα and PGC-1α, combined deletion of STIM1 and STIM2 reduced their levels, implicating STIM2 in transcriptional regulation (Maus et al. 2017). Moreover, lipid accumulation, a hallmark of diabetic cardiomyopathy (Bugger and Abel 2014; Lopaschuk et al. 2021), results from an imbalance between FA uptake and oxidation. STIM1 downregulation increased triglyceride and lipid droplet accumulation (Collins et al. 2019) probably due to reduced expression of lipases that hydrolyze stored lipids (Maus et al. 2017). In this way, lipid overload may suppress STIM1-mediated SOCE via PKC, exacerbating ER stress and lipid accumulation. STIM1 can also be modified by S-acylation, a lipid-dependent process that may serve as a feedback mechanism to restore SOCE under lipid-rich conditions (Collins et al. 2019). These findings highlight STIM1 as a key modulator of cardiac lipid metabolism and can be considered a potential therapeutic target in metabolic heart diseases.

5 Conclusion and Perspectives

Diabetes-induced alterations in Ca^{2+} signaling play a pivotal role in the development of cardiac complications. The evidence demonstrates that SOCE and its molecular components, STIM and/or Orai, regulate not only contractile Ca^{2+} dynamics but also metabolic remodeling, mitochondrial function, and lipid utilization in the diabetic heart. Despite extensive progress, important discrepancies remain regarding whether SOCE is up- or downregulated in diabetic heart, likely reflecting differences in disease stage, animal models, and cell-specific contexts. These findings underscore the need for more systematic and translational studies.

From a therapeutic perspective, targeting Orai1-mediated signaling, STIM1-dependent lipid handling, and their downstream effectors (e.g., CaMKII, calcineurin,

Drp1) represent a promising strategy to mitigate cardiac dysfunction in diabetes. Pharmacological modulation of SOCE may offer cardioprotective benefits, but careful evaluation is required to balance beneficial versus detrimental effects on hypertrophic signaling. Future work should integrate molecular studies with clinical observations to validate SOCE as a therapeutic target in diabetic cardiomyopathy and metabolic heart disease.

Acknowledgments This study is part of the projects PID2022-136279NB-C21 and PID2022-136279NBC22 funded by MICIU/AEI/10.13039/501100011033/, "ERDF A way of making Europe," and Junta de Andalucia [ProyExcel_00530; PI-0020-2024]. CA-M holds a fellowship from FPU program (Ministerio de Ciencia, Innovación y Universidades). CC-S is a "Juan de la Cierva" awardee from Spanish Ministerio de Ciencia, Innovación y Universidades). BD-L and MG-B were supported by contracts from INVESTIGO program (Junta de Andalucia).

References

Ahmad M, Narayanasamy S, Ong HL, Ambudkar I (2022) STIM proteins and regulation of SOCE in ER-PM junctions. Biomolecules 12(8):1152

American Diabetes Association (2011) Standards of medical care in diabetes-2011. Diabetes Care 34:S11–S61

Avagimyan A, Fogacci F, Pogosova N et al (2024) Diabetic cardiomyopathy: 2023 update by the international multidisciplinary Board of Experts. Curr Probl Cardiol 49(1A):10252

Avila-Medina J, Mayoral-Gonzalez I, Galeano-Otero I et al (2020) Pathophysiological significance of store-operated calcium entry in cardiovascular and skeletal muscle disorders and angiogenesis. Adv Exp Med Biol 1131:489–504. (Springer New York LLC)

Baba Y, Hayashi K, Fujii Y, Mizushima A, Watarai H, Wakamori M, Numaga T, Mori Y, Iino M, Hikida M, Kurosaki T (2006) Coupling of STIM1 to store-operated Ca^{2+} entry through its constitutive and inducible movement in the endoplasmic reticulum. Proc Natl Acad Sci U S A 103(45):16704–16709. https://doi.org/10.1073/pnas.0608358103

Bartoli F, Sabourin J (2017) Cardiac remodeling and disease: current understanding of STIM1/Orai1-mediated store-operated Ca2+ entry in cardiac function and pathology. Adv Exp Med Biol 993:523–534. (Springer New York LLC)

Bartoli F, Bailey MA, Rode B et al (2020) Orai1 channel inhibition preserves left ventricular systolic function and Normal Ca2+handling after pressure overload. Circulation 141:199–216

Bers D (2002) Cardiac excitation-contraction coupling. Nature 415:198–215

Bootman MD, Rietdorf K (2017) Tissue specificity: store-operated Ca2+ entry in cardiac myocytes. Adv Exp Med Biol 993:363–387. (Springer New York LLC)

Bugger H, Abel ED (2014) Molecular mechanisms of diabetic cardiomyopathy. Diabetologia 57: 660–671

Cacheux M, Strauss B, Raad N et al (2019) Cardiomyocyte-specific STIM1 (Stromal interaction molecule 1) depletion in the adult heart promotes the development of Arrhythmogenic discordant Alternans. Circ Arrhythm Electrophysiol 12(11):e007382

Calloway N, Owens T, Corwith K et al (2011) Stimulated association of STIM1 and Orai1 is regulated by the balance of PtdIns(4,5)P 2 between distinct membrane pools. J Cell Sci 124: 2602–2610

Chang CL, Chen YJ, Quintanilla CG et al (2018) EB1 binding restricts STIM1 translocation to ER-PM junctions and regulates store-operated Ca2+ entry. J Cell Biol 217:2047–2058

Chaudhari S, Ma R (2016) Store-operated calcium entry and diabetic complications. Exp Biol Med 241:343–352

Chen B, Li T, Wu Y et al (2025) Lipotoxicity: a new perspective in type 2 diabetes mellitus. Diabetes, Metabolic Syndrome and Obesity 18:1223–1237
Collins SR, Meyer T (2011) Evolutionary origins of STIM1 and STIM2 within ancient Ca2+ signaling systems. Trends Cell Biol 21:202–211
Collins HE, Zhu-Mauldin X, Marchase RB, Chatham JC (2013) STIM1/Orai1-mediated SOCE: current perspectives and potential roles in cardiac function and pathology. Am J Physiol Heart Circ Physiol 305:446–458
Collins HE, Pat BM, Zou L et al (2019) Novel role of the ER/SR Ca 2+ sensor, STIM1 in the regulation of cardiac metabolism. Am J Physiol Heart Circ Physiol 316(5):H1014–H1026
Collins HE, Zhang D, Chatham JC (2022) STIM and Orai mediated regulation of calcium signaling in age-related diseases. Front Aging 3:876785
Congur I, Mingrone G, Guan K (2025) Targeting endoplasmic reticulum stress as a potential therapeutic strategy for diabetic cardiomyopathy. Metabolism 162:156062
Coort SLM, Hasselbaink DM, Koonen DPY et al (2004) Enhanced sarcolemmal FAT/CD36 content and triacylglycerol storage in cardiac myocytes from obese zucker rats. Diabetes 53(7):1655–1663
Correll RN, Goonasekera SA, van Berlo JH et al (2015) STIM1 elevation in the heart results in aberrant Ca2+ handling and cardiomyopathy. J Mol Cell Cardiol 87:38–47
Covington ED, Wu MM, Lewis RS (2010) Essential role for the CRAC activation domain in store-dependent oligomerization of STIM1. Mol Biol Cell 21(11):1897–1907. https://doi.org/10.1091/mbc.e10-02-0145
Darenskaya MA, Kolesnikova LI, Kolesnikov SI (2021) Oxidative stress: Pathogenetic role in diabetes mellitus and its complications and therapeutic approaches to correction. Bull Exp Biol Med 171:179–189
DeHaven WI, Smyth JT, Boyles RR, Putney JW (2007) Calcium inhibition and calcium potentiation of Orai1, Orai2, and Orai3 calcium release-activated calcium channels. J Biol Chem 282: 17548–17556
Demuro A, Penna A, Safrina O et al (2011) Subunit stoichiometry of human Orai1 and Orai3 channels in closed and open states. Proc Natl Acad Sci USA 108:17832–17837
Domínguez-Rodríguez A, Mayoral-Gonzalez I, Avila-Medina J et al (2018) Urocortin-2 prevents dysregulation of Ca2+ homeostasis and improves early cardiac remodeling after ischemia and reperfusion. Front Physiol 9:813
Dong Y, Fernandes C, Liu Y et al (2017) Role of endoplasmic reticulum stress signalling in diabetic endothelial dysfunction and atherosclerosis. Diab Vasc Dis Res 14:14–23
Durak A, Olgar Y, Genc K et al (2022) STIM1-Orai1 interaction mediated calcium influx activation contributes to cardiac contractility of insulin-resistant rats. BMC Cardiovasc Disord 22(1):147
Eckstein M, Vaeth M, Aulestia FJ et al (2019) Differential regulation of Ca2+ influx by ORAI channels mediates enamel mineralization. Sci Signal 12(578):eaav4663
Eder P (2017) Cardiac remodeling and disease: SOCE and TRPC signaling in cardiac pathology. Adv Exp Med Biol 993:505–521. (Springer New York LLC)
Eder P, Molkentin JD (2011) TRPC channels as effectors of cardiac hypertrophy. Circ Res 108: 265–272
Emrich SM, Yoast RE, Trebak M (2021) Physiological functions of CRAC channels. Annu Rev Physiol 10(84):355–379
Estrada IA, Donthamsetty R, Debski P et al (2012) STIM1 restores coronary endothelial function in type 1 diabetic mice. Circ Res 111:1166–1175
Fabiato A (1985) Simulated calcium current can both cause calcium loading in and trigger calcium release from the sarcoplasmic reticulum of a skinned canine cardiac purkinje cell. J Gen Physiol 85(2):291–320
Fahrner M, Grabmayr H, Romanin C (2020) Mechanism of STIM activation. Curr Opin Physio 17: 74–79

Falcón D, Calderón-Sánchez EM, Mayoral-González I et al (2024) Inhibition of adenylyl cyclase 8 prevents the upregulation of Orai1 channel, which improves cardiac function after myocardial infarction. Mol Ther 32:646–662

Feske S, Gwack Y, Prakriya M et al (2006) A mutation in Orai1 causes immune deficiency by abrogating CRAC channel function. Nature 441:179–185

Fukushima M, Tomita T, Janoshazi A, Putney JW (2012) Alternative translation initiation gives rise to two isoforms of Orai1 with distinct plasma membrane mobilities. J Cell Sci 125:4354–4361

Gammons J, Trebak M, Mancarella S (2021) Cardiac-specific deletion of orai3 leads to severe dilated cardiomyopathy and heart failure in mice. J Am Heart Assoc 10(8):e019486

Glatz JFC, Nabben M, Young ME et al (2020) re-balancing cellular energy substrate metabolism to mend the failing heart. Biochim Biophys Acta Mol basis Dis 1866(5):165579

Gökçe Y, Erkan O, Savaş K et al (2022) Pharmacological blockade of angiotensin II receptor restores diabetes-associated reduction of store operated Ca2+ entry in adult cardiomyocytes. Biochem Biophys Res Commun 610:56–60

Grabmayr H, Romanin C, Fahrner M (2021) Stim proteins: an ever-expanding family. Int J Mol Sci 22:1–19

He Y, Yang X, He X et al (2025) Mechanisms and therapeutics of insulin signaling transduction genes in diabetic cardiomyopathy: a comprehensive updated review. Front Endocrinol (Lausanne) 16:1589695

Hou X, Pedi L, Diver MM, Long SB (2012) crystal structure of the calcium release-activated calcium channel Orai. Science (1979) 338:1308–1313

Huang GN, Zeng W, Kim JY, Yuan JP, Han L, Muallem S, Worley PF (2006) STIM1 carboxyl-terminus activates native SOC, I(crac) and TRPC1 channels. Nat Cell Biol. 8(9):1003–1010. https://doi.org/10.1038/ncb1454

Hulot J-S, Fauconnier J, Ramanujam D et al (2011) Critical role for stromal interaction molecule 1 in cardiac hypertrophy. Circulation 124(7):796–805

Jardín I, López JJ, Zbidi H et al (2011) Attenuated store-operated divalent cation entry and association between STIM1, Orai1, hTRPC1 and hTRPC6 in platelets from type 2 diabetic patients. Blood Cells Mol Dis 46:252–260

Jardin I, Berna-Erro A, Nieto-Felipe J et al (2022) Similarities and differences between the Orai1 variants: Orai1α and Orai1β. Int J Mol Sci 23(23):14568

Jia G, Hill MA, Sowers JR (2018) Diabetic cardiomyopathy: an update of mechanisms contributing to this clinical entity. Circ Res 122:624–638

Kamath ND, Matreyek KA (2025) Comprehensive mutational characterization of the calcium-sensing STIM1 EF-hand reveals residues essential for structure and function. Genetics 231(2): iyaf146

Kar P, Lin Y-P, Bhardwaj R et al (2021) The N terminus of Orai1 couples to the AKAP79 signaling complex to drive NFAT1 activation by local Ca 2+ entry. Proc Natl Acad Sci USA 118(19): e2012908118

Kawasaki T, Ueyama T, Lange I et al (2010) Protein kinase C-induced phosphorylation of Orai1 regulates the intracellular Ca2+ level via the store-operated Ca2+ channel. J Biol Chem 285: 25720–25730

Kojima A, Kitagawa H, Omatsu-Kanbe M et al (2012) Presence of store-operated Ca2 entry in C57BL/6J mouse ventricular myocytes and its suppression by sevoflurane. Br J Anaesth 109: 352–360

Liang L, Xie Y, Shen Y et al (2017) A rare de novo interstitial duplication at 4p15.2 in a boy with severe congenital heart defects, limb anomalies, hypogonadism, and global developmental delay. Cytogenet Genome Res 150:112–117

Liou J, Fivaz M, Inoue T, Meyer T (2007) Live-cell imaging reveals sequential oligomerization and local plasma membrane targeting of stromal interaction molecule 1 after Ca^{2+} store depletion. Proc Natl Acad Sci U S A 104(22):9301–9306. https://doi.org/10.1073/pnas.0702866104

Lis A, Peinelt C, Beck A et al (2007) CRACM1, CRACM2, and CRACM3 are store-operated Ca2+ channels with distinct functional properties. Curr Biol 17:794–800

Liu HZ, Wu W (2023) Effect of SKF96365 on myocardial fibrosis in type-ii diabetic rats. Front Biosci Landmark 28(9):231
Liu P, Yang Z, Wang Y, Sun A (2023) Role of STIM1 in the regulation of cardiac energy substrate preference. Int J Mol Sci 24(17):13188
Lopaschuk GD, Karwi QG, Tian R et al (2021) Cardiac energy metabolism in heart failure. Circ Res 128:1487–1513
Lopez JJ, Jardín I, Jiménez-Velarde V et al (2025) A subset of Orai1α and Orai1β subunits heteromerizes to form CRAC channels. Cell Commun Signal 23(1):260
Luo X, Hojayev B, Jiang N et al (2012) STIM1-dependent store-operated Ca 2+ entry is required for pathological cardiac hypertrophy. J Mol Cell Cardiol 52:136–147
Luo R, Le Gourriérec P, Antigny F et al (2024) STIM2 variants regulate Orai1/TRPC1/TRPC4-mediated store-operated Ca2+ entry and mitochondrial Ca2+ homeostasis in cardiomyocytes. Cell Calcium 119:102871
Luong TVT, Yang S, Kim J (2025) Lipotoxicity as a therapeutic target in the type 2 diabetic heart. J Mol Cell Cardiol 201:105–121
Maahs DM, West NA, Lawrence JM, Mayer-Davis EJ (2010) Epidemiology of type 1 diabetes. Endocrinol Metab Clin N Am 39:481–497
Maruyama Y, Ogura T, Mio K et al (2009) Tetrameric Orai1 is a teardrop-shaped molecule with a long, tapered cytoplasmic domain. J Biol Chem 284:13676–13685
Maus M, Cuk M, Patel B et al (2017) Store-operated Ca2+ entry controls induction of lipolysis and the transcriptional reprogramming to lipid metabolism. Cell Metab 25:698–712
Młynarska E, Czarnik W, Dzieża N et al (2025) Type 2 diabetes mellitus: new Pathogenetic mechanisms, treatment and the most important complications. Int J Mol Sci 26(3):1094
Nakamura M, Liu T, Husain S et al (2019) Glycogen synthase kinase-3α promotes fatty acid uptake and Lipotoxic cardiomyopathy. Cell Metab 29:1119–1134.e12
Narayanasamy S, Ong HL, Ambudkar IS (2024) A deep dive into the N-terminus of STIM proteins: structure–function analysis and evolutionary significance of the functional domains. Biomolecules 14(10):1200
Nelson HA, Roe MW (2018) Molecular physiology and pathophysiology of stromal interaction molecules. Exp Biol Med 243:451–472
Oritani K, Kincade PW (1996) Identification of stromal cell products that interact with pre-B cells. J Cell Biol 134(3):771–782. https://doi.org/10.1083/jcb.134.3.77
Pang Y, Hunton DL, Bounelis P, Marchase RB (2002) Hyperglycemia inhibits capacitative calcium entry and hypertrophy in neonatal cardiomyocytes. Diabetes 51(12):3461–3467
Penna A, Demuro A, Yeromin AV et al (2008) The CRAC channel consists of a tetramer formed by Stim-induced dimerization of Orai dimers. Nature 456:116–120
Prakriya M, Feske S, Gwack Y et al (2006) Orai1 is an essential pore subunit of the CRAC channel. Nature 443:230–233
Putney J (1986) A model for receptor-regulated calcium entry. Cell Calcium 7(1):1–12
Ren J, Gintant GA, Miller RE, Davidoff AJ (1997) High extracellular glucose impairs cardiac E-C coupling in a glycosylation-dependent manner. Am J Phys 273(6):H2876–H2883
Rivera AA, White CR, Guest LL et al (1995) Hyperglycemia alters cytoplasmic Ca2+ responses to capacitative Ca2+ influx in rat aortic smooth muscle cells. Am J Phys 269(6 Pt 1):C1482–C1488
Romero-García T, Landa-Galvan HV, Pavón N et al (2020) Autonomous activation of CaMKII exacerbates diastolic calcium leak during beta-adrenergic stimulation in cardiomyocytes of metabolic syndrome rats. Cell Calcium 91:102267
Rubler S, Dlugash J, Yuceoglij YZ et al (1972) New type of cardiomyopathy associated with diabetic glomeruloscierosis. Am J Cardiol 30(6):595–602
Sabbioni S, Veronese A, Trubia M et al (1999) Exon structure and promoter identification of STIM1 (alias GOK), a human gene causing growth arrest of the human tumor cell lines G401 and RD. Cytogenet Cell Genet 86(3–4):214–218

Sabourin J, Boet A, Rucker-Martin C et al (2018) Ca2+ handling remodeling and STIM1L/Orai1/TRPC1/TRPC4 upregulation in monocrotaline-induced right ventricular hypertrophy. J Mol Cell Cardiol 118:208–224

Sabourin J, Beauvais A, Luo R et al (2022) The SOCE machinery: an unbalanced knowledge between left and right ventricular pathophysiology. Cells 11(20):3282

Saliba Y, Keck M, Marchand A et al (2015) Emergence of Orai3 activity during cardiac hypertrophy. Cardiovasc Res 105:248–259

Stathopulos PB, Li GY, Plevin MJ, Ames JB, Ikura M (2006) Stored Ca^{2+} depletion-induced oligomerization of stromal interaction molecule 1 (STIM1) via the EF-SAM region: An initiation mechanism for capacitive Ca^{2+} entry. J Biol Chem 281(47):35855–35862. https://doi.org/10.1074/jbc.M608247200

Tarquini R, Lazzeri C, Pala L et al (2011) The diabetic cardiomyopathy. Acta Diabetol 48:173–181

Teo KK, Rafiq T (2021) Cardiovascular risk factors and prevention: a perspective from developing countries. Can J Cardiol 37:733–743

Terrell K, Choi S, Choi S (2023) Calcium's role and signaling in aging muscle, cellular senescence, and mineral interactions. Int J Mol Sci 24(23):17034

Troupes CD, Wallner M, Borghetti G et al (2017) Role of STIM1 in hypertrophy-related contractile dysfunction. Circ Res 121(2):125–136

Tsvilovskyy V, Solís-López A, Schumacher D et al (2018) Deletion of Orai2 augments endogenous CRAC currents and degranulation in mast cells leading to enhanced anaphylaxis. Cell Calcium 71:24–33

Tu C-C, Wan B-Y, Zeng Y (2020) STIM2 knockdown protects against ischemia/reperfusion injury through reducing mitochondrial calcium overload and preserving mitochondrial function. Life Sci 247:116560

Vaeth M, Yang J, Yamashita M et al (2017) ORAI2 modulates store-operated calcium entry and T cell-mediated immunity. Nat Commun 8:14714

Wang J, Fu J, Li J et al (2017) Enhanced store-operated Ca 2+ entry in high glucose-cultured neonatal and adult diabetic rat cardiomyocytes. Int J Clin Exp Pathol 10(2):877–889

Wang QC, Wang X, Tang TS (2018) EB1 traps STIM1 and regulates local store-operated Ca2+ entry. J Cell Biol 217:1895–1897

Wang S, Schianchi F, Neumann D et al (2021) Specific amino acid supplementation rescues the heart from lipid overload-induced insulin resistance and contractile dysfunction by targeting the endosomal mTOR–v-ATPase axis. Mol Metab 53:101293

Willoughby D, Everett KL, Halls ML et al (2012) Direct binding between Orai1 and AC8 mediates dynamic interplay between ca 2+ and cAMP signaling. Sci Signal 5(219):ra29

Wu QR, Zheng DL, Liu PM et al (2021) High glucose induces Drp1-mediated mitochondrial fission via the Orai1 calcium channel to participate in diabetic cardiomyocyte hypertrophy. Cell Death Dis 12(2):216

Wu J, Jia Z, Wu X et al (2025) Early cardioprotective effects of SGLT2i on hypertensive cardiac remodeling via STIM1/Orai1-dependent calcium signaling: beyond blood pressure control. J Bioenerg Biomembr. https://doi.org/10.1007/s10863-025-10067-w

Yoast RE, Emrich SM, Trebak M (2020a) The anatomy of native CRAC channel(s). Curr Opin Physio 17:89–95

Yoast RE, Emrich SM, Zhang X et al (2020b) The native ORAI channel trio underlies the diversity of Ca2+ signaling events. Nat Commun 11(1):2444

Yu F, Hubrack SZ, Chakraborty S et al (2019) Remodeling of ER-plasma membrane contact sites but not STIM1 phosphorylation inhibits Ca2+ influx in mitosis. Proc Natl Acad Sci USA 116: 10392–10401

Zhao X, Liu S, Wang X et al (2022) Diabetic cardiomyopathy: clinical phenotype and practice. Front Endocrinol (Lausanne) 13:1032268

Zheng L, Stathopulos PB, Schindl R et al (2011) Auto-inhibitory role of the EF-SAM domain of STIM proteins in store-operated calcium entry. Proc Natl Acad Sci 108(4):1337–1342

The SERCA Pump: A Key Molecular Target in Calcium Handling of Vascular Smooth Muscle Cells in Metabolic Syndrome

Cristian J. Arriero-Carrillo and Angélica Rueda

Contents

Abstract

The calcium ion (Ca^{2+}) is a fundamental intracellular messenger involved in the transduction of diverse receptor signaling pathways. Transient increases in cytoplasmic Ca^{2+} concentration ($[Ca^{2+}]_{cyt}$) regulate many cellular functions, including the contraction of vascular smooth muscle cells (VSMCs), which are active components of the blood vessels. A key protein in intracellular Ca^{2+} handling is the sarco/endoplasmic reticulum (SR/ER) Ca^{2+} ATPase, or SERCA pump. This transmembrane protein belongs to the P-type ATPase family and uses energy from ATP hydrolysis to transport Ca^{2+} from the cytoplasm into intracellular reservoirs within the SR of VSMCs. By lowering $[Ca^{2+}]_{cyt}$, SERCA activity promotes vasorelaxation. In mammals, three genes, *ATP2A1*, *ATP2A2,* and *ATP2A3,* encode at least twelve SERCA pump isoforms. Alternative mRNA

C. J. Arriero-Carrillo · A. Rueda (✉)
Department of Biochemistry, Center for Research and Advanced Studies (Cinvestav) of the National Polytechnic Institute, México City, Mexico
e-mail: arueda@cinvestav.mx

A. Rueda, M. Nieves-Cintrón (eds.), *Cardiovascular Alterations in Metabolic Diseases*, Handbook of Experimental Pharmacology 293,
https://doi.org/10.1007/164_2026_798

splicing is the primary mechanism for generating most isoforms, leading to tissue-specific expression patterns. In VSMCs from the aorta and mesenteric arteries, the expression of SERCA2a, SERCA2b, and, more recently, SERCA3 has been reported. This chapter will review the structure, mechanism of action, and physiological role of the SERCA pump in the intracellular Ca^{2+} handling of VSMCs, as well as its alterations in metabolic syndrome.

Keywords

Intracellular calcium handling · Metabolic syndrome · SERCA pump isoforms · Vascular smooth muscle cells

1 Introduction

All muscle tissue is composed of cells with the capability to contract and relax, known as myocytes, which transform chemical energy into mechanical force and produce movement. All muscles possess elastic, excitable, and contractile properties, being the major organ effectors in the human body (Shadrin et al. 2016; Sweeney and Hammers 2018; Widmaier et al. 2014). Mammalian muscles are classified into three main types based on the arrangement of contractile proteins and their location in the body: skeletal, cardiac, and smooth (Sweeney and Hammers 2018; Widmaier et al. 2014). Both skeletal and cardiac muscles are referred to as striated muscles due to their organized contractile protein ultrastructure, the sarcomere, which is the basic contractile unit. The sarcomere is organized into distinct regions: two birefringent, isotropic bands (I-bands), abundant in actin (thin filaments), flank the central anisotropic band (A-band), which is darker under polarized light, and enriched in myosin (thick filaments) (Sweeney and Hammers 2018). Unlike cardiac and skeletal muscles, smooth muscle does not exhibit the characteristic sarcomere ultrastructure. However, it contracts to pump blood through the vasculature and to move the contents of hollow organs. Additionally, smooth muscle contraction is characterized by involuntary movements that are under the control of the autonomic nervous system. The layered arrangement of smooth muscle cells (SMCs) allows relaxation and contraction with great elasticity. Smooth muscles are found in the walls of hollow organs, in the eyes, where they adjust the shape of the lens, and in the vasculature, primarily in the arteries, contracting or relaxing to manage blood circulation, participating in blood pressure regulation (Khalil 2010; Webb 2003).

The arteries can be categorized as either conducting arteries (e.g., the aorta and carotids) or resistance arteries, depending on their morphological features and physiological functions. Conducting arteries are those with a vessel diameter greater than 500 μm, and a significant content of elastic fibers, which facilitates their distensibility, presenting low resistance to blood flow (Brown et al. 2018). The resistance or myogenic arteries are blood vessels located before the capillaries (part of the microcirculation system), which control vascular resistance in resting conditions and blood flow in response to mechanical or hormonal stimuli

(Christensen and Mulvany 2001; Sharma and Mcneill 2006). Resistance arteries typically have a maximal internal diameter of 100–500 μm. Like all arteries, they show a characteristic three-layered structure: (1) from the lumen of the vessel, the inner layer, called *tunica intima,* is constituted by a selective-permeable monolayer of endothelial cells (ECs); (2) the *tunica media* is formed by one or two layers of vascular smooth muscle cells (VSMCs) surrounding the ECs, and a reduced amount of elastic fibers; and (3) the outermost layer is the *tunica adventitia*, which forms a connective tissue made of collagen and elastin (Brown et al. 2018; Christensen and Mulvany 2001; Jackson 2021; Sharma and Mcneill 2006).

The arterial myogenic tone and the myogenic response are intrinsic characteristics of resistance arteries; these two mechanisms play a key role in the autoregulation of blood flow in different organs of the body. A gradual increase in intravascular pressure induces an increase in vessel diameter, which generates a plasma membrane (PM) depolarization (VSMCs have a resting membrane potential around −60 mV), favoring a certain level of contraction, returning the vessel to its initial diameter; this mechanism is known as the myogenic response. The basal level of VSMC contraction within a blood vessel is termed myogenic tone. This tone is modulated by vasoconstrictor and vasorelaxation signals, including ions, neurotransmitters, hormones, substances derived from the endothelium, and local metabolites (D'Angelo et al. 1997; Davis 2012; Nelson et al. 1995; Tykocki et al. 2017). Contraction elicited by diverse stimuli, such as mechanical, neuro-humoral, and local factors, along with relaxation, in which the SERCA pump has a key role, relies on the free cytoplasmic Ca^{2+} concentration ($[Ca^{2+}]_{cyt}$) of VSMCs. All these mechanisms actively regulate arterial diameter, thereby affecting blood flow.

2 Role of the SERCA Pumps in the Intracellular Ca^{2+} Handling of Vascular Smooth Muscle Cells

Ca^{2+} in its free form is a crucial intracellular messenger that regulates a vast variety of cellular processes, such as those involved in the contraction and relaxation of VSMCs, among others (Carafoli and Krebs 2016). The resting $[Ca^{2+}]_{cyt}$ in VSMCs ranges 90–110 nM (Ledoux et al. 2006), while the extracellular environment contains ~2 mM. Increases in $[Ca^{2+}]_{cyt}$ within the range of 0.2 to 0.8 μM promote the contraction of VSMCs and thus arterial vasoconstriction. Conversely, relaxation relies on mechanisms that restrict extracellular Ca^{2+} entry and favors Ca^{2+} reuptake into the intracellular Ca^{2+} stores or promotes the Ca^{2+} extrusion toward the extracellular milieu, allowing $[Ca^{2+}]_{cyt}$ to go back to the resting conditions (Berridge et al. 2000; Ledoux et al. 2006; Orallo 1996).

The regulation of the $[Ca^{2+}]_{cyt}$ in VSMCs is orchestrated by a toolkit of proteins in charge of the Ca^{2+} transportation system; for instance, Ca^{2+} entry is mediated by Ca^{2+}-permeable channels at the PM, while Ca^{2+} release is mediated by ionic channels at the intracellular Ca^{2+} stores (Amberg and Navedo 2013; Fernández-Velasco et al. 2014; Orallo 1996). Ca^{2+} influx is predominantly driven by L-type voltage-gated Ca^{2+} channels (LTCCs) such as $Ca_V1.2$, but also by other channels, including T-type voltage-gated Ca^{2+} channels (TTCCs). The intracellular Ca^{2+} signals are also generated by the release of Ca^{2+} from intracellular stores, through intracellular Ca^{2+} channels such as the ryanodine receptor (RyR) and the inositol 1,4,5-trisphosphate receptor (IP_3R). In the control of resting $[Ca^{2+}]_{cyt}$ participates at least two Ca^{2+} extrusion mechanisms across the PM: the plasma membrane Ca^{2+} ATPase (PMCA) and the Na^+/Ca^{2+} exchanger (NCX) (Amberg and Navedo 2013; Chemaly et al. 2018; Fernández-Velasco et al. 2014; Orallo 1996). The sarco/endoplasmic reticulum Ca^{2+}ATPase (SERCA pump) recovers and maintains resting $[Ca^{2+}]_{cyt}$. All these proteins create an intricate system of $[Ca^{2+}]_{cyt}$ regulation. Any alteration in the expression and/or the activity of these proteins might favor abnormal vasoconstriction and can be involved in the increased incidence of cerebrovascular diseases in pathologies such as hypertension (Amberg and Navedo 2013; Fernández-Velasco et al. 2014).

The $[Ca^{2+}]_{cyt}$ plays a key role in both the contraction and the relaxation of small resistance arteries. Ca^{2+} signals favoring contraction can also come from the sarcoplasmic reticulum (SR) Ca^{2+} stores through (1) heterotrimeric G-protein coupled receptors (GPCRs), which trigger the production of the second messenger IP_3. IP_3 binds to its receptor (IP_3R), causing the release of Ca^{2+} from the SR; (2) the activation of the RyR; and (3) the Ca^{2+} entry mechanism that can be started by the depletion of the intracellular Ca^{2+} stores. This mechanism is also known as store-operated Ca^{2+} entry (SOCE), which causes the aggregation of stromal-interaction molecule 1 (STIM1) monomers at the SR membrane, recruiting the Ca^{2+} release-activated Ca^{2+} channel protein 1 (ORAI1) at the PM and allowing the Ca^{2+} influx to cytoplasm. The Ca^{2+} sources for contraction vary depending on the excitation mechanism (Amberg and Navedo 2013; Fernández-Velasco et al. 2014; Marchand et al. 2012).

An increase in $[Ca^{2+}]_{cyt}$ triggers the activation of the contractile machinery of VSMCs, which reduces the lumen of the arteries (a phenomenon known as vasoconstriction) and increases vascular resistance. The contraction of VSMCs is triggered by the binding of Ca^{2+} to calmodulin (CaM). This protein possesses 4 EF-hand domains with the ability to bind Ca^{2+}. The Ca-CaM complex activates the catalytic subunit of myosin light chain kinase (MLCK), which phosphorylates 20 kDa myosin (MLC) at serine 19 (Ser19). This phosphorylation induces a conformational change in the globular domain of MLC, increasing its ATPase activity. Consequently, MLC can interact with actin and function as a molecular motor (Amberg and Navedo 2013; Fernández-Velasco et al. 2014; Ogut and Brozovich 2003).

For relaxation to occur, $[Ca^{2+}]_{cyt}$ must decrease. The removal of Ca^{2+} from the cytoplasm is primarily mediated by the PMCA and the SERCA pump, with the NCX playing a minor role. This reduction in $[Ca^{2+}]_{cyt}$ allows the myosin light chain phosphatase (MLCP) to dephosphorylate the MLC, leading to actin-myosin uncoupling and promoting relaxation (Somlyo 1985). In smooth muscle, relaxation is strongly influenced by the negative feedback generated by the SERCA pump, which recaptures Ca^{2+} from the cytoplasm into the SR. The transient rise in SR Ca^{2+} levels briefly activates clusters of RyRs, producing highly localized and short-lived Ca^{2+} release events, known as Ca^{2+} sparks. These Ca^{2+} sparks activate

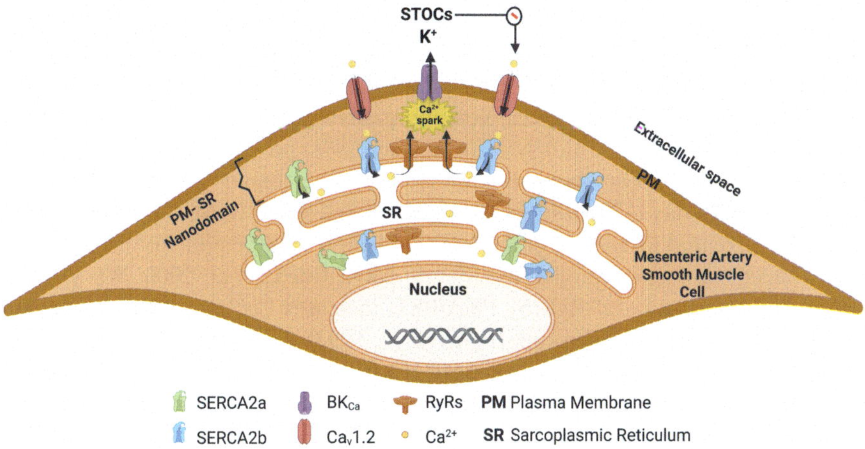

Fig. 1 Intracellular Ca^{2+} handling in vascular smooth muscle cells. Schematic representation of a single VSMC highlighting the main proteins involved in intracellular Ca^{2+} dynamics. The SERCA pump is essential for maintaining resting $[Ca^{2+}]_{cyt}$ and the SR Ca^{2+} load, regulating both relaxation and contraction. PM depolarization increases the *Po* of LTCCs, leading to Ca^{2+} influx. The resulting rise in $[Ca^{2+}]_{cyt}$ activates the contractile machinery and triggers contraction. Elevated $[Ca^{2+}]_{cyt}$ also stimulates SERCA2a and SERCA2b, augmenting SR Ca^{2+} levels. This activates clusters of RyRs, producing Ca^{2+} sparks. These Ca^{2+} events occur at the subplasmalemmal nanodomain between the PM and SR, where they activate BK_{Ca} channels, generating transient and spontaneous K^+ currents (STOCs), causing PM hyperpolarization, which reduces the *Po* of LTCCs and promotes vasorelaxation. (Figure created in BioRender.com)

large-conductance Ca^{2+}-activated K^+ channels (BK_{Ca} channels), generating spontaneous and transient outward K^+ currents (STOCs) that hyperpolarize the PM. As a result, the open probability (*Po*) of LTCCs decreases, further lowering $[Ca^{2+}]_{cyt}$ and ultimately leading to vasorelaxation (Fig. 1) (Essin and Gollasch 2009; Fernández-Velasco et al. 2014; Jaggar et al. 2000; Rueda et al. 2013).

VSMCs express the three known RyR isoforms: RyR1, RyR2, and RyR3, each with distinct subcellular distributions (Clark et al. 2010; Essin and Gollasch 2009; Kaßmann et al. 2019; Vaithianathan et al. 2010). This differential distribution has been observed in VSMCs from both cerebral and pulmonary arteries (Clark et al. 2010; Vaithianathan et al. 2010). In cerebral arteries, RyR1 is mainly located in the cytoplasm (or extra-perinuclear region) and, to a lesser extent, between the subplasmalemmal (or PM-SR nanodomain) and perinuclear regions. RyR2 is the most abundant isoform, primarily localized in the PM-SR nanodomain. It is also found in the extra-perinuclear region and, in smaller amounts, in the perinuclear region. Finally, RyR3 is present in the cytoplasm and perinuclear regions, but is almost absent from the subplasmalemmal region (Vaithianathan et al. 2010). The precise functional significance of these distributions in VSMCs is not fully understood. What we do know is that RyR1 and RyR2 mediate the generation of Ca^{2+} sparks, whereas RyR3 contributes minimally (Essin and Gollasch 2009). Ca^{2+} sparks are characterized by their spatiotemporal properties: frequency (events/s), duration (ms), size (μm), and amplitude (F/F_0). These properties depend on the number of RyRs within clusters, their *Po*, and the SR Ca^{2+} load (Cheng and Lederer 2008; Jaggar et al. 2000; Liu et al. 2009). RyR activity is regulated by Ca^{2+} on both the cytoplasmic and luminal sides; post-translational modifications such as phosphorylation, oxidation, and nitrosylation; and accessory proteins in both cytoplasmic and luminal sides. On the cytoplasmic side, we found proteins from the immunophilin family (12 and 12.6 kDa; FKBP12 and FKBP12.6), CaM, and sorcin, which stabilize the closed state of RyRs. Dissociation of these proteins increases the *Po* and alters Ca^{2+} spark properties (Ji et al. 2004; Rueda et al. 2006; Wang et al. 2004). Phosphorylation of RyR by PKA/PKG increases Ca^{2+} spark frequency and STOCs, promoting vasorelaxation (Porter et al. 1998). In contrast, PKC activation reduces both Ca^{2+} spark frequency and STOCs, thereby diminishing vasorelaxation (Bonev et al. 1997). Pharmacological inhibition of RyRs further demonstrates their role in vasorelaxation (Jaggar et al. 1998b, 2000; Knot et al. 1998). Importantly, Ca^{2+} spark frequency and amplitude are directly correlated with the SR Ca^{2+} content and the SERCA pump activity (Jaggar et al. 1998a; Wellman et al. 2001; Zhuge et al. 1999). This highlights the need to better understand how SERCA pump expression and activity are regulated in VSMCs.

3 General Characteristics of the SERCA Pump

The SERCA pump is a key protein for maintaining Ca^{2+} homeostasis in VSMCs. Its functions include (1) promoting relaxation by regulating resting $[Ca^{2+}]_{cyt}$ and (2) restoring SR Ca^{2+} load required for G-protein-coupled receptor-induced vasoconstriction (Salazar-Enciso et al. 2022; Wright et al. 2013). The SERCA pump actively transports Ca^{2+} from the cytoplasm into the SR against its electrochemical gradient, a process that requires energy from ATP hydrolysis (approximately 39–42 kJ/mol). For each molecule of ATP hydrolyzed, the SERCA pump moves two Ca^{2+} ions, thereby maintaining a 10,000-fold difference between $[Ca^{2+}]_{cyt}$ (in the nM range) and the SR luminal Ca^{2+} (in the μM range) under resting conditions. This enzyme is highly efficient, with optimal coupling between chemical energy and ion transport, making it a pump of remarkable thermodynamic effectiveness (Kabashima et al. 2020; Møller et al. 2005; Toyoshima 2009).

The SERCA pump belongs to the P-type ATPase family because of its ability to undergo auto-phosphorylation at Aspartic Acid 351 (Asp351). This property enables the pump to transport Ca^{2+} by alternating the affinity and accessibility of Ca^{2+} binding sites through conformational changes (Kabashima et al. 2020; Kühlbrandt 2004; Møller et al. 2005; Toyoshima et al. 2000). The catalytic cycle of the SERCA pump involves several conformational states, which are not precisely defined because they may vary across isoforms. The SERCA cycle is based on the transition between two main conformational states, known as E1 and E2. In the E1 conformation, the two Ca^{2+}-binding sites have high affinity and face the cytoplasm. In the E2 conformation, the Ca^{2+}-binding sites have low affinity and are oriented toward the SR lumen. In the E1 state, cytosolic Ca^{2+} and ATP bind to the pump, forming the

$2Ca^{2+}$-E1-ATP complex. Auto-phosphorylation then converts this complex into the $2Ca^{2+}$-E1-P form, a high-energy state in which the cations are trapped. A subsequent conformational change produces the $2Ca^{2+}$-E2-P state, a low-energy state where the Ca^{2+} binding sites shift to a low-affinity orientation toward the SR lumen. The cycle concludes with the release of Ca^{2+} into the lumen, which is exchanged for 2–3 protons. Following dephosphorylation, these protons are translocated back to the cytosolic side, driving the conformational change from E2 to E1state (Kabashima et al. 2020; Møller et al. 2005; Olesen et al. 2007; Toyoshima 2008; Tsunekawa et al. 2018; Wuytack et al. 2002).

The SERCA pump consists of a single polypeptide chain of ~1,000 amino acid residues (aa's) with a *M*r ~ 110 kDa (Toyoshima 2008, 2009). The first 3D structure was determined for SERCA1a, purified from rabbit skeletal muscle (Toyoshima et al. 2000). This isoform has been extremely helpful for characterizing the 3D structure and mechanism of action of SERCA, as it shares a high identity with the other isoforms. Structurally, the SERCA pump is organized into four domains. Three are cytoplasmic domains, corresponding to the upper part of the enzyme: the nucleotide-binding domain (N), the site of ATP binding; the actuator domain (A), involved in occlusion and dephosphorylation; and the phosphorylation domain (P), which contains the critical Asp351 residue (auto-phosphorylation site) and the Mg^{2+} coordination site. The fourth domain is the transmembrane domain, typically composed of ten α-transmembrane helices (M1-M10); the exception is SERCA2b, which has eleven α-transmembrane helices (M1-M11) and an additional luminal loop, which increases Ca^{2+} affinity but reduces the maximum turnover rate (Olesen et al. 2004; Toyoshima 2008, 2009; Toyoshima et al. 2000; Vandecaetsbeek et al. 2011; Wuytack et al. 2002).

The SERCA pump has two Ca^{2+} binding sites (sites I and II) positioned side by side and separated by approximately 5.7 Å. Site I lies between α-transmembrane helices M5 and M6, with additional contributions from helix M8 in a distal position. Site II is formed by helix M4, which is partially uncoiled, allowing the oxygen atoms of its side chains to align within the same plane. The binding and release of Ca^{2+} at its binding sites depend on the phosphorylation and dephosphorylation of SERCA, which drive conformational changes that shift the protein between high- and low-affinity states. This regulation is mediated through structural communication between the Ca^{2+} binding sites and the phosphorylation site. Specifically, the cytoplasmic regions of helices M5 and M4 are attached to the P domain near the Asp351 residue. As a result, conformational changes in the P domain induced by phosphorylation are mechanically transmitted to the transmembrane sites, modulating Ca^{2+} binding and release (Møller et al. 2005; Toyoshima 2008, 2009; Toyoshima et al. 2000).

3.1 SERCA Pump Isoforms

In mammals, three genes (*ATP2A1*, *ATP2A2*, and *ATP2A3*) have been identified, which encode up to twelve isoforms of the SERCA pump through alternative mRNA splicing (Gélébart et al. 2003; Lipskaia et al. 2013b; Xu and Van Remmen 2021).

The *ATP2A1* gene is located on chromosome 16p11.2, spans 26 kb, and includes 24 exons. This gene produces two isoforms: SERCA1a and SERCA1b. The splicing of this gene is developmentally regulated. SERCA1b is expressed during early fetal development, later replaced by SERCA1a as fetal growth progresses. SERCA1a is expressed in fast-twitch skeletal muscle and has been detected in the heart, though not predominantly (Gélébart et al. 2003; Lipskaia et al. 2013b; Periasamy and Kalyanasundaram 2007).

The *ATP2A2* gene is located on chromosome 12, locus q24.11, spans 70 kb, and contains 21 exons. This gene generates four isoforms: SERCA2a, SERCA2b, SERCA2c, and SERCA2d. SERCA2a is highly expressed in cardiac muscle, with lower levels in skeletal and smooth muscle. SERCA2b is encoded by three mRNA subclasses that differ only in the 3′ untranslated region. It is expressed ubiquitously with tissue-dependent variation. SERCA2c has been detected at the mRNA level in epithelial, mesenchymal, and hematopoietic cell lines. The SERCA2c protein has been confirmed in primary human mast cells and cardiomyocytes. Finally, SERCA2d is the least studied isoform and is identified only at the mRNA level (including intron 19) as a novel splicing variant in human skeletal muscle. Its existence as an endogenous protein has not been described. Interestingly, its expression is reduced in type 1 diabetes (DM1) muscles (Dally et al. 2006; Gélébart et al. 2003; Kimura et al. 2005; Lipskaia et al. 2013b).

Finally, the *ATP2A3* gene is located on chromosome 17p13.2, spans 41 kb, and contains 25 exons. This gene produces six isoforms by alternative splicing, giving rise to the largest SERCA family: SERCA3a, SERCA3b, SERCA3c, SERCA3d, SERCA3e, and SERCA3f. SERCA3a, SERCA3d, and SERCA3f are ubiquitously expressed and often co-expressed with SERCA2b in specific tissues, including colon, gastric epithelium, vascular endothelium, β-pancreatic cells, and Purkinje cells. Although the mRNA of these isoforms is detectable, protein levels are low or undetectable (Chemaly et al. 2013).

3.2 Isoforms of the SERCA Pump in Vascular Smooth Muscle Cells

The predominant SERCA pump isoforms in VSMCs are SERCA2a and SERCA2b (Table 1). These two SERCA isoforms differ from each other in the number of aa's encoding them: SERCA2a comprises 997 aa's, while SERCA2b contains 1,042 aa's. The first 993 aa's are identical in both isoforms. In SERCA2b, the last four aa's of SERCA2a are replaced by an additional 49 aa's (Fransen et al. 2020; Verboomen et al. 1992). These extra residues generate unique structural features: an additional cytosolic loop (L10/11, aa's 994–1012) between transmembrane helices 10 and 11; an additional transmembrane α-helix (M11, aa's 1013–1030), and a luminal

Table 1 SERCA isoforms in arteries

Vascular smooth muscle tissue	SERCA isoforms expressed	Detection method	References
Aorta	SERCA2a SERCA2b SERCA3	IH, qPCR, WB	Fransen et al. (2020), Levitsky et al. (1993), Searls et al. (2010), Wu et al. (2001)
Pulmonary artery	SERCA2a SERCA2b	IH, qPCR, WB	Clark et al. (2010)
Mesenteric artery	SERCA2a SERCA2b	IC	Lagaud et al. (1999)
Carotid artery	SERCA2a SERCA2b	IC, WB	Jang et al. (2016)
Mammary artery	SERCA2a SERCA2b	IC, WB	Lipskaia et al. (2013a)
Femoral artery	SERCA2 SERCA3	WB	Searls et al. (2010)
Cerebral artery	SERCA2	WB, qPCR	Miranda-Saturnino et al. (2014)

IH immunohistochemistry, *qPCR* quantitative polymerase chain reaction, *WB* Western blot, *IC* immunocytochemistry

extension tail (LE, aa's 1031–1042). These elements confer distinct functional properties through interactions with other regions of the pump (Zhang et al. 2020) (Fig. 2).

For example, Phe1018 (M11) interacts with Trp927 (cytosolic loop 8/9) via van der Waals forces. Val1029 (M11) interacts with Leu967, Leu970, and Lys971 (M10) (Inoue et al. 2019). Cryo-EM studies revealed the LE approaches M7, promoting interactions with the luminal loop between M7 and M8 (L7/8). Together, M11 and LE stabilize conformational states of SERCA2b, modifying its kinetic properties compared to isoforms lacking these extensions (Inoue et al. 2019). In functional analyses, SERCA2b shows a 2.3-fold lower Vmax than SERCA2a (SERCA2b = 1.8×10^2 min^{-1} vs. SERCA2a = 4.2×10^2 min^{-1}). SERCA2b has a lower Kd for Ca^{2+} binding (0.21 μM) compared to SERCA2a (0.35 μM). Likely, the Ca^{2+} uptake activity ($K_{0.5}$) of SERCA2b was lower (0.17 μM) than that of SERCA2a (0.31 μM) (Verboomen et al. 1992). Overall, SERCA2b exhibits lower ATPase activity but higher Ca^{2+} affinity, despite near-identical sequence similarity with SERCA2a (Inoue et al. 2019). Interestingly, when a synthetic peptide emulating the LE fragment of SERCA2b was exogenously added to SERCA2a, it inhibited the ATPase activity of SERCA2a and increased its affinity for Ca^{2+}. This suggests the LE fragment directly interacts with SERCA2a and modulates its Ca^{2+} affinity (Vandecaetsbeek et al. 2009; Zhang et al. 2020). On the other hand, SERCA3 isoforms have much lower Ca^{2+} affinity than SERCA2b, and up to tenfold lower than SERCA1a (Lipskaia et al. 2013b), suggesting that they are active only at very

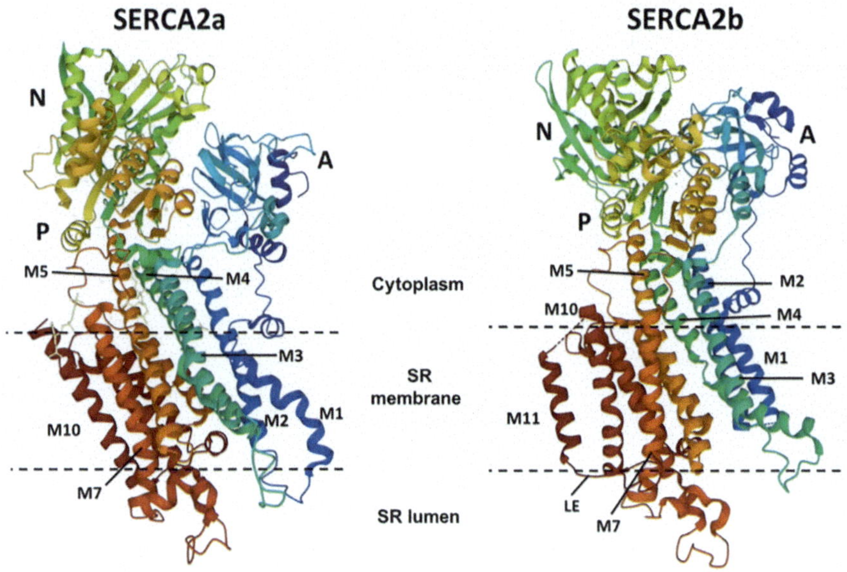

Fig. 2 3D structure of SERCA2a and SERCA2b. SERCA2a and SERCA2b are the predominant SERCA pump isoforms in VSMCs. Structurally, the SERCA pump consists of four domains. Three cytoplasmic domains: nucleotide binding domain (N), phosphorylation domain (P), and actuator domain (A). The fourth domain is embedded in the SR membrane and consists of 10 transmembrane α-helices (M1-M10) for SERCA2a (*left*) and 11 (M1-M11) in the SERCA2b (*right*). SERCA2a is composed of 997 amino acid residues (Uniprot ID: P16615-2) while SERCA2b has 1,042 residues (canonical isoform P16615-1). Both isoforms share high sequence identity, with the first 993 residues identical. The additional 49 amino acids in SERCA2b at the C-terminal region form an extra cytosolic loop between M10 and M11. This structural extension distinguishes SERCA2b from SERCA2a and contributes to its functional differences

high $[Ca^{2+}]_{cyt}$. Nevertheless, SERCA3 isoforms display a markedly faster turnover rate (~100 s^{-1}) (Lipskaia et al. 2013b).

The subcellular distribution of SERCA isoforms in VSMCs remains poorly understood. Evidence from pulmonary artery VSMCs has shown that SERCA2a and SERCA2b are found at distinct intracellular localizations, resulting in functional segregation of SR Ca^{2+} stores (Clark et al. 2010). SERCA2b is predominantly localized in the subplasmalemmal region within the PM-SR nanodomain (~72%), whereas SERCA2a was restricted to the perinuclear region (~90%). This spatial segregation suggests heterogeneity in intracellular Ca^{2+} mobilization in a stimulus-specific manner (Clark et al. 2010). In the aorta from the transgenic mouse lacking SERCA2a and expressing only SERCA2b (SERCA2b/b), phenylephrine-induced contraction was greater than in control aortas (SERCA2a/b). Notably, this effect persisted even when Ca^{2+} influx was blocked with diltiazem, an LTCC antagonist of the benzodiazepine subclass that inhibits LTCC in the resting state. These findings support the hypothesis that SERCA2b plays a critical role in coupling intracellular

Ca^{2+} release to contraction, consistent with its differential subcellular localization compared to SERCA2a (Fransen et al. 2020).

3.3 Functional Role of the SERCA Pump in the Subplasmalemmal Ca^{2+} Buffering System in Vascular Smooth Muscle Cells

Intracellular Ca^{2+} is not uniformly distributed in VSMCs. The idea of a subplasmalemmal Ca^{2+} buffering system, in which the SERCA pump plays a key role, originates from the seminal observations of Devine et al. (1972). They showed the presence of a superficial SR closely apposed to the PM, particularly caveolae (Devine et al. 1972). In these specialized regions – now referred to as PM-SR nanodomains – the superficial SR is found within 10–100 nm of the PM. This proximity enables tight regulation of $[Ca^{2+}]_{cyt}$ through the preferential localization of Ca^{2+} transport proteins, including the SERCA pump (Devine et al. 1972; Essin and Gollasch 2009; Rembold and Chen 1998; van Breemen et al. 1995). The functional importance of the PM-SR nanodomain was unveiled by Van Breemen's experiments using rabbit aortic rings. He showed that norepinephrine- or high K^+-induced contraction could be modulated by lanthanum chloride, which blocks Ca^{2+} channels, thereby regulating Ca^{2+} influx and contraction (Rembold and Chen 1998; Van Breemen 1977). Importantly, Van Breemen observed a dissociation between the rate of $^{45}Ca^{2+}$ influx and smooth muscle contraction, proposing that extracellular Ca^{2+} first accumulates in the subplasmalemmal region before diffusing into the deeper cytoplasm (Van Breemen 1977). According to this hypothesis, VSMCs contain at least two functional Ca^{2+} domains: (1) a contractile domain, covering most of the cytoplasm, where Ca^{2+} activates the contractile filaments via the Ca^{2+}/CaM complex and (2) a subplasmalemmal nanodomain formed by the cytoplasm space between the SR and the PM, which can manage $[Ca^{2+}]_{cyt}$ equal to or greater than the contractile domain but does not directly trigger contraction. The Ca^{2+} barrier between these domains facilitates Ca^{2+} uptake into the SR while reduces $[Ca^{2+}]_{cyt}$ in the deep regions due to restricted Ca^{2+} diffusion (Evans et al. 2016; Rembold and Chen 1998). This hypothesis proposes the existence of a fenestrated superficial SR, where incoming Ca^{2+} is partly extruded by PMCA and NCX before reaching the deeper cytoplasm. Crucially, in this PM-SR nanodomain, the SERCA pump recaptures Ca^{2+} directly into the superficial SR, forming a barrier that limits Ca^{2+} influx. Contraction occurs only when Ca^{2+} reaches the deeper cytoplasm, where contractile myofilaments reside (Chen and van Breemen 1993; Van Breemen et al. 2013). This subplasmalemmal Ca^{2+} buffering system allows temporally uncoupling of Ca^{2+} influx from force development, supported by the observation that SR Ca^{2+} release stimulates contraction more effectively than Ca^{2+} influx (Casteels and Droogmans 1981). Overall, this theory underscores the critical role of the SERCA pump and superficial SR in controlling $[Ca^{2+}]_{cyt}$ and contractile activity (Evans 2017).

The contribution of the SERCA pump to SR Ca^{2+} loading, Ca^{2+} spark generation, and vasorelaxation is supported by further evidence from the phospholamban

(PLN)-deficient transgenic mouse, where loss of PLN regulation enhanced SR Ca^{2+} loading, increased Ca^{2+} spark frequency, and STOCs in VSMCs from middle cerebral arteries (Wellman et al. 2001).

In carotid and mesenteric arteries from spontaneously hypertensive rats (SHR), SERCA inhibition with thapsigargin (TGN) and cyclopiazonic acid (CPA) reduces SR Ca^{2+} buffering capacity. These studies showed that Ca^{2+} influx during rest or norepinephrine stimulation is strongly buffered by the superficial SR, likely linked to the increased SERCA2 expression of SERCA2 in SHR mesenteric arteries (Nomura and Asano 2002). Using SERCA pump inhibitors in smooth muscle cells has revealed the necessity of the SERCA pump as a participant in this Ca^{2+} buffering mechanism triggered by Ca^{2+} influx via LTTCs (Janssen et al. 1999; Kim et al. 1997). A study performed in our laboratory allowed us to obtain data reflecting the involvement of the SERCA pump in the Ca^{2+} buffering barrier in VSMs of mesenteric arteries. We demonstrated that the SERCA pump limits the Ca^{2+} entry in VSMCs of mesenteric arteries, even under conditions in which Ca^{2+} influx could be exacerbated by aldosterone-induced LTCC increased expression (Salazar-Enciso et al. 2022).

All these data support the theory of the subplasmalemmal Ca^{2+} buffering system in VSMCs and strongly suggest that the SERCA pump is an essential component of a functional unit that regulates $[Ca^{2+}]$ through its key participation in Ca^{2+} reuptake in SR surface-localized reservoirs (Jones et al. 2005).

4 SERCA Pump Dysfunction in Experimental Models of Metabolic Syndrome

Metabolic syndrome (MetS) is a cluster of interrelated physiological and biochemical alterations that increase the risk of cardiovascular disease and metabolic disorders such as type 2 diabetes (DM2) (Romero-García et al. 2025). MetS is diagnosed when at least three of the following criteria occur simultaneously: central obesity, hypertriglyceridemia, arterial hypertension, impaired fasting glucose, insulin resistance, and decreased high-density lipoprotein (HDL) (Alberti et al. 2009; Romero-García et al. 2025). MetS is now considered a major public health problem worldwide (Bartkowiak et al. 2024; Jamali et al. 2024). Approximately 20–30% of adults globally are affected (Jamali et al. 2024; Li et al. 2023; Noubiap et al. 2022).

In Mexico, MetS prevalence reaches 45.3% (43.7% in men and 46.8% in women) (Campos-Nonato et al. 2025). In the United States, the prevalence is 34.7% (35.1% in men and 34.3% in women) (Hirode and Wong 2020). Individuals with MetS are predisposed to vascular diseases, which may be related to disruptions in Ca^{2+} handling. Altered Ca^{2+} handling protein expression or activity may lead to impaired myogenic tone and vascular reactivity (Romero-García et al. 2025).

The SERCA pump has become a target in prediabetic conditions because its dysfunction has been reported in several experimental models of MetS (Davies 2015; Romero-García et al. 2025). To study MetS, researchers often use hypercaloric diets (high in fat or sugar, e.g., sucrose or fructose) in animal models

(Wong et al. 2016; Romero-García et al. 2025). Neeb et al. reported that a high-fat diet induced MetS features in Ossabaw pigs, which was a better MetS model than the one developed in Yucatan pigs with the same diet. The Ossabaw pig model of MetS showed impaired coronary blood flow. The coronary artery smooth muscle cells of Ossabaw pigs with MetS showed reduced SR Ca^{2+} release due to decreased SERCA pump activity (Neeb et al. 2010).

An experimental MetS model using male C57BL/6 J mice (characterized by increased fat mass, glucose intolerance, hypertension, and hyperinsulinemia) showed impaired endothelium-dependent aortic relaxation (Weisbrod et al. 2013). This vascular dysfunction was linked to reduced SERCA pump activity caused by oxidation of the cysteine-674 residue (C674-SO_3H) and suppression of SERCA responsiveness to nitric oxide (NO). In subsequent cultures of VSMC from MetS and control mice, MetS myocytes showed elevated production of ROS, leading to irreversible SERCA oxidation and diminished capacity of NO to inhibit cell migration. Notably, overexpression of the SERCA2b isoform restored NO-dependent inhibition of VSMC migration (Qin et al. 2014).

McKenney et al. developed a MetS model in Ossabaw pigs fed a high fat, atherogenic diet. MetS pigs exhibited coronary artery disease (CAD), classified as either "mild" or "severe." Mild CAD was associated with an increase in SR Ca^{2+} load, whereas severe CAD showed reduced steady-state SR Ca^{2+} levels. These changes correlated with changes in SERCA pump activity: increased in mild disease but dramatically decreased in severe disease (McKenney-Drake et al. 2016). Similarly, Badin et al. induced MetS in young Ossabaw pigs by feeding them an atherogenic diet for 11 months. These animals exhibited increased body weight, hypercholesterolemia, and glucose intolerance. MetS pigs developed CAD associated with dysregulated intracellular Ca^{2+} handling in VSMCs, driven by reduced SERCA pump activity (Badin et al. 2018).

Climent et al. studied obese Zucker rats (OZR), which carry an autosomal recessive mutation in the leptin receptor gene. These rats displayed increased body weight, hyperglycemia, mild hyperinsulinemia, and elevated cholesterol and triglyceride levels. Their coronary arteries showed altered intracellular Ca^{2+} dynamics. Although SERCA expression was unchanged, prior work had demonstrated SERCA oxidation in VSMCs from the coronary arteries of MetS rats. These oxidation events were phenotypically linked to impaired Ca^{2+} handling in OZR coronary arteries (Climent et al. 2020).

Finally, Lee et al. generated a MetS model in male Sprague-Dawley rats fed a high-fructose diet (60%). Despite no increase in body weight, these rats developed hyperinsulinemia, hyperlipidemia and increased glycemia. MetS rats exhibited contractile dysfunction in mesenteric lymphatic vessels, driven by dysregulated intracellular Ca^{2+} handling. This dysfunction was associated with altered SERCA pump expression, specifically reduced SERCA2a isoform levels, which impaired Ca^{2+} buffering capacity in VSMCs (Lee et al. 2020).

Collectively, these findings highlight the importance of the SERCA pump as a critical molecular target in MetS-induced vascular dysfunction. However, further investigation is needed to clarify whether MetS exerts transcriptional effects on

SERCA and whether these effects are isoform-specific. SERCA2a and SERCA2b are the most abundant isoforms in VSMCs, each with distinct roles in intracellular Ca^{2+} handling due to their different subcellular distribution (Clark et al. 2010). Thus, elucidating the precise impact of MetS on SERCA expression and activity remains an important research priority.

The SERCA pump is finely modulated by a family of transmembrane micropeptides called regulins, which include phospholamban (PLN), sarcolipin (SLN), myoregulin (MLN), endoregulin (ELN), other regulin (ALN), and the micropeptide encoded by a dwarf open reading frame (DWORF). All these peptides, except for DWORF, exert an inhibitory effect on SERCA activity through direct interaction; DWORF, in contrast, promotes its activation by displacing inhibitory peptides (Anderson et al. 2016; Rathod et al. 2021). In VSMCs, PLN is the only member of this family whose expression has been clearly confirmed (Wellman et al. 2001). Although ALN has been described as a ubiquitously expressed peptide, its specific presence in VSMCs has not been validated (Anderson et al. 2016). PLN phosphorylation constitutes a key regulatory mechanism, as it reduces its affinity for SERCA, thus allowing an increase in pump activity (Rathod et al. 2021).

The impact of MetS on the expression or activity of these regulins has been poorly explored. The literature is mostly limited to cardiomyocytes in MetS rats, in which no significant changes in PLN expression have been reported, but alterations in its phosphorylation status have been reported. These modifications may have relevant functional consequences by indirectly modulating SERCA activity and intracellular Ca^{2+} signaling. No studies have been conducted to evaluate the role of these regulins as functional or adaptive targets in response to systemic metabolic alterations, such as MetS (Okatan et al. 2016; Romero-García et al. 2020). However, changes in SERCA activity have been documented under MetS conditions, suggesting the possibility of regulation mediated by these peptides. Therefore, there is an urgent need to investigate whether changes in the expression, function, or regulation of these peptides occur in VSMCs in the context of MetS, to elucidate their contribution in the Ca^{2+} handling dysfunction observed in MetS.

5 SERCA Pump as a Therapeutic Target

The SERCA pump plays a fundamental role in regulating intracellular Ca^{2+} homeostasis. Dysfunction of SERCA has been linked to a wide range of pathologies, including metabolic disorders, cardiovascular diseases, and cancer. In VSMCs, SERCA dysfunction contributes to the development of vascular diseases, making the SERCA pump a promising therapeutic target. However, no studies to date provide direct evidence for pharmacological modulators of this pump in VSMCs (Yu and Tian 2025). In oncology, SERCA modulation has been extensively studied, as its activation or inhibition influences cell proliferation and apoptosis. This evidence has led to the development of SERCA pump modulators as potential anticancer drugs (Casemore and Xing 2015).

Recently, a machine learning-based study screened a large database of natural products, identifying activators of the SERCA2a pump isoform. The study highlighted ten structurally related compounds derived from *Zingiber officinale*, *Aframomum melegueta*, *Alpinia officinarum*, *Alpinia oxyphylla*, and *Capsicum* as activators of SERCA2a. ATPase assays confirmed that seven of these compounds activate SERCA at low concentrations. Among them, yakuchinone A and alpinoid D, showed compelling concentration-dependent ATPase activity, efficient lipid bilayer binding, and favorable permeation in molecular dynamics simulations (Cruz-Cortés et al. 2025). In addition, structure-activity relationship (SAR) studies identified small molecules analogous to indoline, benzofuran, and benzodioxole as potent SERCA2a activators, increasing pump activity by ~57% (Ard et al. 2025).

Regarding metabolic diseases, pharmacological activation of SERCA2b by the allosteric compound CDN1163 has shown beneficial effects in animal models of DM2. This activator improves glucose tolerance, lowers fasting glucose, and reduces hepatic steatosis. These effects are attributed to the restoration of Ca^{2+} homeostasis in the ER/SR, activation of the AMPK pathway, and improved mitochondrial biogenesis (Kang et al. 2016). Furthermore, natural polyphenols such as resveratrol, gingerol, green tea polyphenols, and luteolin have been identified as SERCA activators with therapeutic potential in conditions associated with ER stress. These compounds modulate Ca^{2+} signaling and protect cells from metabolic damage (Viskupicova and Rezbarikova 2022). Overall, these studies highlight structural features that govern SERCA modulation and provide a strong conceptual framework for designing next-generation therapeutic strategies targeting specific SERCA isoforms.

Disclosure All scientific content, interpretations, and conclusions are the responsibility of the authors.

References

Alberti KGMM, Eckel RH, Grundy SM, Zimmet PZ, Cleeman JI, Donato KA, Fruchart JC, James WPT, Loria CM, Smith SC (2009) Harmonizing the metabolic syndrome: a joint interim statement of the international diabetes federation task force on epidemiology and prevention; National heart, lung, and blood institute; American heart association; World heart federation; International atherosclerosis society; And international association for the study of obesity. Circulation 120(16):1640–1645. https://doi.org/10.1161/CIRCULATIONAHA.109.192644

Amberg GC, Navedo MF (2013) Calcium dynamics in vascular smooth muscle. Microcirculation (New York, N.Y.: 1994) 20(4):281–289. https://doi.org/10.1111/micc.12046

Anderson DM, Makarewich CA, Anderson KM, Shelton JM, Bezprozvannaya S, Bassel-Duby R, Olson EN (2016) Widespread control of calcium signaling by a family of SERCA-inhibiting micropeptides. Sci Signal 9(457). https://doi.org/10.1126/SCISIGNAL.AAJ1460/SUPPL_FILE/9_RA119_SM.PDF

Ard A, Cruz-Cortés C, Gan X, Guerrero-Serna G, White AD, Clasby MC, Espinoza-Fonseca LM (2025) SAR-guided development of small-molecule SERCA2a activators: discovery of potent indoline, benzofuran, and benzodioxole analogs for cardiovascular applications. J Med Chem. https://doi.org/10.1021/ACS.JMEDCHEM.5C01192

Badin JK, Bruning RS, Sturek M (2018) Effect of metabolic syndrome and aging on Ca 2+ dysfunction in coronary smooth muscle and coronary artery disease severity in Ossabaw miniature swine. Exp Gerontol 108:247–255. https://doi.org/10.1016/j.exger.2018.04.024

Bartkowiak K, Bartkowiak M, Jankowska-Steifer E, Ratajska A, Kujawa M, Aniołek O, Niderla-Bielińska J (2024) Metabolic syndrome and cardiac vessel remodeling associated with vessel rarefaction: a possible underlying mechanism may result from a poor Angiogenic response to altered VEGF signaling pathways. In J Vasc Res 61(4):151–159. S. Karger AG. https://doi.org/10.1159/000538361

Berridge MJ, Lipp P, Bootman MD (2000) The versatility and universality of calcium signalling. Nat Rev 1(October):11–21. https://doi.org/10.1038/35036035

Bonev AD, Jaggar JH, Rubart M, Nelson MT (1997) Activators of protein kinase C decrease Ca2+ spark frequency in smooth muscle cells from cerebral arteries. Am J Phys 273(6 Pt 1):C2090–C2095

Brown IAM, Diederich L, Good ME, Leon J, Murphy SA, Cortese-krott MM, Hall JL, Le H, Isakson BE (2018) Vascular smooth muscle remodeling in conductive and resistance arteries in hypertension: VSMC in hypertension. Arterioscler Thromb Vasc Biol 38(9):1969–1985. https://doi.org/10.1161/ATVBAHA.118.311229.Vascular

Campos-Nonato I, Ramírez-Villalobos M, Monterrubio-Flores E, Mendoza-Herrera K, Aguilar-Salinas C, Pedroza-Tobías A, Simón B (2025) Prevalence of metabolic syndrome and combinations of its components: findings from the Mexican National Health and Nutrition Survey, 2021. Metab Syndr Relat Disord 23(4):193–204. https://doi.org/10.1089/met.2024.0179

Carafoli E, Krebs J (2016) Why calcium? How calcium became the best communicator. J Biol Chem 291(40):20849–20857. https://doi.org/10.1074/jbc.R116.735894

Casemore D, Xing C (2015) Integrative cancer science and therapeutics SERCA as a target for cancer therapies. Integr Cancer Sci Therap 2(2):100–103. https://doi.org/10.15761/ICST.1000122

Casteels R, Droogmans G (1981) Exchange characteristics of the noradrenaline-sensitive calcium store in vascular smooth muscle cells or rabbit ear artery. J Physiol 317(1):263–279. https://doi.org/10.1113/jphysiol.1981.sp013824

Chemaly E, Bobe R, Adnot S, Hajjar RJ, Lipskaia L (2013) Sarco (Endo) plasmic reticulum calcium ATPases (SERCA) isoforms in the normal and diseased cardiac, vascular and skeletal muscle. J Cardiovasc Dis Diagn 01(04):1–6. https://doi.org/10.4172/2329-9517.1000113

Chemaly ER, Troncone L, Lebeche D (2018) SERCA control of cell death and survival. Cell Calcium 69:46–61. https://doi.org/10.1016/j.ceca.2017.07.001

Chen Q, van Breemen C (1993) The superficial buffer barrier in venous smooth muscle: sarcoplasmic reticulum refilling and unloading. Br J Pharmacol 109(2):336–343. https://doi.org/10.1111/j.1476-5381.1993.tb13575.x

Cheng H, Lederer WJ (2008) Calcium sparks. Physiol Rev 88(4):1491–1545. https://doi.org/10.1152/physrev.00030.2007

Christensen KL, Mulvany MJ (2001) Location of resistance arteries. J Vasc Res 38(1):1–12. https://doi.org/10.1159/000051024

Clark JH, Kinnear NP, Kalujnaia S, Cramb G, Fleischer S, Jeyakumar LH, Wuytack F, Evans AM (2010) Identification of functionally segregated sarcoplasmic reticulum calcium stores in pulmonary arterial smooth muscle. J Biol Chem 285(18):13542–13549. https://doi.org/10.1074/jbc.M110.101485

Climent B, Santiago E, Sánchez A, Muñoz-Picos M, Pérez–Vizcaíno F, García-Sacristán A, Rivera L, Prieto D (2020) Metabolic syndrome inhibits store-operated Ca2+ entry and calcium-induced calcium-release mechanism in coronary artery smooth muscle. Biochem Pharmacol 182. https://doi.org/10.1016/j.bcp.2020.114222

Cruz-Cortés C, Fernández-de Gortari E, Aguayo-Ortiz R, Šeflová J, Ard A, Clasby M, Anumonwo J, Michel Espinoza-Fonseca L (2025) Machine learning-driven discovery of structurally related natural products as activators of the cardiac calcium pump SERCA2a.

ChemMedChem 20(9):e202400913. https://doi.org/10.1002/CMDC.202400913; REQUESTEDJOURNAL:JOURNAL:18607187;PAGE:STRING:ARTICLE/CHAPTER
D'Angelo G, Davis MJ, Meininger GA (1997) Calcium and mechanotransduction of the myogenic response. Am J Physiol Heart Circ Physiol 273:H175–H182. https://doi.org/10.1152/ajpheart.1997.273.1.h175
Dally S, Bredoux R, Corvazier E, Andersen JP, Clausen JD, Dode L, Fanchaouy M, Gelebart P, Monceau V, Del Monte F, Gwathmey JK, Hajjar R, Chaabane C, Bobe R, Raies A, Enouf J (2006) Ca2+-ATPases in non-failing and failing heart: evidence for a novel cardiac sarco/endoplasmic reticulum Ca2+-ATPase 2 isoform (SERCA2c). Biochem J 395(2):249–258. https://doi.org/10.1042/BJ20051427
Davies MG (2015) New insights on the role of SERCA during vessel remodeling in metabolic syndrome. Diabetes 64(9):3066–3068. https://doi.org/10.2337/DB15-0761
Davis MJ (2012) Perspective: physiological role(s) of the vascular myogenic response. Microcirculation 19(2):99–114. https://doi.org/10.1111/j.1549-8719.2011.00131.x
Devine CE, Somlyo AV, Somlyo AP (1972) Sarcoplasmic reticulum and excitation-contraction coupling in mammalian smooth muscles. J Cell Biol 52(3):690–718. https://doi.org/10.1083/jcb.52.3.690
Essin K, Gollasch M (2009) Role of ryanodine receptor subtypes in initiation and formation of calcium sparks in arterial smooth muscle: comparison with striated muscle. J Biomed Biotechnol 2009(1). https://doi.org/10.1155/2009/135249
Evans AM (2017) Nanojunctions of the sarcoplasmic reticulum deliver site- and function-specific calcium signaling in vascular smooth muscles. In: Advances in pharmacology, vol 78, 1st edn. Elsevier Inc. https://doi.org/10.1016/bs.apha.2016.10.001
Evans AM, Fameli N, Ogunbayo OA, Duan J, Navarro-Dorado J (2016) From contraction to gene expression: nanojunctions of the sarco/endoplasmic reticulum deliver site- and function-specific calcium signals. Sci China Life Sci 59(8):749–763. https://doi.org/10.1007/s11427-016-5071-0
Fernández-Velasco M, Ruiz-Hurtado G, Gómez AM, Rueda A (2014) Ca2+ handling alterations and vascular dysfunction in diabetes. Cell Calcium 56(5):397–407. https://doi.org/10.1016/j.ceca.2014.08.007
Fransen P, Chen J, Vangheluwe P, Guns PJ (2020) Contractile behavior of mouse aorta depends on SERCA2 isoform distribution: effects of replacing SERCA2a by SERCA2b. Front Physiol 11 (March):1–13. https://doi.org/10.3389/fphys.2020.00282
Gélébart P, Martin V, Enouf J, Papp B (2003) Identification of a new SERCA2 splice variant regulated during monocytic differentiation. Biochem Biophys Res Commun 303(2):676–684. https://doi.org/10.1016/S0006-291X(03)00405-4
Hirode G, Wong RJ (2020) Trends in the prevalence of metabolic syndrome in the United States, 2011-2016. JAMA 323(24):2526. https://doi.org/10.1001/JAMA.2020.4501
Inoue M, Sakuta N, Watanabe S, Zhang Y, Yoshikaic K, Tanaka Y, Ushioda R, Kato Y, Takagi J, Tsukazaki T, Nagata K, Inaba K (2019) Structural basis of Sarco/endoplasmic reticulum ca 2+ -ATPase 2b regulation via transmembrane helix interplay. Cell Rep 27(4):1221–1230. https://doi.org/10.1016/j.celrep.2019.03.106
Jackson WF (2021) Myogenic tone in peripheral resistance arteries and arterioles: the pressure is on! Front Physiol 12(July):699517. https://doi.org/10.3389/fphys.2021.699517
Jaggar JH, Stevenson A, Nelson MT (1998a) Voltage dependence of Ca2+ sparks in intact cerebral arteries. Am J Phys 274(6):C1755–C1761. https://doi.org/10.1152/ajpcell.1998.274.6.C1755
Jaggar JH, Wellman GC, Heppner TJ, Porter VA, Perez GJ, Gollasch M, Kleppisch T, Rubart M, Stevenson AS, Lederer WJ, Knot HJ, Bonev AD, Nelson MT (1998b) Ca2+ channels, ryanodine receptors and Ca(2+)-activated K+ channels: a functional unit for regulating arterial tone. Acta Physiol Scand 164(4):577–587. https://doi.org/10.1046/j.1365-201X.1998.00462.x
Jaggar JH, Porter VA, Jonathan Lederer W, Nelson MT (2000) Calcium sparks in smooth muscle. Am J Physiol Cell Physiol 278:C235–C256. https://doi.org/10.1152/ajpcell.2000.278.2.c235

Jamali Z, Ayoobi F, Jalali Z, Bidaki R, Lotfi MA, Esmaeili-Nadimi A, Khalili P (2024) Metabolic syndrome: a population-based study of prevalence and risk factors. Sci Rep 14(1). https://doi.org/10.1038/s41598-024-54367-4

Jang SP, Oh JG, Kang DH, Kang JY, Kang SW, Hajjar RJ, Park WJ (2016) A decoy peptide targeted to protein phosphatase 1 attenuates degradation of SERCA2a in vascular smooth muscle cells. PLoS One 11(10):e0165569. https://doi.org/10.1371/journal.pone.0165569

Janssen LJ, Betti PA, Netherton SJ, Walters DK (1999) Superficial buffer barrier and preferentially directed release of Ca2+ in canine airway smooth muscle. Am J Physiol Lung Cell Mol Physiol 276(5). https://doi.org/10.1152/ajplung.1999.276.5.l744

Ji G, Feldman ME, Greene KS, Sorrentino V, Xin H, Kotlikoff MI (2004) RYR2 proteins contribute to the formation of Ca2+ Sparks in smooth muscle. J Gen Physiol 123:377–386. https://doi.org/10.1085/jgp.200308999

Jones AW, Smith JM, Edwards JM, Neeb ZP, Alloosh MA, Long X, Bratz IN, Peller CR, Byrd JP, Kumar S, Obukhov AG, Sturek M, Schäfer N, Lohmann C, Winnik S, van Tits LJ, Miranda MX, Vergopoulos A, Ruschitzka F et al (2005) Calcium-activated potassium channels and the regulation of vascular tone. Circ Res 85(2):411–425. https://doi.org/10.1016/S0140-6736(15)00257-3

Kabashima Y, Ogawa H, Nakajima R, Toyoshima C (2020) What ATP binding does to the Ca2+ pump and how nonproductive phosphoryl transfer is prevented in the absence of Ca2. Proc Natl Acad Sci USA 117(31):18448–18458. https://doi.org/10.1073/pnas.2006027117

Kang S, Dahl R, Hsieh W, Shin A, Zsebo KM, Buettner C, Hajjar RJ, Lebeche D (2016) Small molecular allosteric activator of the sarco/endoplasmic reticulum Ca2+-ATPase (SERCA) attenuates diabetes and metabolic disorders. J Biol Chem 291(10):5185–5198. https://doi.org/10.1074/JBC.M115.705012/ASSET/5184A26E-8834-480B-9FAF-82D1A480783E/MAIN.ASSETS/GR7.JPG

Kaßmann M, Szijártó IA, García-Prieto CF, Fan G, Schleifenbaum J, Anistan YM, Tabeling C, Shi Y, le Noble F, Witzenrath M, Huang Y, Markó L, Nelson MT, Gollasch M (2019) Role of ryanodine type 2 receptors in elementary Ca2+ signaling in arteries and vascular adaptive responses. J Am Heart Assoc 8(9):e010090. https://doi.org/10.1161/JAHA.118.010090

Khalil RA (2010) Regulation of vascular smooth muscle function. Colloq Ser Integr Syst Physiol: Mol Funct 2(1):1–62. https://doi.org/10.4199/c00012ed1v01y201005isp007

Kim SJ, Ahn SC, Kim JK, Kim YC, So I, Kim KW (1997) Changes in intracellular Ca2+ concentration induced by L-type Ca2+ channel current in Guinea pig gastric myocytes. Am J Physiol Cell Physiol 273(6 42-6):1947–1956. https://doi.org/10.1152/ajpcell.1997.273.6.c1947

Kimura T, Nakamori M, Lueck JD, Pouliquin P, Aoike F, Fujimura H, Dirksen RT, Takahashi MP, Dulhunty AF, Sakoda S (2005) Altered mRNA splicing of the skeletal muscle ryanodine receptor and sarcoplasmic/endoplasmic reticulum Ca2+-ATPase in myotonic dystrophy type 1. Hum Mol Genet 14(15):2189–2200. https://doi.org/10.1093/hmg/ddi223

Knot HJ, Standen NB, Nelson MT (1998) Ryanodine receptors regulate arterial diameter and wall [Ca2+] in cerebral arteries of rat via Ca2+-dependent K+ channels. J Physiol 508(1):211–221. https://doi.org/10.1111/j.1469-7793.1998.211br.x

Kühlbrandt W (2004) Biology, structure and mechanism of P-type ATPases. Nat Rev Mol Cell Biol 5(4):282–295. https://doi.org/10.1038/nrm1354

Lagaud GJ, Randriamboavonjy V, Roul G, Stoclet JC, Andriantsitohaina R (1999) Mechanism of Ca2+ release and entry during contraction elicited by norepinephrine in rat resistance arteries. Am J Phys 276(1 Pt 2):H300–H308

Ledoux J, Werner ME, Brayden JE, Nelson MT (2006) Calcium-activated potassium channels and the regulation of vascular tone. Physiology 21:69–79. https://doi.org/10.1152/physiol.00040.2005

Lee Y, Chakraborty S, Muthuchamy M (2020) Roles of sarcoplasmic reticulum Ca2+ ATPase pump in the impairments of lymphatic contractile activity in a metabolic syndrome rat model. Sci Rep 10(1). https://doi.org/10.1038/s41598-020-69196-4

Levitsky D, Clergue M, Lambert F, Souponitskayas V, Jemtelfl, Le TH, Lecarpentier Y, Lomprell A-M (1993) Sarcoplasmic reticulum calcium transport and Ca2+ -ATPase gene expression in thoracic and abdominal aortas of normotensive and spontaneously hypertensive rats. J Biol Chem 268(11):8325–8331. https://doi.org/10.1016/s0021-9258(18)53099-4

Li W, Qiu X, Ma H, Geng Q (2023) Incidence and long-term specific mortality trends of metabolic syndrome in the United States. Front Endocrinol 13. https://doi.org/10.3389/fendo.2022.1029736

Lipskaia L, Hadri L, Le Prince P, B E, Atassi F, Liang L, Glorian M, Limon I, Lompre A, Lehoux S, Hajjar RJ (2013a) SERCA2a gene transfer prevents intimal proliferation in an organ culture of human internal mammary artery. Gene Ther 20(4):396–406. https://doi.org/10.1038/gt.2012.50. SERCA2a

Lipskaia L, Hadri L, Lopez J, Hajjar RJ, Bobe R (2013b) Benefit of SERCA2a gene transfer to vascular endothelial and smooth muscle cells: a new aspect in therapy of cardiovascular diseases. Curr Vasc Pharmacol 11(4):465–479

Liu Q-H, Zheng Y-M, Korde AS, Yadav VR, Rathore R, Wess J, Wang Y-X (2009) Membrane depolarization causes a direct activation of G protein-coupled receptors leading to local Ca2+ release in smooth muscle. Proc Natl Acad Sci USA 106(27):11418–11423. https://doi.org/10.1073/pnas.0813307106

Marchand A, Abi-Gerges A, Saliba Y, Merlet E, Lompré AM (2012) Calcium signaling in vascular smooth muscle cells: from physiology to pathology. Adv Exp Med Biol 740:795–810. https://doi.org/10.1007/978-94-007-2888-2_35

McKenney-Drake ML, Rodenbeck SD, Owen MK, Schultz KA, Alloosh M, Tune JD, Sturek M (2016) Biphasic alterations in coronary smooth muscle Ca2+ regulation in a repeat cross-sectional study of coronary artery disease severity in metabolic syndrome. Atherosclerosis 249:1–9. https://doi.org/10.1016/j.atherosclerosis.2016.03.032

Miranda-Saturnino MJ, de Alba-Aguayo DR, Mercado-Morales M, Guerrero-Hernández A, Rueda A (2014) Increased Serca pump expression is associated with slow termination of calcium sparks and delayed local recovery in vascular smooth muscle cells of hyperthyroid rats. Biophys J 106(2):321a. https://doi.org/10.1016/j.bpj.2013.11.1854

Møller JV, Nissen P, Sørensen TLM, Le Maire M (2005) Transport mechanism of the sarcoplasmic reticulum Ca2+-ATPase pump. Curr Opin Struct Biol 15(4):387–393. https://doi.org/10.1016/j.sbi.2005.06.005

Neeb ZP, Edwards JM, Alloosh M, Long X, Mokelke EA, Sturek M (2010) Metabolic syndrome and coronary artery disease in Ossabaw compared with Yucatan swine. Comp Med 60(4):300. https://pmc.ncbi.nlm.nih.gov/articles/PMC2930329/

Nelson MT, Cheng H, Rubart M, Santana LF, Bonev AD, Knot HJ, Lederer WJ (1995) Relaxation of arterial smooth muscle by calcium sparks. Science 270(5236):633–637. https://doi.org/10.1126/science.270.5236.633

Nomura Y, Asano M (2002) Increased Ca2+ buffering function of sarcoplasmic reticulum in small mesenteric arteries from spontaneously hypertensive rats. Hypertens Res 25(2):231–239. https://doi.org/10.1291/hypres.25.231

Noubiap JJ, Nansseu JR, Lontchi-Yimagou E, Nkeck JR, Nyaga UF, Ngouo AT, Tounouga DN, Tianyi FL, Foka AJ, Ndoadoumgue AL, Bigna JJ (2022) Geographic distribution of metabolic syndrome and its components in the general adult population: a meta-analysis of global data from 28 million individuals. In: Diabetes research and clinical practice, vol 188. Elsevier Ireland Ltd. https://doi.org/10.1016/j.diabres.2022.109924

Ogut O, Brozovich FV (2003) Regulation of force in vascular smooth muscle. J Mol Cell Cardiol 35(4):347–355. https://doi.org/10.1016/S0022-2828(03)00045-2

Okatan EN, Durak AT, Turan B (2016) Electrophysiological basis of metabolic-syndrome-induced cardiac dysfunction. Can J Physiol Pharmacol 94(10):1064–1073. https://doi.org/10.1139/CJPP-2015-0531;WGROUP:STRING:CSP

Olesen C, Sørensen TLM, Nielsen RC, Møller JV, Nissen P (2004) Dephosphorylation of the calcium pump coupled to counterion occlusion. Science 306(5705):2251–2255. https://doi.org/10.1126/science.1106289
Olesen C, Picard M, Winther AML, Gyrup C, Morth JP, Oxvig C, Møller JV, Nissen P (2007) The structural basis of calcium transport by the calcium pump. Nature 450(7172):1036–1042. https://doi.org/10.1038/nature06418
Orallo F (1996) Regulation of cytosolic calcium levels in vascular smooth muscle. Pharmacol Ther 69(3):153–171. https://doi.org/10.1016/0163-7258(95)02042-X
Periasamy M, Kalyanasundaram A (2007) SERCA pump isoforms: their role in calcium transport and disease. Muscle Nerve 35(4):430–442. https://doi.org/10.1002/mus.20745
Porter V a, Bonev a D, Knot HJ, Heppner TJ, Stevenson a S, Kleppisch T, Lederer WJ, Nelson MT (1998) Frequency modulation of Ca2+ sparks is involved in regulation of arterial diameter by cyclic nucleotides. Am J Phys 274:C1346–C1355
Qin Z, Hou X, Weisbrod RM, Seta F, Cohen RA, Tong X (2014) Nox2 mediates high fat high sucrose diet-induced nitric oxide dysfunction and inflammation in aortic smooth muscle cells. J Mol Cell Cardiol 72:56–63. https://doi.org/10.1016/j.yjmcc.2014.02.019
Rathod N, Bak JJ, Primeau JO, Fisher ME, Espinoza-fonseca LM, Lemieux MJ, Young HS (2021) Nothing regular about the regulins: distinct functional properties of SERCA transmembrane peptide regulatory subunits. Int J Mol Sci 22(16):8891. https://doi.org/10.3390/IJMS22168891/S1
Rembold CM, Chen XL (1998) The buffer barrier hypothesis, [Ca2+](i) homogeneity, and sarcoplasmic reticulum function in swine carotid artery. J Physiol 513(2):477–492. https://doi.org/10.1111/j.1469-7793.1998.477bb.x
Romero-García T, Landa-Galvan HV, Pavón N, Mercado-Morales M, Valdivia HH, Rueda A (2020) Autonomous activation of CaMKII exacerbates diastolic calcium leak during beta-adrenergic stimulation in cardiomyocytes of metabolic syndrome rats. Cell Calcium 91:102267. https://doi.org/10.1016/J.CECA.2020.102267
Romero-García T, Vázquez-Jiménez JG, Sánchez-Hernández R, Olivares-Reyes JA, Rueda A (2025) Insulin resistance, Ca2+ signaling alterations and vascular dysfunction in prediabetes and metabolic syndrome. Front Physiol 16. Frontiers Media SA. https://doi.org/10.3389/fphys.2025.1535153
Rueda A, Song M, Toro L, Stefani E, Valdivia HH (2006) Sorcin modulation of Ca2+ sparks in rat vascular smooth muscle cells. J Physiol 576(3):887–901. https://doi.org/10.1113/jphysiol.2006.113951
Rueda A, Fernández-Velasco M, Benitah J-P, Gómez AM (2013) Abnormal Ca2+ spark/STOC coupling in cerebral artery smooth muscle cells of obese type 2 diabetic mice. PLoS One 8(1):e53321. https://doi.org/10.1371/journal.pone.0053321
Salazar-Enciso R, Guerrero-Hernández A, Gómez AM, Benitah JP, Rueda A (2022) Aldosterone-induced Sarco/endoplasmic reticulum Ca2+ pump upregulation counterbalances Cav1.2-mediated Ca2+ influx in mesenteric arteries. Front Physiol 13:834220. https://doi.org/10.3389/fphys.2022.834220
Searls YM, Loganathan R, Smirnova IV, Stehno-Bittel L (2010) Intracellular Ca2+regulating proteins in vascular smooth muscle cells are altered with type 1 diabetes due to the direct effects of hyperglycemia. Cardiovasc Diabetol 9:1–17. https://doi.org/10.1186/1475-2840-9-8
Shadrin I, Khodabukus A, Bursac N (2016) Striated muscle function, regeneration, and repair. Cell Mol Life Sci 73(22):4175–4202. https://doi.org/10.1007/s00018-016-2285-z
Sharma V, Mcneill JH (2006) The etiology of hypertension in the metabolic syndrome part three: the regulation and dysregulation of blood pressure. Curr Vasc Pharmacol 4(4):305–320. http://www.ncbi.nlm.nih.gov/pubmed/17073700
Somlyo AP (1985) Excitation-contraction coupling and the ultrastructure of smooth muscle. Circ Res 57(4):497–507. https://doi.org/10.1161/01.RES.57.4.497
Sweeney H, Hammers D (2018) Muscle contraction. Cold Spring Harb Perspect Biol 10:a023200. https://doi.org/10.1101/cshperspect.a023200

Toyoshima C (2008) Structural aspects of ion pumping by Ca2+-ATPase of sarcoplasmic reticulum. Arch Biochem Biophys 476(1):3–11. https://doi.org/10.1016/j.abb.2008.04.017

Toyoshima C (2009) How Ca2+-ATPase pumps ions across the sarcoplasmic reticulum membrane. Biochim Biophys Acta, Mol Cell Res 1793(6):941–946. https://doi.org/10.1016/j.bbamcr.2008.10.008

Toyoshima C, Nakasako M, Nomura H, Ogawa H (2000) Crystal structure of the calcium pump of sarcoplasmic reticulum at 2.6 Å resolution. Nature 405(6787):647–655. https://doi.org/10.1038/35015017

Tsunekawa N, Ogawa H, Tsueda J, Akiba T, Toyoshima C (2018) Mechanism of the E2 to E1 transition in Ca2+ pump revealed by crystal structures of gating residue mutants. Proc Natl Acad Sci USA 115(50):12722–12727. https://doi.org/10.1073/pnas.1815472115

Tykocki NR, Boerman EM, Jackson WF (2017) Smooth muscle ion channels and regulation of vascular tone in resistance arteries and arterioles. Compr Physiol 7(2):485–581. https://doi.org/10.1002/cphy.c160011

Vaithianathan T, Narayanan D, Asuncion-Chin MT, Jeyakumar LH, Liu J, Fleischer S, Jaggar JH, Dopico AM (2010) Subtype identification and functional characterization of ryanodine receptors in rat cerebral artery myocytes. Am J Physiol Cell Physiol 299:C264–C278. https://doi.org/10.1152/ajpcell.00318.2009

Van Breemen C (1977) Calcium requirement for activation of intact aortic smooth muscle. J Physiol 272(2):317–329. https://doi.org/10.1113/jphysiol.1977.sp012046

van Breemen C, Chen Q, Laher I (1995) Superficial buffer barrier function of smooth muscle sarcoplasmic reticulum. Trends Pharmacol Sci 16(3):98–105. https://doi.org/10.1016/S0165-6147(00)88990-7

Van Breemen C, Fameli N, Evans AM (2013) Pan-junctional sarcoplasmic reticulum in vascular smooth muscle: nanospace Ca2+ transport for site- and function-specific Ca2+ signalling. J Physiol 591(8):2043–2054. https://doi.org/10.1113/jphysiol.2012.246348

Vandecaetsbeek I, Trekels M, De Maeyer M, Ceulemans H, Lescrinier E, Raeymaekers L, Wuytack F, Vangheluwe P (2009) Structural basis for the high Ca2+ affinity of the ubiquitous SERCA2b Ca2+ pump. Proc Natl Acad Sci USA 106(44):18533–18538. https://doi.org/10.1073/pnas.0906797106

Vandecaetsbeek I, Vangheluwe P, Raeymaekers L, Wuytack F, Vanoevelen J (2011) The Ca2+ pumps of the endoplasmic reticulum and Golgi apparatus. Cold Spring Harb Perspect Biol 3(5). https://doi.org/10.1101/cshperspect.a004184

Verboomen H, Wuytack F, De Smedt H, Himpens B, Casteels R (1992) Functional difference between SERCA2a and SERCA2b Ca2+ pumps and their modulation by phospholamban. Biochem J 286(2):591–595. https://doi.org/10.1042/bj2860591

Viskupicova J, Rezbarikova P (2022) Natural polyphenols as SERCA activators: role in the endoplasmic reticulum stress-related diseases. Molecules 27(16):5095. https://doi.org/10.3390/MOLECULES27165095

Wang Y-X, Zheng Y-M, Mei Q-B, Wang Q-S, Collier ML, Fleischer S, Xin H-B, Kotlikoff MI (2004) FKBP12.6 and cADPR regulation of Ca2+ release in smooth muscle cells. Am J Physiol Cell Physiol 286(3):C538–C546. https://doi.org/10.1152/ajpcell.00106.2003

Webb RC (2003) Smooth muscle contraction and relaxation. Am J Physiol - Adv Physiol Educ 27(1–4):201–206. https://doi.org/10.1152/advan.00025.2003

Weisbrod RM, Shiang T, Al Sayah L, Fry JL, Bajpai S, Reinhart-King CA, Lob HE, Santhanam L, Mitchell G, Cohen RA, Seta F (2013) Arterial stiffening precedes systolic hypertension in diet-induced obesity. Hypertension 62(6):1105. https://doi.org/10.1161/HYPERTENSIONAHA.113.01744

Wellman GC, Santana LF, Bonev AD, Nelson MT (2001) Role of phospholamban in the modulation of arterial Ca2+ sprks and Ca2+-activated K+ channels by cAMP. Am J Physiol Cell Physiol 281(3). https://doi.org/10.1152/AJPCELL.2001.281.3.C1029/ASSET/IMAGES/LARGE/H00910645007.JPEG

Widmaier EP, Raff H, Strang KT, Vander AJ (2014) Vander's human physiology: the mechanisms of body function, 13th edn. McGraw-Hill Higher Education

Wong SK, Chin KY, Suhaimi FH, Fairus A, Ima-Nirwana S (2016) Animal models of metabolic syndrome: a review. Nutr Metab 13(1):65. https://doi.org/10.1186/S12986-016-0123-9

Wright DB, Tripathi S, Sikarwar A, Santosh KT, Perez-Zoghbi J, Ojo OO, Irechukwu N, Ward JPT, Schaafsma D (2013) Regulation of GPCR-mediated smooth muscle contraction: implications for asthma and pulmonary hypertension. Pulm Pharmacol Ther 26(1):121–131. https://doi.org/10.1016/j.pupt.2012.06.005

Wu K, Bungard D, Lytton J, Lyt- J (2001) Regulation of SERCA Ca 2 + pump expression by cytoplasmic [Ca 2 +] in vascular smooth muscle cells Regulation of SERCA Ca 2 ℰ pump expression by cytoplasmic [Ca 2 ℰ] in vascular smooth muscle cells. Am J Physiol Cell Physiol 280:C843–C851

Wuytack F, Raeymaekers L, Missiaen L (2002) Molecular physiology of the SERCA and SPCA pumps. Cell Calcium 32(5–6):279–305. https://doi.org/10.1016/S0143416002001847

Xu H, Van Remmen H (2021) The SarcoEndoplasmic Reticulum Calcium ATPase (SERCA) pump: a potential target for intervention in aging and skeletal muscle pathologies. Skelet Muscle 11(1):1–9. https://doi.org/10.1186/s13395-021-00280-7

Yu Q, Tian W (2025) The role of SERCA in vascular diseases, a potential therapeutic target. Cell Calcium 129:103039. https://doi.org/10.1016/J.CECA.2025.103039

Zhang Y, Inoue M, Tsutsumi A, Watanabe S, Nishizawa T, Nagata K, Kikkawa M, Inaba K (2020) Cryo-EM structures of SERCA2b reveal the mechanism of regulation by the luminal extension tail. Sci Adv 6(33):1–12. https://doi.org/10.1126/sciadv.abb0147

Zhuge R, Tuft RA, Fogarty KE, Bellve K, Fay FS, Walsh JV (1999) The influence of sarcoplasmic reticulum Ca2+ concentration on Ca2+ Sparks and spontaneous transient outward currents in single smooth muscle cells. J Gen Physiol 113:215–228

Oxidative Modifications in Cardiac Mitochondrial and Ca^{2+} Handling Proteins in Obesity and Metabolic Syndrome: Antioxidant Alternatives

Karla Carvajal, David Julian Arias-Chávez, Patrick Mailloux-Salinas, Guadalupe Bravo, and Norma Leticia Gómez-Viquez

Contents

Abstract

Obesity and its related comorbidities, collectively defined as metabolic syndrome (MetS), represent a major health concern due to their strong association with increased cardiometabolic risk. A defining feature of obesity and MetS is the

K. Carvajal
Laboratorio de Nutrición experimental, Instituto Nacional de Pediatría, Ciudad de México, México

D. J. Arias-Chávez
Escuela de Dietética y Nutrición Dr. José Quintín Olascoaga Moncada, ISSSTE, Ciudad de México, México

P. Mailloux-Salinas
Laboratorio de Compuestos Bioactivos, Departamento de Ingeniería Bioquímica, Escuela Nacional de Ciencias Biológicas-IPN, Unidad Profesional Adolfo López Mateos, Ciudad de México, Mexico

G. Bravo · N. L. Gómez-Viquez (✉)
Departamento de Farmacobiología, Centro de Investigación y de Estudios Avanzados del IPN, Ciudad de México, Mexico
e-mail: nogomez@cinvestav.mx

A. Rueda, M. Nieves-Cintrón (eds.), *Cardiovascular Alterations in Metabolic Diseases*, Handbook of Experimental Pharmacology 293,
https://doi.org/10.1007/164_2026_794

excessive production of reactive oxygen species and reactive nitrogen species, resulting in systemic oxidative stress (OS) and nitrosative stress (NS). In the heart, OS and NS induce structural and conformational alterations in proteins, referred to as oxidative post-translational modifications (oxPTMs). These modifications disrupt protein function, thereby impairing essential cellular processes and ultimately contributing to diastolic and systolic dysfunction. Several proteins critical for cardiac function have been identified as targets of oxPTMs in the context of obesity and MetS. Among the most studied are mitochondrial proteins such as dynamin-related protein 1 (Drp1), respiratory chain complexes I, II, and IV, and creatine kinase, as well as Ca^{2+}-handling proteins including sarcoplasmic reticulum Ca^{2+}-ATPase (SERCA2a) and ryanodine receptors (RyR2). This chapter summarizes current knowledge on the mechanisms underlying cardiac dysfunction in obesity and MetS, with a particular emphasis on OS and its damaging effects on mitochondrial metabolism and Ca^{2+} handling. Finally, we provide an update on recent findings regarding natural antioxidants and mitochondria-targeted antioxidant therapies, highlighting their potential as treatment strategies for cardiovascular diseases associated with obesity and MetS.

Keywords

Heart · Metabolic syndrome · Mitochondria · Nitration · Obesity · Oxidative post-translational modifications · RyR2 · SERCA2a · S-nitrosylation

1 Introduction

Obesity is a serious medical condition and a major global health challenge, driven by its increasing prevalence and strong association with cardiovascular diseases (CVD) that compromise both quality of life and life expectancy (World Health Organization n.d.; Caballero 2007; Carvajal et al. 2014; Chen et al. 2022). In 2022, an estimated 2.5 billion adults (≥18 years) were classified as overweight, of whom 890 million were living with obesity. Additionally, over 390 million children and adolescents aged 5 to 19 years were overweight, including 160 million affected by obesity (World Health Organization n.d.).

Central obesity is a key driver of a cluster of well-established risk factors for the development of type 2 diabetes (T2DM) and heart failure (HF), including insulin resistance (IR), hypertension, dyslipidemia (characterized by hypertriglyceridemia and reduced HDL-cholesterol levels), and impaired glucose tolerance. These clinical and biochemical abnormalities are tightly interconnected and collectively define metabolic syndrome (MetS) (Jia et al. 2016; Colak and Pap 2021; Ren et al. 2021; Ilkun and Boudina 2013; Masenga et al. 2023). While each component of MetS contributes to cardiac dysfunction individually, their coexistence confers an even greater cardiovascular risk (Ilkun and Boudina 2013).

At the molecular level, metabolic disturbances associated with obesity and MetS are linked to systemic low-grade inflammation, as well as elevated levels of reactive oxygen species (ROS) and reactive nitrogen species (RNS) that lead to a state of oxidative stress (OS) and nitrosative stress (NS) (Colak and Pap 2021; Ilkun and Boudina 2013; Masenga et al. 2023). In the heart, local OS and NS can generate lipotoxicity and trigger oxidative post-translational modifications (oxPTMs) in various proteins, resulting in abnormal protein function. These alterations lead to disrupted mitochondrial metabolism, activation of pro-apoptotic signaling pathways, impaired Ca^{2+} handling, hypertrophy, fibrosis, and changes in substrate utilization, among other effects, all of which contribute to cardiac dysfunction and, over time, the development of HF (Carvajal et al. 2014; Chen et al. 2022; Ilkun and Boudina 2013; Masenga et al. 2023).

In this chapter, we review recent advances in the study of oxPTMs in mitochondrial and Ca^{2+}-handling proteins, as well as their role in impaired cardiac function associated with obesity and MetS. We also discuss emerging antioxidant therapies aimed at treating these alterations.

2 Mechanisms Contributing to Systemic OS in Obesity and MetS

Obesity, defined as an excessive accumulation of body fat, is the core component of MetS, which can induce systemic OS through different mechanisms. During obesity, the excessive oxidation of substrates, such as glucose, lipids, and saturated fatty acids, particularly trans-fatty acids, stimulates specific intracellular pathways that promote OS in adipose tissue. These pathways include O_2^- generation via oxidative phosphorylation, glyceraldehyde autoxidation, protein kinase C activation, and stimulation of the polyol and hexosamine pathways (Colak and Pap 2021). Additionally, increased visceral fat accumulation is associated with low-grade chronic inflammation, driven by hypertrophied adipose tissue and the activation of immune cells. Hypertrophied adipocytes exhibit an altered secretory profile, characterized by a reduced production of anti-inflammatory adipokines, such as adiponectin, and an increased secretion of pro-inflammatory adipokines, including TNF-α, IL-1β, IL-6, and leptin. Adipose tissue expansion also enhances chemokine release, promoting macrophage recruitment and activation, which further amplifies inflammation and increases ROS and RNS production, thereby exacerbating OS and NS (Carvajal et al. 2014; Colak and Pap 2021; Masenga et al. 2023). Additionally, local OS in adipocytes increases the synthesis of TNF-α, IL-1β, and IL-6 by inducing the activation of pro-inflammatory transcription factors, such as NF-κB and activator protein-1 (AP-1). These cytokines further amplify ROS production by promoting inflammation and IR in adipocytes and other peripheral tissues, including the heart, which increases lipolysis and leads to the excessive release and accumulation of free fatty acids (FFAs), ultimately causing mitochondrial DNA damage and lipotoxicity (Colak and Pap 2021; Ren et al. 2021; Gutiérrez-Cuevas et al. 2021).

3 Mechanisms Contributing to Cardiac OS in Obesity and MetS

Growing evidence indicates that obesity promotes cardiac dysfunction by inducing OS within the myocardium through mechanisms involving both inflammation and IR in this tissue. Specifically, IL-6 has been reported to impair cardiac glucose metabolism and promote IR by potentiating suppressor of cytokine signaling-3 (SOCS3)-mediated inhibition of insulin receptor substrate-1 (IRS-1) and by reducing AMP-activated protein kinase (AMPK) activity (Carvajal et al. 2014). Decreased AMPK also results in decreased SIRT-1/nuclear factor-erythroid factor 2-related factor 2 (Nrf2) signaling that mediates genetic transcription of antioxidants such as superoxide dismutase (SOD), glutathione peroxidase (GPx), and catalase (CAT) (Hammad et al. 2023). Impaired glucose utilization due to IR favors a metabolic shift toward increased mitochondrial oxidation of FFAs, which elevates mitochondrial oxygen consumption and enhances ROS production. In addition, cardiac IR favors lipoprotein lipase activity, leading to increased FFAs and triglycerides release and augmented FFAs supply (Pulinilkunnil and Rodrigues 2006). FFAs-induced ROS generation causes oxidative damage of mitochondrial proteins, promotes mitochondrial uncoupling, and ultimately impairs ATP synthesis and further exacerbates ROS production (Carvajal et al. 2014; Colak and Pap 2021; Ilkun and Boudina 2013; Masenga et al. 2023; Gutiérrez-Cuevas et al. 2021). Furthermore, intermediates from lipid metabolism, including ceramides, diacylglycerol, and fatty acyl CoA, can also worsen IR by increasing serine phosphorylation of IRS-1 (Carvajal et al. 2014). These findings show that elevated ROS production and mitochondrial dysfunction in the heart are tightly interconnected to IR, forming a complex network and a vicious cycle of cellular mechanisms whose initiating event remains uncertain. All these mechanisms have been implicated in impairment of cardiac efficiency and contractility in obesity.

4 OS and Cardiac Dysfunction in Obesity and MetS

ROS and RNS, while essential for physiological processes such as cellular signaling and immune defense, become highly detrimental at elevated concentrations. Under physiological conditions, ROS and RNS production is balanced by antioxidant systems, and act as key signaling molecules that mediate oxPTMs in proteins, thereby regulating critical cardiac processes, such as excitation–contraction coupling (ECC), mitochondrial function, Ca^{2+} handling, and the expression of genes involved in cardiac remodeling and survival (Chen et al. 2022; Masenga et al. 2023; Zima and Blatter 2006; Perjés et al. 2012). However, excessive ROS and RNS production disrupts this redox balance and has been implicated in the development of cardiac dysfunction in different pathological conditions, including obesity and MetS, diabetes, aging, ischemia, and HF (Carvajal et al. 2014; Chen et al. 2022; Colak and Pap 2021; Ilkun and Boudina 2013; Masenga et al. 2023; Gutiérrez-Cuevas et al. 2021; Wende 2016; Hajam et al. 2022; Seitz et al. 2024; Liu et al. 2022).

In obesity and MetS, this redox balance is disrupted due to mitochondrial dysfunction, increased activity of ROS-generating enzymes such as NADPH oxidase, and reduced levels of endogenous antioxidants, leading to OS (Chen et al. 2022; Colak and Pap 2021; Ilkun and Boudina 2013; Hajam et al. 2022). Excess ROS exerts direct toxic effects on cardiac cells, causing oxidative damage not only to mitochondria but also to other cellular components. They are implicated in maladaptive events such as endoplasmic reticulum stress, membrane lipid alterations, apoptosis, abnormal remodeling, and impaired Ca^{2+} handling, all of which contribute to diastolic and systolic dysfunction and increase susceptibility to HF (Carvajal et al. 2014; Chen et al. 2022; Ilkun and Boudina 2013; Gutiérrez-Cuevas et al. 2021). Moreover, chronic ROS overload, together with IR and lipotoxicity, exacerbates oxPTMs and accelerates myocardial deterioration (Li et al. 2022a).

Pathological oxPTMs include carbonylation, tyrosine nitration, S-glutathionylation, and thiol oxidation, among others, which impair the structure and function of proteins essential for myocardial contraction, mitochondrial metabolism, and intracellular signaling (Zima and Blatter 2006; Wende 2016; Santos et al. 2016; Tomin et al. 2019). At the mitochondrial level, these modifications reduce electron transport chain efficiency, decrease ATP synthesis, and promote cytochrome c release, ultimately leading to cardiomyocyte apoptosis (Wallace and Fan 2010). Furthermore, redox modifications of proteins involved in Ca^{2+} handling can directly impair cardiac contractility (Carvajal et al. 2014; Zima and Blatter 2006; Vincent et al. 2001). Therefore, identifying oxPTMs as molecular biomarkers and preventing excessive ROS production through antioxidant strategies may offer therapeutic benefits for preserving cardiac function.

5 oxPTMs in Mitochondrial Proteins That Contribute to Cardiac Dysfunction in Obesity and MetS

Since mitochondria are the primary source of energy in myocardial tissue, accounting for more than 90% of ATP production under physiological resting conditions, their coordinated function and adequate energy supply are essential for preserving cardiac performance. Growing evidence implicates mitochondrial dysfunction in the development of various cardiac diseases, including hypertrophy, ischemia, and HF (Li et al. 2022b). Representing over 30% of the heart's volume, mitochondria are also the major, although not exclusive, source of ROS in the heart, primarily generated through electron transfer during oxidative phosphorylation. Consequently, any disturbance in mitochondrial components can enhance ROS production, with the first targets of this excess ROS being the protein complexes involved in mitochondrial metabolism.

Excessive mitochondrial ROS impairs protein function by oxidizing critical amino acid residues that are essential for catalysis and structural integrity. These modifications, named oxPTMs, can disturb protein function in a reversible and irreversible mode, compromising ATP production and, by extension, cardiac

Table 1 oxPTMs in cardiac mitochondrial and Ca^{2+}-handling proteins reported in obesity and MetS

Protein	Modification	Effect on protein	Affected function	Reference
Drp 1	S-nitrosylation	Activation	Mitochondrial fission	Jin et al. (2021)
Drp 1	Acetylation	Stimulation	Mitochondrial fission	Hu et al. (2020)
Complex I	S-nitrosylation	Inhibition	MPTP opening	Haynes et al. (2004)
Complex II	S-nitrosylation	Inhibition	MPTP opening	Valdez et al. (2005)
Complex IV	Nitration	Inhibition	Electron transfer	Haynes et al. (2004)
mitCK	S-nitrosylation	Dimerization	MPTP opening	Brdiczka et al. (2006)
SERCA2a	Free-thiol oxidation	Inhibition	Diastolic dysfunction	Balderas-Villalobos et al. (2013)
SERCA2a	Carbonylation	Inhibition	Diastolic dysfunction	Li et al. (2006)
RyR2	Free-thiol oxidation	Inhibition/ Activation	Systolic dysfunction	Gómez-Viquez et al. (2023)/ Sánchez et al. (2018)
RyR2	Carbonylation	Activation	Systolic dysfunction	Roussel et al. (2015)
RyR2	S-nitrosylation	Activation	Systolic dysfunction	Roussel et al. (2015)

performance. oxPTMs include S-glutathionylation, S-nitrosylation, N-sulfenylation, and disulfide bond formation, among others, which occur at reactive cysteine residues, and nitration in tyrosine. In parallel, non-oxidative lysine acylations, including propionylation, crotonylation, and butyrylation, although not directly caused by oxidative mechanisms, can alter mitochondrial metabolism and potentially contribute to subsequent oxidative protein damage within these organelles (Marquez et al. 2016; Fang et al. 2025).

Some of the mechanisms in mitochondria that are dysregulated due to oxPTMs range from mitochondrial dynamics, Ca^{2+} homeostasis, ROS signaling, and protein-protein interaction (Table 1). These alterations lead to structural and functional impairments in the heart, ultimately resulting in a decline in cardiac performance. In MetS, cardiac mitochondria can enter a self-perpetuating cycle of OS, in which increased ROS production not only damages proteins but also affects other cellular components, such as lipids and DNA, driving the cell toward apoptosis and eventual death (Hu et al. 2022).

Mitochondrial dynamics comprise mitochondrial fission and fusion, movements relaying the turnover of these organelles. These processes can be altered by the S-nitrosylation of dynamin-related protein 1 (Drp1), a protein that induces mitochondrial fission and leads to mitochondrial fragmentation. Excessive fission caused by S-nitrosylation of Drp1 causes dysfunctional small mitochondria with fragmented cristae, contributing to the loss of energy that supports the electrogenic potential and contractile performance of cardiomyocytes (Jin et al. 2021). Furthermore, functional Drp1 has been demonstrated to be necessary for canonical Agt7-mediated mitochondrial mitophagy, which preserves mitochondrial function in the hearts of obese rats fed with a high-fat diet (HFD) (Xi Fang and Gustafsson 2023). Thus, PTMs of Drp1 may critically define its role in regulating mitochondrial autophagy. Indeed, in the early stages of HFD-induced obesity, phosphorylation of Drp1 at Ser 616 promotes its association with mitochondrial membranes, activating an alternative autophagy pathway mediated by Ulk1/Rab9, which may protect the heart from obesity-induced damage. By contrast, Drp1 acetylation at lysine 642 (K642) is increased in hearts from HFD-fed mice and cardiomyocytes exposed to palmitate. Concomitant with Drp1 acetylation, hearts from HFD-fed mice exhibit hypertrophy, fibrosis, IR, and cell death. Thus, excessive lipid supply appears to promote Drp1 acetylation, stimulating pathological mitochondrial fission and ultimately leading to cardiac dysfunction (Hu et al. 2020).

In obesity and MetS-related cardiomyopathy, mitochondrial nitric oxide synthase (NOS) is activated by low-grade inflammation and OS, leading to excessive mitochondrial NO production, which in turn promotes the overproduction of RNS, such as ·NO and $ONOO^-$ (Dedkova and Blatter 2009; Lacza et al. 2009; Ghafourifar and Sen 2007; Haynes et al. 2004; Valdez et al. 2005). RNS mediates oxPTMs through S-nitrosylation, which triggers the pathological formation of misfolded proteins, disrupts mitochondrial dynamics, and activates apoptotic pathways, ultimately causing disturbances in target vital organs (Nakamura and Lipton 2011). S-nitrosylation is proven to inhibit Complex I, which influences Ca^{2+}-dependent opening of the mitochondrial permeability transition pore (MPTP) that occurs as a cause or consequence of events such as ischemia/reperfusion episodes and inflammatory responses in the heart (Brdiczka et al. 2006).

Opening of MPTP occurs when protein-protein interactions among the complexes that build mitochondrial contact sites, junctions where the inner and outer mitochondrial membranes converge, undergo structural and conformational changes (Brdiczka et al. 2006). These changes disrupt contact site integrity and lead to the formation of non-selective pits, allowing the uncontrolled release of signaling molecules that serve as death triggers and disturb the proton gradient that maintains ATP production. These events prompt the signaling pathways of mitophagy, apoptosis, and necrosis. Among the proposed proteins involved in the opening of the cardiac MPTP under excessive ROS are cyclophylin D (CypD), voltage-dependent anion channel (VDAC), mitochondrial adenine nucleotide translocase (ANT), mitochondrial F1/F0 ATP synthase (F1/F0ATPase), mitochondrial phosphate carrier (PiC), mitochondrial creatine kinase (mCK), mitochondrial hexokinase II (mHk), and 18 kDa translocator protein (TSPO) (Alves-Figueiredo et al. 2021). Notably, nitration of ANT, VDAC, and F1/F0 ATPase, as well as S-nitrosylation of F1/F0 ATPase and CypD, have been reported to impact the opening of MPTP, resulting from a loss of protein interactions during cardiac ischemia/reperfusion

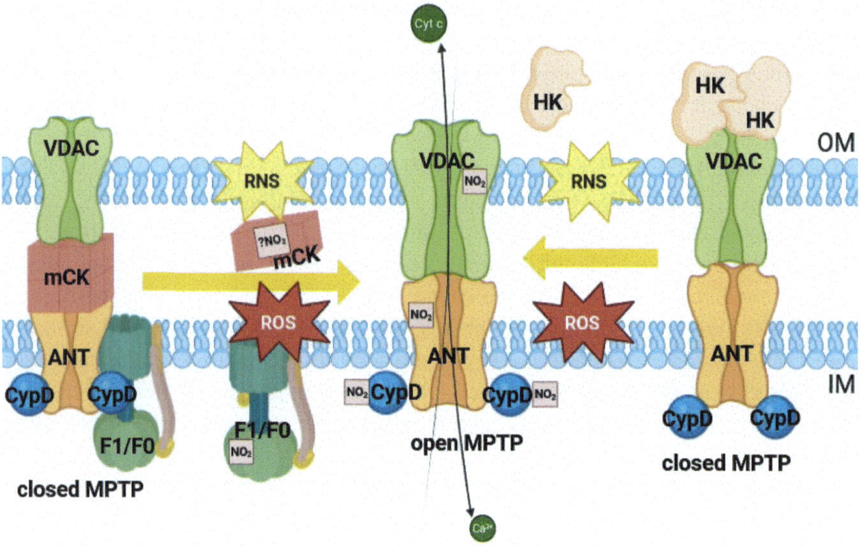

Fig. 1 Cardiac mitochondrial complexes involved in the formation of the mitochondrial permeability transition pore (MPTP). Under physiological conditions, contact sites between the outer membrane (OM) and inner membrane (IM) prevent MPTP opening by maintaining protein–protein interactions. These interactions are disrupted by the action of reactive oxygen species (ROS) and reactive nitrogen species (RNS), which induce oxidative post-translational modifications (oxPTMs) and trigger MPTP opening, ultimately leading to apoptosis and cell death. CypD cyclophylin D, VDAC voltage-dependent anion channel, ANT mitochondrial adenine nucleotide translocase, F1/F0 mitochondrial F1/F0 ATP synthase, mCK mitochondrial creatine kinase, HK hexokinase type II

injury and aging (Alves-Figueiredo et al. 2021; Cheng et al. 2010; Yang et al. 2019; Haynes et al. 2010; Das et al. 2012) (Fig. 1).

Some proteins of the mitochondrial electron transport chain have been identified as targets of S-nitrosylation. In addition to the previously documented inhibition of cytochrome c oxidase, Complexes I and IV are also inhibited by NO. While inhibition of Complex IV is easily reversible, inhibition of Complex I remains irreversible. Other cardiac metabolic enzymes are also susceptible to this oxidative modification, such as aconitase and several dehydrogenases from the Krebs cycle (Piantadosi 2012). The net effect on cardiac function is a decline in energy production, which compromises the ability of the obese and MetS heart to cope with harmful insults such as ischemia, increased workload, high energetic demands, or metabolic overcharge.

On the other hand, the decreased activity of mitochondrial complex II found in the hearts from rats fed a HFD has been related to reversible oxidation of Cys 89 and 231 in the SDHA subunit and Cys 100, 103, and 115 in the SDHB subunit (Sverdlov et al. 2015). Similarly, in a rat model of MetS induced by a high-sucrose diet (HSD), cardiac mitochondrial mCK activity was diminished and could be partially restored by dithiothreitol, a reducing agent. In addition to the enzymatic impairment, isolated hearts from HSD-fed rats exhibited reduced cardiac performance and diastolic dysfunction. Moreover, functional mCK in contact sites was disrupted (Carvajal et al. 2003; Carvajal et al. 2005). Although these studies did not identify specific oxPTMs in mCK, it is now clear that reversible and irreversible reduced activity of cardiac mitochondrial enzymes and electron transport complexes may result from oxidation of susceptible residues driven by excessive ROS and RNS during obesity and MetS.

6 oxPTMS in Ca^{2+} Handling Proteins That Contribute to Cardiac Dysfunction in Obesity and MetS

Mitochondrial OS in obesity and MetS not only impairs energy production but can also alter the function of cytosolic proteins, such as kinases, phosphatases, ion channels, and transporters, that are critical for intracellular Ca^{2+} homeostasis, thereby linking metabolic injury to mechanical dysfunction (Chen et al. 2022; Zima and Blatter 2006; Hajam et al. 2022; Arias-Chávez et al. 2022; Arias-Chávez et al. 2023a). In this context, studies in obese patients and experimental models of obesity and MetS have reported diastolic mechanical abnormalities in the heart characterized by prolonged relaxation. These studies also showed the presence of a subclinical systolic dysfunction manifested by a slight to moderately reduced ejection fraction and decreased fractional shortening (Carvajal et al. 2014; Ren et al. 2021; Gutiérrez-Cuevas et al. 2021). Although multiple factors contribute to both diastolic and systolic dysfunction, abnormal function of Ca^{2+} handling proteins is among the most relevant, with oxPTMs potentially playing a key role in these impairments (Table 1).

As is well established, ECC involves the activation of voltage-gated L-type Ca^{2+} channels (LCCs) during the action potential, generating an inward Ca^{2+} current (I_{Ca}) that triggers the opening of ryanodine receptor 2 (RyR2) channels in the sarcoplasmic reticulum (SR). RyR2-mediated SR Ca^{2+} release increases cytosolic Ca^{2+} concentration ($[Ca^{2+}]_c$), named the systolic Ca^{2+} transient, initiating contraction. Relaxation occurs as $[Ca^{2+}]_c$ returns to baseline, primarily via reuptake into the SR by SR Ca^{2+}-ATPase 2a (SERCA2a) and extrusion through the sarcolemma Na^+/Ca^{2+} exchanger (NCX) (Bers 2002). Notably, during diastole, RyR2 exhibits basal activity manifested as spontaneous Ca^{2+} sparks, which constitute a diastolic SR Ca^{2+} leak that is balanced by SERCA2a-mediated SR Ca^{2+} reuptake to determine the steady-state SR Ca^{2+} load and the amount of Ca^{2+} available for subsequent contraction (Shannon et al. 2002).

It has been shown that the activity of RyR2 and SERCA2a can be modulated by oxPTMs (Zima and Blatter 2006; Qin et al. 2014; Zima and Mazurek 2016), thereby placing these proteins under the regulatory influence of physiological levels of ROS and RNS to fine-tune cardiac performance. Indeed, elevated ROS production associated with increased cardiac demand has been suggested to augment systolic SR Ca^{2+} release, implying that oxPTMs in RyR2 may serve as a mechanism for positive inotropy in the healthy heart (Heinzel et al. 2006). Similarly, physiological

ROS levels can induce S-glutathionylation of SERCA2a, enhancing its activity and thereby improving both systolic and diastolic cardiomyocyte function (Qin et al. 2014). Consistent with this, we recently reported that basal ROS production in cardiomyocytes optimizes SR Ca^{2+} signaling during ECC by maintaining RyR2 and SERCA2a function (Gómez-Viquez et al. 2023).

By contrast, excessive ROS and RNS production in obesity and MetS can induce oxPTMs in Ca^{2+} handling proteins, disrupting their function and leading to diastolic and systolic cardiac dysfunction (Carvajal et al. 2014; Chen et al. 2022; Gómez-Viquez et al. 2023; Balderas-Villalobos et al. 2013; Li et al. 2006; Dong et al. 2006). Evidence from animal models of obesity and MetS has shown that diastolic dysfunction, characterized by prolonged systolic Ca^{2+} transients and delayed cell relaxation, is associated with decreased SERCA2a activity resulting from its oxidation (Carvajal et al. 2014; Chen et al. 2022; Balderas-Villalobos et al. 2013; Li et al. 2006). In this context, Li and coworkers reported that in ob/ob mice, impaired relaxation is linked to reduced SERCA2a activity due to augmented irreversible carbonyl oxidation (Li et al. 2006). Similarly, in cardiomyocytes from HSD-fed rats, we observed that decreased SERCA2a activity is associated with a reduced number of free thiol residues, as demonstrated by labeling with biotinylated iodoacetamide (Balderas-Villalobos et al. 2013). Collectively, these findings suggest that under pathological conditions, SERCA2a is susceptible to multiple oxPTMs that impair its activity. Indeed, in HF and aging, reduced SERCA2a activity has been associated with sulfonylation at Cys 674, nitration at Tyr 294/295, as well as decreased free thiol content (Carvajal et al. 2014; Qin et al. 2014). Whether these specific residues in SERCA2a are modified in obesity and MetS remains to be determined.

Systolic cardiac dysfunction in obesity and MetS is characterized by blunted cell shortening, which in some studies has been linked to reduced amplitude of systolic Ca^{2+} transients (Carvajal et al. 2014; Balderas-Villalobos et al. 2013). Although the role of ROS and RNS in systolic dysfunction under these diseases has been less extensively studied, some reports suggest that it may involve abnormal RyR2 activity due to oxPTMs (Gómez-Viquez et al. 2023; Sánchez et al. 2018; Roussel et al. 2015). In this context, we provided evidence that OS in ventricular myocytes from HSD-fed rats contributes not only to a depressed amplitude of systolic Ca^{2+} transients but also to decreased frequency of diastolic Ca^{2+} sparks. In the same work, we found that these alterations were accompanied by diminished RyR2 activity linked to decreased levels of free reactive thiols in the channel (Gómez-Viquez et al. 2023). These findings suggest that OS in obesity and MetS may blunt SR Ca^{2+} release by inducing oxPTMs in Cys residues of RyR2, ultimately leading to reduced channel function. In contrast, another study reported that triggering of cardiac arrhythmias in HFD-fed mice is associated with increased RyR2 activity, which coincided with a marked reduction in free thiol residues in the channel, suggesting that oxPTMs were responsible for its hyperactivation (Sánchez et al. 2018). The reasons for these discrepancies remain unclear but may be related to differences in the experimental model, species, or stage of cardiomyopathy progression. Nevertheless, further detailed investigations are required to identify the specific oxPTMs and amino acids that impair RyR2 function in obesity and MetS. In this regard,

S-nitrosylation, S-glutathionylation, and disulfide oxidation have been described as modulators of RyR2 activity, with the latter being the predominant modification involved in the abnormal increase in RyR2 activity observed in HF (Carvajal et al. 2014; Zima and Blatter 2006; Zima and Mazurek 2016). Indeed, S-nitrosylation of RyR2 appears to exert a protective effect against OS by preventing irreversible oxidation of Cys residues within these channels (Zima and Mazurek 2016). Notably, incubation of cardiomyocytes with palmitoyl-carnitine increases RyR2 carbonylation and S-nitrosylation, leading to increased SR Ca^{2+} leak, which contributes to reduced systolic Ca^{2+} transient amplitude and SR Ca^{2+} load (Roussel et al. 2015).

7 Emerging Antioxidant Therapies

Given the central role of OS in the development of cardiac dysfunction associated with obesity and MetS, antioxidants represent a promising therapeutic strategy. Among natural antioxidants, polyphenols such as resveratrol, quercetin, and curcumin have demonstrated in preclinical models the capacity to activate the Nrf2 pathway, downregulate pro-inflammatory genes, and enhance mitochondrial bioenergetics (Savova et al. 2025; Mohib et al. 2018).

Lycopene, a carotenoid abundant in tomatoes, is recognized as one of the most potent dietary antioxidants (Arias-Chávez et al. 2023b). Its strong capacity to scavenge ROS, particularly peroxyl radicals and singlet oxygen, protects lipid membranes from oxidative damage. Evidence indicates that lycopene improves endothelial function, attenuates systemic inflammation, and modulates antioxidant protein expression through Nrf2 activation in animal models of MetS (Albrahim and Robert 2022; Gajendragadkar et al. 2014; Cheng et al. 2017). From a clinical perspective, the administration of lycopene at doses $\geq$25 mg per day has been shown to effectively reduce LDL cholesterol levels by approximately 10%, an effect comparable to that of low-dose statins in patients with mild hypercholesterolemia. In addition, a significant reduction in systolic blood pressure has been documented, further supporting its potential as a cardioprotective agent (Ried and Fakler 2011). Furthermore, lycopene inhibits cardiac hypertrophy through the suppression of ROS-dependent mechanisms. In in vitro models (neonatal Sprague-Dawley rat cardiomyocytes) and in vivo models (C57BL/6 mice), it has been shown to significantly block pressure overload–induced hypertrophy, reverse the increase in ROS generation during the hypertrophic process, and delay the activation of pro-hypertrophic signaling pathways mediated by MAPK and Akt (Zeng et al. 2019).

Legume sprouts, including lentils, chickpeas, beans, and soybeans, are characterized by a marked enrichment in phenolic compounds and enzymatic antioxidants. On the other hand, it has been reported in diabetic murine models that legume sprouts such as faba bean (*Vicia faba L.*), lentil (*Lens esculenta L.*), chickpea (*Cicer arietinum L.*), and fenugreek (*Trigonella foenum-graecum L.*) exert a hypoglycemic effect, decrease triglycerides and LDL cholesterol, increase HDL cholesterol, and have a potential antioxidant effect by enhancing SOD and GSH activity and reducing malondialdehyde (MDA) levels (Farag et al. 2022). These effects are attributed to the presence of flavonoids, isoflavones, and antioxidant enzymes such as SOD, which mitigate oxPTMs in cardiac proteins. Moreover, sprouted legumes activate endogenous antioxidant defenses through the Keap1/Nrf2/ARE axis, thereby reinforcing mitochondrial resilience and promoting cardiomyocyte survival under OS (Khang et al. 2016; Zhou et al. 2021).

Resveratrol can modulate the Nrf2/ARE pathway, reduce H_2O_2 production, and inhibit MAPK, leading to improvements in insulin sensitivity, lipolysis, and endothelial function (Zhou et al. 2021). However, its clinical translation is limited by low bioavailability. Selenium, an essential trace element, constitutes a key component of antioxidant enzymes such as GPx and thioredoxin reductase (TrxR) (Arias-Chávez et al. 2023b). Selenium deficiency has been linked to increased risk of cardiomyopathy, hypertension, and IR. Its supplementation restores mitochondrial antioxidant activity, reduces cardiac inflammation, and contributes to favorable ventricular remodeling in obesity models (Bhattarai et al. 2024). However, meta-analyses and systematic reviews have shown that, in both preclinical and clinical studies, exposure to high levels of selenium was associated with an increased risk of diabetes and prediabetes (Shao et al. 2022). Other trace elements such as zinc, manganese, and magnesium also play important roles in ROS neutralization and mitochondrial DNA protection, with evidence supporting their preventive roles against OS-induced cardiac damage (Cai et al. 2023; Hasani et al. 2024; Bo and Pisu 2008; Boden et al. 2012).

Coenzyme Q10, although an effective antioxidant, exhibits limited mitochondrial penetration. In contrast, mitochondria-targeted derivatives such as MitoQ have demonstrated superior efficacy. Preclinical studies show that MitoQ reduces adiposity, dyslipidemia, hyperglycemia, and oxidative DNA damage in HFD models, while improving mitochondrial metabolism, attenuating hypertrophy, and preventing cardiomyocyte apoptosis (Feillet-Coudray et al. 2014; Mercer et al. 2012; Rossman et al. 2018). In obese rats, MitoQ prevented cardiac hypertrophy and fibrosis, restored glucose reuptake, and normalized mitochondrial proteins, including complexes I/II and fumarase. Clinical trials in humans reported improvements in endothelial function and reductions in LDL oxidation and systolic blood pressure, although outcomes remain inconsistent. Similarly, SkQ-type analogs (plastoquinones conjugated with triphenylphosphonium, TPP^+) demonstrate enhanced mitochondrial accumulation and provide sustained protection of mitochondrial DNA and function (Feillet-Coudray et al. 2014; Mercer et al. 2012; Rossman et al. 2018; Jia et al. 2025).

Despite these advances, the clinical utility of antioxidants remains limited by factors such as poor bioavailability, instability, and lack of molecular specificity. Therefore, antioxidant therapy should be integrated with lifestyle interventions, including a balanced diet, regular physical activity, and strict glycemic control. Furthermore, systematic monitoring of OS biomarkers such as oxPTMs, MDA, DNA oxidative damage markers, and systemic inflammation mediators is essential to assess therapeutic efficacy and optimize antioxidant-based strategies for individualized patient care.

8 Conclusion

Recent advances in biochemical research on proteins, particularly high-resolution mass spectrometry, redox proteomics approaches (such as biotin-switch assays and resin-assisted capture), and structural methods including cryo-electron microscopy, have enabled the precise identification of specific amino acid residues modified in key proteins that regulate cardiac function, mostly those targeted by ROS and RNS. The consequences of these modifications have been characterized at the molecular, cellular, and organ levels in various experimental models. Nevertheless, their direct contribution to cardiac dysfunction in the context of obesity and MetS remains poorly defined. Mitochondrial and Ca^{2+}-handling proteins are especially critical for sustaining myocardial performance and constitute primary sites of injury that may extend beyond the heart to other vital organs. Addressing these gaps requires further investigation to design strategies that restore health in the setting of the global obesity and MetS pandemic. Within this framework, antioxidant-based therapies represent a promising and continuously evolving approach to counteract the deleterious effects of oxPTMs on cardiac function. The future of this field will depend on the integration of combination therapies, the application of molecular biomarkers, and the personalization of treatments according to each patient's metabolic profile.

Acknowledgments We thank the Instituto Nacional de Pediatría for its support through program E022 (INP 2018/038).

Conflict of Interest Authors declare no conflict of interest.

References

Albrahim T, Robert AA (2022) Lycopene effects on metabolic syndrome and kidney injury in rats fed a high-fat diet: an experimental study. ACS Omega 7(35):30930–30938

Alves-Figueiredo H, Silva-Platas C, Lozano O, Vázquez-Garza E, Guerrero-Beltrán CE, Zarain-Herzberg A, García-Rivas G (2021) A systematic review of post-translational modifications in the mitochondrial permeability transition pore complex associated with cardiac diseases. Biochim Biophys Acta Mol basis Dis 1867(1):165992

Arias-Chávez DJ, Mailloux-Salinas P, Altamirano J, Huang F, Gómez-Viquez NL, Bravo G (2022) Consumption of combined fructose and sucrose diet exacerbates oxidative stress, hypertrophy and $CaMKII_{\delta}$ oxidation in hearts from rats with metabolic syndrome. Mol Cell Biochem 477(4). 1309–1320

Arias-Chávez DJ, Mailloux-Salinas P, Aparicio JL, Bravo G, Gómez-Viquez NL (2023a) Combined fructose and sucrose consumption from an early age aggravates cardiac oxidative damage and causes a dilated cardiomyopathy in SHR rats. J Clin Biochem Nutr 73(3):205–213

Arias-Chávez DJ, Mailloux-Salinas P, Ledesma-Aparicio J, Campos-Pérez E, Medina-Campos ON, Pedraza-Chaverri J, Bravo G (2023b) Selenium in combination with a tomato lipid extract as a therapy for benign prostatic hyperplasia and its alterations in rats with induced BPH. J Cell Mol Med 27(20):3147–3156

Balderas-Villalobos J, Molina-Muñoz T, Mailloux-Salinas P, Bravo G, Carvajal K, Gómez-Viquez NL (2013) Oxidative stress in cardiomyocytes contributes to decreased SERCA2a activity in rats with metabolic syndrome. Am J Physiol Heart Circ Physiol 305(9):H1344–H1353

Bers DM (2002) Cardiac excitation-contraction coupling. Nature 415:198–205

Bhattarai U, Xu R, He X, Pan L, Niu Z, Wang D, Zeng H, Chen JX, Clemmer JS, Chen Y (2024) High selenium diet attenuates pressure overload-induced cardiopulmonary oxidative stress, inflammation, and heart failure. Redox Biol 76:103325

Bo S, Pisu E (2008) Role of dietary magnesium in cardiovascular disease prevention, insulin sensitivity and diabetes. Curr Opin Lipidol 19(1):50–56

Boden MJ, Brandon AE, Tid-Ang JD, Preston E, Wilks D, Stuart E, Cleasby ME, Turner N, Cooney GJ, Kraegen EW (2012) Overexpression of manganese superoxide dismutase ameliorates high-fat diet-induced insulin resistance in rat skeletal muscle. Am J Physiol Endocrinol Metab 303(6):E798–E805

Brdiczka DG, Zorov DB, Sheu SS (2006) Mitochondrial contact sites: their role in energy metabolism and apoptosis. Biochim Biophys Acta 1762(2):148–163

Caballero B (2007) The global epidemic of obesity, an overview. Epidemiol Rev 29:1–5

Cai L, Tan Y, Watson S, Wintergerst K (2023) Diabetic cardiomyopathy - zinc preventive and therapeutic potentials by its anti-oxidative stress and sensitizing insulin signaling pathways. Toxicol Appl Pharmacol 477:116694

Carvajal K, Baños G, Moreno-Sánchez R (2003) Impairment of glucose metabolism and energy transfer in the rat heart. Mol Cell Biochem 249:157165

Carvajal K, El Hafidi M, Marin-Hernández A, Moreno-Sánchez R (2005) Structural and functional changes in heart mitochondria from sucrose-fed hypertriglyceridemic rats. Biochim Biophys Acta 1709(3):231–239

Carvajal K, Balderas-Villalobos J, Bello-Sanchez MD, Phillips-Farfán B, Molina-Muñoz T, Aldana-Quintero H, Gómez-Viquez NL (2014) Ca^{2+} mishandling and cardiac dysfunction in obesity and insulin resistance: role of oxidative stress. Cell Calcium 56:408–415

Chen Z, Jin ZX, Cai J, Li R, Deng KQ, Ji YX, Lei F, Li HP, Lu Z, Li H (2022) Energy substrate metabolism and oxidative stress in metabolic cardiomyopathy. J Mol Med 100:1721–1739

Cheng Q, Sedlic F, Pravdic D, Bosnjak ZJ, Kwok WM (2010) Biphasic effect of nitric oxide on the cardiac voltage-dependent anion channel. FEBS Lett 585:328–334

Cheng HM, Koutsidis G, Lodge JK, Ashor A, Siervo M, Lara J (2017) Tomato and lycopene supplementation and cardiovascular risk factors: a systematic review and meta-analysis. Atherosclerosis 257:100–108

Colak E, Pap D (2021) The role of oxidative stress in the development of obesity and obesity-related metabolic disorders. J Med Biochem 40(1):1–9

Das S, Steenbergen C, Murphy E (2012) Does the voltage dependent anion channel modulate cardiac ischemia-reperfusion injury? Biochim Biophys Acta 1818(6):1451–1456

Dedkova EN, Blatter LA (2009) Characteristics and function of cardiac mitochondrial nitric oxide synthase. J Physiol 587(4):851–872

Dong F, Fang CX, Yang X, Zhang X, Lopez FL, Ren J (2006) Cardiac overexpression of catalase rescues cardiac contractile dysfunction induced by insulin resistance: role of oxidative stress, protein carbonyl formation and insulin sensitivity. Diabetologia 49(6):1421–1433

Fang J, Wu S, Zhao H, Zhou C, Xue L, Lei Z, Li H, Shan Z (2025) New types of post-translational. Modification of proteins in cardiovascular diseases. J Cardiovasc Transl Res 18:634–649

Farag MA, Naser AF, Zayed A, Sharaf El-Dine MG (2022) Comparative insights into four major legume sprouts efficacies for diabetes management and its complications: untargeted versus targeted NMR biochemometrics approach. Metabolites 13(1):63

Feillet-Coudray C, Fouret G, Ebabe-Elle R, Rieusset J, Bonafos B, Chabi B, Crouzier D, Zarkovic K, Zarkovic N, Ramos J, Badia E, Murphy MP, Cristol JP, Coudray C (2014) The mitochondrial-targeted antioxidant MitoQ ameliorates metabolic syndrome features in obesogenic diet-fed rats better than Apocynin or allopurinol. Free Radic Res 48(10):1232–1246

Gajendragadkar PR, Hubsch A, Mäki-Petäjä KM, Serg M, Wilkinson IB, Cheriyan J (2014) Effects of oral lycopene supplementation on vascular function in patients with cardiovascular disease and healthy volunteers: a randomised controlled trial. PLoS One 9(6):e99070

Ghafourifar P, Sen CK (2007) Mitochondrial nitric oxide synthase. Front Biosci 12:1072–1078

Gómez-Viquez NL, Balderas-Villalobos J, Bello-Sánchez MD, Mayorga-Luna M, Mailloux-Salinas P, García-Castañeda M, Ríos-Pérez EB, Mártinez-Ávila MA, Camacho-Castillo LDC, Bravo G, Ávila G, Altamirano J, Carvajal K (2023) Oxidative stress in early metabolic syndrome impairs cardiac RyR2 and SERCA2a activity and modifies the interplay of these proteins during Ca^{2+} waves. Arch Physiol Biochem 129(5):1058–1070

Gutiérrez-Cuevas J, Sandoval-Rodriguez A, Meza-Rios A, Monroy-Ramírez HC, Galicia-Moreno-M, García-Bañuelos J, Santos A, Armendariz-Borunda J (2021) Molecular mechanisms of obesity-linked cardiac dysfunction: an up-date on current knowledge. Cells 10:629

Hajam YA, Rani R, Ganie SY, Sheikh TA, Javaid D, Qadri SS, Pramodh S, Alsulimani A, Alkhanani MF, Harakeh S et al (2022) Oxidative stress in human pathology and aging: molecular mechanisms and perspectives. Cells 11(3):552

Hammad M, Raftari M, Cesario R, Salma R, Godoy P, Emami S, Haghdoost S (2023) Roles of oxidative stress and Nrf2 signaling in pathogenic and non-pathogenic cells. A possible general mechanism of resistance to therapy. Antioxidants 12(7):1371

Hasani M, Monfared V, Aleebrahim-Dehkordi E, Jafari A, Agh F, Khazdouz M, Vahid F, Vafa M (2024) The effect of selenium, zinc, and their combined supplementation on cardiometabolic biomarkers-comparing their effects in the energy restriction and high-fat diet methods in obese rats. Curr Mol Med 24(10):1307–1315

Haynes V, Elfering S, Traaseth N, Giulivi C (2004) Mitochondrial nitric-oxide synthase: enzyme expression, characterization, and regulation. J Bioenerg Biomembr 36(4):341–346

Haynes V, Traaseth NJ, Elfering S, Fujisawa Y, Giulivi C (2010) Nitration of specific tyrosines in F0F1 ATP synthase and activity loss in aging. Am J physiol Endocrinol Metab 298(5):E978–E987

Heinzel FR, Luo Y, Dodoni G, Boengler K, Petrat F, Di Lisa F, de Groot H, Schulz R, Heusch G (2006) Formation of reactive oxygen species at increased contraction frequency in rat cardiomyocytes. Cardiovasc Res 71(2):374–382

Hu Q, Zhang H, Gutiérrez-Cortés N, Wu D, Wang P, Zhang J, Mattison JA, Smith E, Bettcher LF, Wang M, Lakatta EG, Sheu SS, Wang W (2020) Increased Drp1 acetylation by lipid overload induces cardiomyocyte death and heart dysfunction. Circ Res 126(4):456–470

Hu J, Wen X, Long P, Xiong S, Lui H, Cai L, Deng H, Zhang Z (2022) The role of post-translational modifications in driving abnormal cardiovascular complications at high altitude. Front Cardiovasc Med 9:886300

Ilkun O, Boudina S (2013) Cardiac dysfunction and oxidative stress in the metabolic syndrome: an update on antioxidant therapies. Curr Pharm Des 19(27):4806–4817

Jia G, Jia Y, Sowers JR (2016) Contribution of maladaptive adipose tissue expansion to development of cardiovascular disease. Compr Physiol 7:253–262

Jia H, Song Y, Hua Y, Li K, Li S, Wang Y (2025) Molecular mechanism of aerobic exercise ameliorating myocardial mitochondrial injury in mice with heart failure. Int J Mol Sci 26(5):2136

Jin JY, Wei XX, Zhi XL, Wang XH, Meng D (2021) Drp1-dependent mitochondrial fission in cardiovascular disease. Acta Pharmacol Sin 42(5):655–664

Khang DT, Dung TN, Elzaawely AA, Xuan TD (2016) Phenolic profiles and antioxidant activity of germinated legumes. Foods 5(2):27

Lacza Z, Pankotai E, Busija DW (2009) Mitochondrial nitric oxide synthase: current concepts and controversies. Front Biosci (Landmark Edition) 14(12):4436–4443

Li SY, Yang X, Ceylan-Isik AF, Du M, Sreejayan N, Ren J (2006) Cardiac contractile dysfunction in Lep/Lep obesity is accompanied by NADPH oxidase activation, oxidative modification of sarco(endo)plasmic reticulum Ca^{2+}-ATPase and myosin heavy chain isozyme switch. Diabetologia 49(6):1434–1446

Li A, Zheng N, Ding X (2022a) Mitochondrial abnormalities: a hub in metabolic syndrome-related cardiac dysfunction caused by oxidative stress. Heart Fail Rev 27(4):1387–1394

Li J, Li J, Chen Y, Hu W, Gong X, Qiu H, Chen H, Xin Y, Li H (2022b) The role of mitochondria in metabolic syndrome-associated cardiomyopathy. Oxidative Med Cell Longev 2022:9196232

Liu YP, Zhang TN, Wen R, Liu CF, Yang N (2022) Role of posttranslational modifications of proteins in cardiovascular disease. Oxid Med Cell Longev 2022:1–16

Marquez J, Lee SR, Kim N, Han J (2016) Post-translational modifications of cardiac mitochondrial proteins in cardiovascular disease: not lost in translation. Korean Circ J 46:1

Masenga SK, Kabwe LS, Chakulya M, Kirabo A (2023) Mechanisms of oxidative stress in metabolic syndrome. Int J Mol Sci 24:7898

Mercer JR, Yu E, Figg N, Cheng KK, Prime TA, Griffin JL, Masoodi M, Vidal-Puig A, Murphy MP, Bennett MR (2012) The mitochondria-targeted antioxidant MitoQ decreases features of the metabolic syndrome in ATM+/−/ApoE−/− mice. Free Radic Biol Med 52(5):841–849

Mohib M, Afnan K, Paran TZ, Khan S, Sarker J, Hasan N, Hasan I, Sagor AT (2018) Beneficial role of citrus fruit polyphenols against hepatic dysfunctions: a review. J Diet Suppl 15(2):223–250

Nakamura T, Lipton SA (2011) S-Nitrosylation of critial protein thiols mediates protein misfolding and mitochondrial dysfunction in neurodegenerative diseases. Antioxid Redox Signal 14(8): 1479–1492

Perjés Á, Kubin AM, Kónyi A, Szabados S, Cziráki A, Skoumal R, Ruskoaho H, Szokodi I (2012) Physiological regulation of cardiac contractility by endogenous reactive oxygen species. Acta Physiol 205(1):26–40

Piantadosi C (2012) Regulation of mitochondrial processes by protein S-nitrosyltion. Biochim Biophys Acta 1820:712–721

Pulinilkunnil T, Rodrigues B (2006) Cardiac lipoprotein lipase: metabolic basis for diabetic heart disease. Cardiovasc Res 69(2):329–340

Qin F, Cohen RA, Colucci WS (2014) Regulation of SERCA via oxidative modifications: implications for the pathophysiology of diastolic dysfunction in the aging heart. In: Jugdutt B (ed) Aging and heart failure. Springer, New York

Ren J, Wu NN, Wang S, Sowers JR, Zhang Y (2021) Obesity cardiomyopathy: evidence, mechanisms, and therapeutic implications. Physiol Rev 101(4):1745–1807

Ried K, Fakler P (2011) Protective effect of lycopene on serum cholesterol and blood pressure: meta-analyses of intervention trials. Maturitas 68(4):299–310

Rossman MJ, Santos-Parker JR, Steward CAC, Bispham NZ, Cuevas LM, Rosenberg HL, Woodward KA, Chonchol M, Gioscia-Ryan RA, Murphy MP, Seals DR (2018) Chronic supplementation with a mitochondrial antioxidant (MitoQ) improves vascular function in healthy older adults. Hypertension 71(6):1056–1063

Roussel J, Thireau J, Brenner C, Saint N, Scheuermann V, Lacampagne A, Le Guennec JY, Fauconnier J (2015) Palmitoyl-carnitine increases RyR2 oxidation and sarcoplasmic reticulum Ca^{2+} leak in cardiomyocytes: role of adenine nucleotide translocase. Biochim Biophys Acta 1852(5):749–758

Sánchez G, Araneda F, Peña JP, Finkelstein JP, Riquelme JA, Montecinos L, Barrientos G, Llanos P, Pedrozo Z, Said M, Bull R, Donoso P (2018) High-fat-diet-induced obesity produces spontaneous ventricular arrhythmias and increases the activity of ryanodine receptors in mice. Int J Mol Sci 19(2):533

Santos CXC, Raza S, Shah AM (2016) Redox signaling in the cardiomyocyte: from physiology to failure. Int J Biochem Cell Biol 74:145–151

Savova MS, Todorova MN, Binev BK, Georgiev MI, Mihaylova LV (2025) Curcumin enhances the anti-obesogenic activity of orlistat through SKN-1/NRF2-dependent regulation of nutrient metabolism in Caenorhabditis elegans. Int J Obes 49(3):516–526

Seitz A, Busch M, Kroemer J, Schneider A, Simon S, Jungmann A, Katus HA, Most P, Ritterhoff J (2024) S100A1's single cysteine is an indispensable redox switch for the protection against diastolic calcium waves in cardiomyocytes. Am J Physiol Heart Circ Physiol 327(1):H275–H286

Shannon TR, Ginsburg KS, Bers DM (2002) Quantitative assessment of the SR Ca^{2+} leak-load relationship. Circ Res 91:594–600

Shao R, Su L, Li L, Wu J, He X, Mao D, Cheng Y, Liu J, Chen C, Jin Y, Gao S (2022) Higher selenium was associated with higher risk of diabetes: consistent evidence from longitudinal and cross-sectional studies based on nail and serum selenium measures. Sci Total Environ 840: 156618

Sverdlov AL, Elezaby A, Behring JB, Bachschmid MM, Luptak I, Tu VH, Siwik DA, Miller EJ, Liesa M, Shirihai OS, Pimentel DR, Cohen RA, Colucci WS (2015) High fat, high sucrose diet causes cardiac mitochondrial dysfunction due in part to oxidative post-translational modification of mitochondrial complex II. J Mol Cell Cardiol 78:165–173

Tomin T, Schittmayer M, Honeder S, Heininger C, Birner-Gruenberger R (2019) Irreversible oxidative post-translational modifications in heart disease. Expert Rev Proteomics 16(8): 681–693

Valdez LB, Zaobornyj T, Boveris A (2005) Functional activity of mitochondrial nitric oxide synthase. Methods Enzymol 396:444–455

Vincent HK, Powers SK, Dirks AJ, Scarpace PJ (2001) Mechanism for obesity-induced increase in myocardial lipid peroxidation. Int J Obes 25:378–388

Wallace DC, Fan W (2010) Energetics, epigenetics, mitocondrial genetics. Mitochondrion 10(1): 12–31

Wende AR (2016) Post-translational modifications of the cardiac proteome in diabetes and heart failure. Proteomics Clin Appl 10(1):25–38

World Health Organization (n.d.) Obesity and Overweight. Web site. Available online: https://www.who.int/news-room/fact-sheets/detail/obesity-and-overweight

Xi Fang X, Gustafsson AB (2023) DRP1-mediated mitophagy: safeguarding obese hearts from cardiomyopathy. Circ Res 133:22–24

Yang M, Xu Y, Heisner JS, Sun J, Stowe DF, Kwok WM, Camara AKS (2019) Peroxynitrite nitrates adenine nucleotide translocase and voltage-dependent anion channel 1 and alters their interactions and association with hexokinase II in mitochondria. Mitochondrion 46:380–392

Zeng J, Zhao J, Dong B, Cai X, Jiang J, Xue R, Yao F, Dong Y, Liu C (2019) Lycopene protects against pressure overload-induced cardiac hypertrophy by attenuating oxidative stress. J Nutr Biochem 66:70–78

Zhou Z, Fan Z, Meenu M, Xu B (2021) Impact of germination time on resveratrol, phenolic acids, and antioxidant capacities of different varieties of Peanut (*Arachis hypogaea* Linn.) from China. Antioxidants 10(11):1714

Zima A, Blatter LA (2006) Redox regulation of cardiac calcium channels and transporters. Cardiovasc Res 71(2):310–321

Zima A, Mazurek SR (2016) Functional impact of ryanodine receptor oxidation on intracellular calcium regulation in the heart. Rev Physiol Biochem Pharmacol 171:39–62

Role of Innate Immune Receptors in Cardiac Damage Linked to Metabolic Disorders

Almudena Val-Blasco, Marta Gil-Fernández, Andrea Bueno-Sen, Paula Cantolla-Pablo, María Fernández-Velasco, and Patricia Prieto

Contents

Abstract

This chapter underscores the pivotal role of immune receptors, particularly Toll-like receptors (TLRs) and NOD-like receptors (NLRs), in the intricate interplay between metabolic diseases and their associated cardiovascular comorbidities. Their involvement extends beyond mere initiation, profoundly influencing the progression of these complex conditions. The recognition of TLRs and NLRs as promising therapeutic targets is a significant advancement, offering potential avenues for intervention in both metabolic disorders and their cardiovascular sequels.

The significance of these pattern recognition receptors (PRRs) lies in their capacity to orchestrate inflammatory responses, a critical factor in the pathogenesis of metabolic diseases. Dysregulation of these pathways contributes to chronic,

A. Val-Blasco (✉) · M. Gil-Fernández (✉) · A. Bueno-Sen · P. Cantolla-Pablo · M. Fernández-Velasco
Instituto de Investigación Hospital Universitario la PAZ, IdiPAZ, Madrid, Spain

P. Prieto (✉)
Departamento de Farmacología, Farmacognosia y Botánica, Facultad de Farmacia, Universidad Complutense de Madrid, Madrid, Spain
e-mail: patpri02@ucm.es

A. Rueda, M. Nieves-Cintrón (eds.), *Cardiovascular Alterations in Metabolic Diseases*, Handbook of Experimental Pharmacology 293,
https://doi.org/10.1007/164_2026_793

low-grade inflammation, a hallmark of conditions such as obesity and type 2 diabetes. This persistent inflammation, in turn, fuels the development of cardiovascular complications such as atherosclerosis, hypertension, and heart failure.

Targeting TLRs and NLRs presents a strategic approach to modulate these inflammatory cascades. By selectively inhibiting or modulating the activity of these receptors, it may be possible to mitigate the detrimental effects of chronic inflammation and prevent or delay the onset of associated comorbidities. However, this approach requires a thorough understanding of the specific TLR and NLR subtypes involved in various disease processes, as well as the intricate signaling pathways they activate.

Furthermore, the development of therapeutic strategies targeting PRRs must consider the potential for off-target effects and the need for personalized medicine. Given the diverse expression patterns and functional roles of TLRs and NLRs across various cell types and tissues, a tailored approach is essential to maximize efficacy and minimize adverse effects. Consequently, ongoing research is focused on identifying specific ligands and inhibitors that can selectively target these receptors, paving the way for novel therapeutic interventions.

Keywords

Cardiovascular problems · *Diabetes mellitus* · Innate immune response · Nucleotide oligomerization-like receptor · Toll-like receptor

1 Introduction

The innate immune system serves as a fundamental defense mechanism against pathogens and cellular damage. This response is orchestrated through pattern recognition receptors (PRRs), which recognize both pathogen-associated molecular patterns (PAMPs) and cell damage-associated molecular patterns (DAMPs) (Kawai and Akira 2010). As a consequence of cellular damage, the innate immune response is activated through these receptors, triggering various signaling cascades that initiate inflammatory responses. However, dysregulation of these pathways may contribute to the development of autoimmune and chronic inflammatory diseases (Midwood and Piccinini 2010), as well as increase the risk of infections by impairing the immune system's capacity to recognize and respond appropriately to both pathogens and endogenous danger signals.

PRRs are widely expressed in immune cells, including macrophages, dendritic cells, neutrophils, as well as non-immune cells such as cardiomyocytes, vascular endothelial cells, and intestinal epithelial cells. They are located both on the cell surface and intracellularly, enabling the detection of extracellular and intracellular pathogens. PRRs are classified into four different families: Toll-like receptors (TLRs), C-type lectin receptors (CLRs), nucleotide-binding oligomerization domain (NOD)-like receptors (NLRs), and retinoic acid-inducible gene (RIG)-like receptors

(RLRs) (Brubaker et al. 2015; Takeuchi and Akira 2010). In addition, it has been described that non-canonical PRRs, such as the receptors for advanced glycation end products (RAGE), bind to advanced glycation end products and other DAMPs, and the cyclic GMP-AMP synthase (cGAS), the principal intracellular DNA sensors in vertebrates (Cross et al. 2024; Dvorkin et al. 2024). The RAGE are multiligand immunoglobulins that are widely expressed across all organs but are especially abundant in the lungs. RAGE activation triggers the signaling pathways of STAT and MAPK (Cross et al. 2024). Related to cGAS PRRs, they are a member of the nucleotidyltransferase family that binds to double-stranded DNA in a sequence-independent fashion, activating the stimulator of IFN genes (STING) and triggering the NF-κB transcription factor to induce the expression of proinflammatory cytokines and chemokines (Dvorkin et al. 2024).

Among all PRRs, TLRs are one of the best characterized. These class I transmembrane proteins are expressed on the plasma membrane and within intracellular compartments such as endosomes and lysosomes. TLRs consist of an N-terminal domain primarily composed of leucine-rich repeats (LRRs) for ligand recognition, a transmembrane segment, and a cytoplasmic Toll/interleukin-1 (IL-1) receptor (TIR) homology domain, essential for downstream signaling (Kawai and Akira 2010; McGettrick and O'Neill 2007). Pathogen recognition by TLRs initiates a signaling cascade that activates transcription factors such as nuclear factor-kappa B (NF-κB) and interferon regulatory factors (IRFs) (Yuk and Jo 2011), resulting in the production of pro-inflammatory cytokines and type I interferons.

Another key family of PRRs is the NLR family, which includes intracellular receptors that detect invading pathogens and initiate immune responses (Nakamura et al. 2014). NLRs share a standard structure consisting of an N-terminal protein-binding motif, a central nucleotide-binding domain (NACHT domain), and a C-terminal LRR domain. Based on their N-terminal region, NLRs are subdivided into four subfamilies. The NLRC subfamily comprises NOD receptors, which harbor caspase activation and recruitment domains (CARDs) that drive the transcriptional activation of inflammatory mediators. The NLRP subfamily, which includes NLRP3, harbors a pyrin domain and plays a pivotal role in inflammasome formation, thereby regulating caspase-1 activation. Although initially characterized in immune cells such as macrophages and monocytes, recent research has revealed NLR expression in specialized cell types, including cardiomyocytes, vascular endothelial cells, and adipocytes, among others (Harati et al. 2024; González-Ramos et al. 2019; Sharma et al. 2021b; Li and Shang 2024).

Beyond their significant role in immunity, both TLRs and NLRs are involved in several pathological processes, including metabolic disorders, such as obesity and type 2 diabetes (T2D). Extensive research has linked these PRRs to inflammation-induced insulin resistance (IR) and diabetes-related cardiac complications (Prajapati et al. 2014).

2 TLR2 and TLR4 in Diabetic Cardiomyopathy

As previously mentioned, TLRs are critical mediators of innate immunity and inflammation (Fitzgerald and Kagan 2020). Dysregulated TLR signaling has been implicated in numerous diseases, including inflammatory bowel diseases (e.g., Crohn's disease, ulcerative colitis), allergic conditions (e.g., asthma, dermatitis), and metabolic diseases such as diabetes (Fukata et al. 2009; Prajapati et al. 2014). In diabetes, abnormal TLR-mediated innate immunity has been broadly related to the development of IR, mainly due to gut microbiota alterations that result in excessive PAMPs levels (Prajapati et al. 2014). Among TLRs, most evidence suggests that TLR2 and TLR4 are key players in diabetes-related complications.

TLR2 is a plasma membrane receptor that recognizes microbial PAMPs and undergoes dimerization upon ligand binding. It can form heterodimers with TLR1, which detect triacylated lipoproteins from Gram-negative bacteria or mycoplasmas, or TLR6, recognizing diacylated lipoproteins from Gram-positive bacteria and mycoplasmas. TLR2 is currently considered a highly versatile receptor since it can also interact with other TLRs, such as TLR4 or TLR10, expanding its PAMP recognition capacity (Oliveira-Nascimento et al. 2012). Although several lines of evidence suggest the existence of TLR2 homodimers, their function remains controversial since their activation appears to be cofactor-dependent (Colleselli et al. 2023). Beyond microbial ligands, TLR2 can also recognize endogenous DAMPs, such as high mobility group box 1 protein (HMGB1), heat shock proteins (HSPs), and alarmins, triggering intracellular signaling cascades that culminate in NF-kB activation (Table 1). TLR4 is another critical mediator in diabetes. This receptor recognizes various PAMPs and DAMPs through its co-receptor myeloid differentiation factor 2 (MD2), forming a ligand-MD2/TLR4 complex that dimerizes and activates intracellular pro-inflammatory cascades, primarily mediated by NF-kB and activator protein 1 (AP-1) (Kim et al. 2023).

In diabetes, both TLR2 and TLR4 have been shown to play critical roles in the development of cardiac complications, particularly diabetic cardiomyopathy (DCM), by detecting hyperglycemia-induced DAMPs. Their activation triggers pro-inflammatory cascades, promoting adverse cardiac remodeling and fibrosis, ultimately leading to heart dysfunction. NF-kB, a key downstream mediator of both receptors, is considered a key factor in the development and progression of DCM (Liu et al. 2024) (Fig. 1).

The involvement of TLR2 and TLR4 in DCM has been demonstrated in knockout (KO) murine models. Studies using preclinical diabetes models reveal that TLR2- or TLR4-deficient mice exhibit reduced adverse cardiac remodeling and improved heart functionality. This protection has been associated with both increased cardiomyocyte survival and improved calcium handling, resulting in better left ventricular function compared to wild-type (WT) mice (Lei et al. 2018; Ye et al. 2021).

In humans, sustained hyperglycemia in diabetic patients activates TLR2- and TLR4-mediated signaling pathways by inducing cellular damage and releasing various DAMPs. These molecules are recognized by TLRs, inducing

Table 1 Major DAMPs implicated in diabetes

DAMP	Source	Relevance in diabetes	References
Advanced Glycation End-products (AGEs)	Formed through non-enzymatic glycation of proteins and lipids under hyperglycemic conditions	Accumulate in diabetic tissues; bind to RAGE, activating inflammatory pathways (e.g., NF-κB), leading to oxidative stress, vascular stiffness, and atherosclerosis	Chen et al. (2017), Cross et al. (2024), Dvorkin et al. (2024), Jangde et al. (2020), Le Bagge et al. (2020), Nogueira-Machado et al. (2011), and Zhao et al. (2025b)
ATP	Cytoplasm (released during cell injury)	Activates NLRP3 inflammasome; contributes to insulin resistance and β-cell dysfunction	Srivastava et al. (2025), Villafan-Bernal et al. (2024), Wei et al. (2024), and Zhang et al. (2024)
Circulating cell-free DNA (cfDNA)	Necrotic/apoptotic cells	Stimulates innate immunity; associated with diabetic complications like nephropathy	Belinda et al. (2025), Li et al. (2025), and Pollastri et al. (2025)
Heat Shock Proteins (e.g., HSP70)	Cytoplasmic chaperones (released under stress)	Activate innate immunity through TLRs; elevated in diabetic patients	Esmaeilzadeh et al. (2023), Hashemi et al. (2024), Irfan et al. (2024), Timofeev et al. (2023), and Zimbone et al. (2023)
HMGB1	Nucleus (released by necrotic or stressed cells)	Elevated in type 2 diabetes; promotes inflammation via TLR4 and RAGE activation	Nogueira-Machado et al. (2011), Rando et al. (2022), Thinschmidt et al. (2016), and Villafan-Bernal et al. (2024)
Mitochondrial DNA (mtDNA)	Mitochondria (released during cell stress or death)	Activates TLR9 and inflammasomes; linked to systemic inflammation in type 2 diabetes	Ahmed et al. (2024), Iheagwam et al. (2025), and Praveen et al. (2025)
S100 proteins (e.g., S100A8/A9)	Cytoplasm of neutrophils and monocytes	Engage RAGE and TLRs; associated with chronic inflammation in obesity and diabetes	Deng et al. (2024), Gonzalez et al. (2020), Lim et al. (2024), Michetti et al. (2024), and Wan et al. (2025)
Uric acid	Purine metabolism (released as crystals)	Promotes inflammation and metabolic syndrome; linked to insulin resistance	Wang and Wang (2025), Yang et al. (2025), and Zhao et al. (2025a)

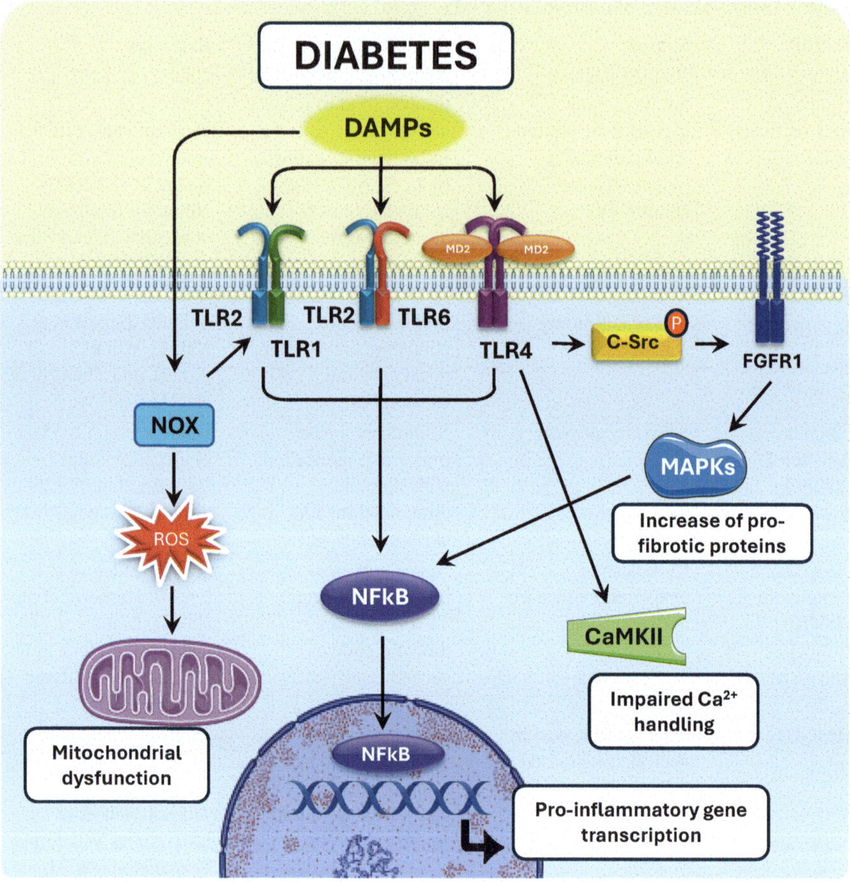

Fig. 1 Scheme of TLR activation and signaling pathways in diabetes. DAMPs released in diabetic patients activate mainly TLR2 and TLR4 in the membrane of cardiac cells, inducing a downstream intracellular signaling that involves NFkB-mediated pro-inflammatory gene transcription, ROS production associated to mitochondrial dysfunction and impaired calcium handling. Moreover, FGFR1 transactivation can drive to increased fibrosis and inflammation. DAMPS Damage-associated molecular patterns, TLR Toll-like receptors, NOX NAPDH oxidases, ROS Reactive oxygen species, NfkB Nuclear factor kB, FGFR Fibroblast growth factor receptor, MAPKs Mitogen-activated protein kinases, CaMKII Calcium/calmodulin-dependent protein kinase II

pro-inflammatory cascades that exacerbate cardiac injury (Nackiewicz et al. 2014). Specifically, for TLR4, glucose itself or advanced glycation end products (AGEs) generated by hyperglycemia can bind to its co-receptor MD2, triggering its activation (Wang et al. 2020a). In the context of diabetes, RAGE receptors have been shown to be involved in angiogenesis and vascular inflammation in diabetic retinopathy (Goldin et al. 2006; Oshitari 2023). Moreover, soluble RAGE expression has been found to be higher in both diabetes I and II (Eleazu et al. 2019), and its activation by AGEs participates in NLRP3 upregulation and neuroinflammation by activating pro-inflammatory macrophages (Chen et al. 2017; Teissier and Boulanger 2019; Jangde et al. 2020). In cardiomyocytes, hyperglycemia-associated TLR4 activation induces Src phosphorylation, which transactivates fibroblast growth factor receptor 1 (FGFR1) and activates mitogen-activated protein kinase (MAPK) signaling pathways, ultimately leading to NF-κB activation. Various studies have highlighted the importance of FGFR1 in diabetes-associated cardiac damage, supported by studies using FGFR1 KO models and pharmacological inhibitors (Chen et al. 2024). Moreover, hyperglycemia induces increased expression of TLR2 and TLR4, at both mRNA and protein levels, further amplifying their deleterious effects (Bernal-Lopez et al. 2013).

In the heart, overactivation of TLR2 and TLR4 pathways induces the release of high levels of several NF-kB-dependent pro-inflammatory mediators, such as interleukin-6 (IL-6), interleukin-1β (IL-1β), and tumor necrosis factor-alpha (TNFα), which have been found at elevated plasma concentrations in T2D patients (Tuttle et al. 2004). This results in a series of deleterious effects on the organ, leading to ventricular dysfunction and hypertrophy, or even promoting the development of atherosclerosis, key hallmarks of DCM (Fig. 1).

Additionally, oxidative stress plays a pivotal role in this process. Reactive oxygen species (ROS) released leads to mitochondrial respiratory chain dysfunction, thereby impairing the functionality of this organelle. Among the major sources of ROS in the cardiovascular system, the NADPH oxidase (NOX) family plays a crucial role. In the context of DCM, NOX1-induced ROS stimulates TLR2 activation, which, in turn, activates NF-κB, exacerbating inflammation and contributing to diabetes-associated cardiac damage (Zhang et al. 2022). Excessive ROS also disrupts calcium handling within cardiomyocytes, primarily due to the overactivation of calcium/calmodulin-dependent protein kinase II (CaMKII), leading to the death of these contractile cells and contributing to severe heart dysfunction (Fig. 1).

The activation of these TLRs significantly contributes to the development of cardiac fibrosis, a key feature of adverse remodeling in DCM patients. For instance, TLR2 activation by DAMPs such as HMGB1 in cardiac fibroblasts reduces their autophagic capacity, causing collagen and actin accumulation that leads to fibrosis (Wu et al. 2018). TLR4 activation induces the overexpression of hypertrophic proteins in cardiomyocytes, mediated by AP-1, which also contributes to the development of cardiac hypertrophy (Frieler and Mortensen 2015). At the endothelial level, TLR2 and TLR4 activation not only triggers immune cell recruitment, mainly monocytes, but also directly damages endothelial cells themselves, compromising vascular integrity and contributing to atheroma plaque formation. Indeed, increased TLR2 mRNA levels have been detected in vascular biopsies of atheroma plaques from T2D and atherosclerosis patients (Rosa et al. 2012). Furthermore, TLR4 activation can also contribute to cardiac metabolic dysfunction by altering lipid metabolism. For instance, studies in type 1 diabetes (T1D) murine models show that TLR4 deficiency reduces lipid accumulation in the heart, thereby mitigating DCM progression (Dong et al. 2012).

An intricate crosstalk between TLRs and NLRs pathways has been described, mainly mediated by NF-κB activation and high ROS levels following stimulation of TLR2 and TLR4. These signals contribute to the activation of NLRs through various mechanisms (Fuentes-Antrás et al. 2014).

3 NLRS in Cardiometabolic Disease

3.1 Nucletotide-Binding Oligometization Domain Type 1 and 2 Receptors

In the absence of infection, several DAMPs can activate NOD receptors, initiating a process known as "sterile inflammation." Upon DAMP recognition by the C-terminal LRR domains, NOD receptors undergo conformational changes, triggering self-oligomerization and the recruitment of CARD-containing effector molecules (Inohara et al. 1999). Consequently, NOD1 and NOD2 interact with the serine-threonine kinase RIP2, activating downstream signaling cascades that involve MAPKs and NF-κB, which drive the transcription of pro-inflammatory cytokines (Inohara et al. 1999; Kanneganti et al. 2007).

Despite their structural similarity, NOD1 and NOD2 exhibit distinct cellular distributions and disease associations. While NOD2 polymorphisms have been implicated in several inflammatory conditions such as Crohn's disease, NOD1 has not been associated with such disorders (Caruso et al. 2014). However, NOD1 activation has been associated with epithelial barrier disruption, cardiomyocyte calcium dysregulation, and metabolic dysfunction. Together, NOD1 and NOD2 have been reported to contribute to the pathophysiology of metabolic diseases, particularly IR. In response to IR, pancreatic β-cells compensate by increasing insulin secretion to maintain normoglycemia; however, chronic hyperinsulinemia predisposes individuals to T2D.

Obesity is the primary cause of IR worldwide (Saltiel and Olefsky 2017) and is strongly associated with chronic, subacute inflammation, particularly in adipose tissue and the liver. Obesity promotes immune cell infiltration into metabolically active tissues, increasing the number of local monocyte-derived macrophages (Liang et al. 2022; Wentworth et al. 2010) within adipose tissue. Following high-fat diet (HFD) feeding in mice models, their macrophages shift toward a pro-inflammatory status (Frieler et al. 1917), correlating with IR progression (Fink et al. 2014; Frieler et al. 1917).

NOD receptors serve as crucial mediators at the interface between immunity and metabolism, with NOD1 playing a significant role in immune cell infiltration, macrophage polarization, and IR development. Schertzer et al. first demonstrated that NOD1/2 double KO mice are protected from HFD-induced insulin intolerance (Schertzer et al. 2011). Similarly, NOD1-deficient mice display improved metabolic outcomes under HFD conditions (Amar et al. 2011), whereas NOD2-deficient mice exhibit worsened insulin tolerance under HFD conditions (Denou et al. 2015). Nevertheless, the precise contribution of NOD1 to obesity-related inflammation remains controversial. Some preclinical studies suggest that NOD1 deficiency protects against obesity-induced inflammation and IR (Botchlett et al. 2017), while others report worsened metabolic outcomes, including accelerated diet-induced obesity and hepatic steatosis in HFD-fed mice (Botchlett et al. 2017).

Beyond IR, NOD1 activation also influences adipocyte lipolysis, further exacerbating metabolic dysfunction. NOD1-dependent signaling enhances basal adipocyte lipolysis, increasing circulating free fatty acids (FFAs), which in turn contribute to ectopic lipid accumulation and impaired insulin signaling (Sharma et al. 2019). Furthermore, NOD receptors have been implicated in endoplasmic reticulum (ER) stress, a key factor in the pathogenesis of IR and T2D (Pagliassotti et al. 2016). Elevated FFAs levels in obesity induce lipotoxicity and chronic inflammation, exacerbating ER stress (Zcan et al. 2004). T2D is frequently associated with DCM, involving myocyte loss, fibrosis, and contractile dysfunction (Haffner et al. 1998; Maya and Villarreal 2010). Emerging evidence suggests that diabetes-related inflammation and NOD1 signaling contribute to cardiac pathology. Prieto et al. first demonstrated increased NOD1 expression in cardiomyocytes of diabetic *db/db* mice and human T2D myocardium, correlating with increased apoptosis (Prieto et al. 2014). Selective NOD1 activation increases TNF-α and IL-6 expression, exacerbating inflammation and fibrosis (Pickup et al. 1997; Prieto et al. 2014). Human cardiac fibroblasts from T2D patients, as well as from *db/db* mice, present sustained NOD1 activation, further promoting fibrotic remodeling (Val-Blasco et al. 2017). Notably, NF-kB inhibition mitigates NOD1-driven fibrosis, highlighting a potential therapeutic avenue (Edfeldt et al. 2002; Val-Blasco et al. 2017) (Fig. 2).

Overall, NOD1 and NOD2 contribute to the pathogenesis of DCM at multiple levels, from IR and lipolysis to cardiac fibrosis and apoptosis. Given their central role in metabolic inflammation and cardiac remodeling, targeting NOD receptors represents a promising therapeutic strategy for mitigating cardiac dysfunction in patients with diabetes.

3.2 NOD-Like Receptor Protein 3

Within the NLR subfamily, NOD-like receptor protein 3 (NLRP3) has been extensively studied for its role in inflammasome activation, particularly in various inflammatory and metabolic diseases (He et al. 2016).

Inflammasomes are cytosolic multiprotein complexes formed by PRRs in response to physiological or pathogenic stimuli, triggering innate immune responses that eliminate pathogens and damaged cells (Deets and Vance 2021). Their primary function is to detect infectious or noxious stimuli and serve as platforms for the activation of specific pro-inflammatory caspase proteases, primarily caspase-1, but also caspase-8, caspase-11 (in mice), and caspase-4/5 (in humans) (Rathinam and Fitzgerald 2016). Each inflammasome complex contains a unique sensor protein that mediates responses to specific stimuli, with assembly dictated by a unique PRR in response to PAMPs or DAMPs (Table 1).

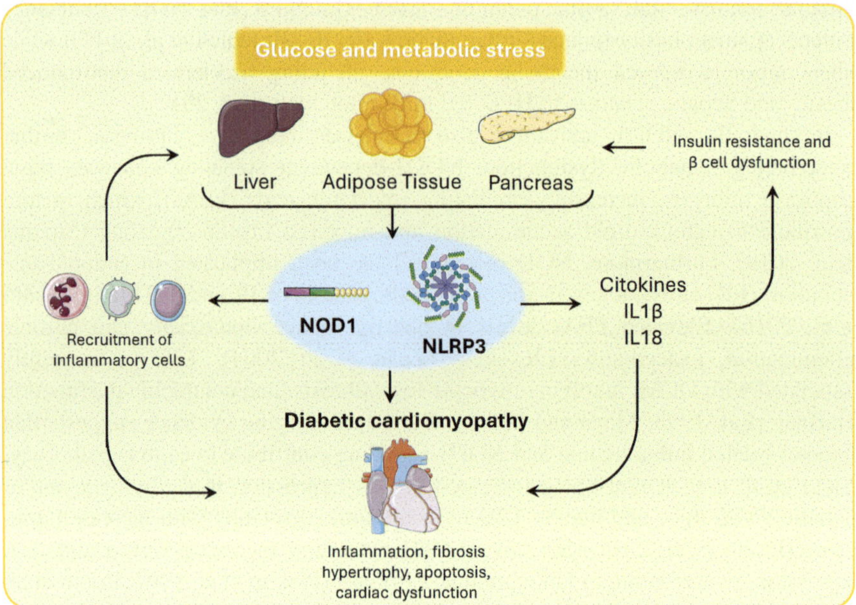

Fig. 2 Scheme of NOD1 and NLRP3 implication in diabetic cardiomyopathy. Upon glucose and metabolic stress in different organs, NOD1 and NLRP3 are activated triggering the expression of pro-inflammatory cytokines such as IL1β and IL18 that leads to insulin resistance and lipolysis in metabolic organs, and to cardiac dysfunction and fibrosis in the heart. NOD1 and NLRP3 activation also enhances the recruitment of immune cells that exacerbate the inflammatory response in the heart, liver, and adipose tissue among others, driving to a vicious cycle. NOD Nucleotide-binding oligomerization domain, NLRP3 NOD-like receptor protein 3, IL interleukin

NLRP3 is the most extensively studied inflammasome due to its significant role in regulating the innate immune system and its involvement in various inflammatory and autoimmune diseases, including arthritis, Alzheimer's disease, and inflammatory bowel disease (Ma et al. 2019; Mao et al. 2018; Santos-García et al. 2025; Walle et al. 2014). Unlike other inflammasomes that are activated by specific agonists, NLRP3 responds to a diverse array of stimuli (Lamkanfi and Dixit 2012; Y. Zhang et al. 2021).

NLRP3 inflammasome activation has been implicated in oxidative stress, vascular and endothelial dysfunction, and the progression of cardiovascular diseases. This activation occurs in two distinct steps: priming and activation. The priming step is initiated by the recognition of PAMPs or DAMPs through TLRs or cytokine receptors (Habas et al. 2022; Shen et al. 2022), triggering downstream signaling pathways such as MAPK and NF-κB pathways, leading to upregulation of NLRP3 and pro-Il-1β expression (Escartín-Gutiérrez et al. 2023). The activation step is then initiated by a secondary stimulus, often potassium efflux, which promotes NLRP3 oligomerization and the recruitment of the adaptor protein ASC (apoptosis-associated speck-like protein containing a CARD), which facilitates the formation of the catalytically active protease caspase-1 and the assembly of the NLRP3 inflammasome complex (Wang et al. 2020b). Activated caspase-1 initiates downstream responses, including the cleavage of IL-1β and IL-18 into their mature forms, which are subsequently released to amplify the inflammatory response. Additionally, NLRP3 inflammasome activation induces pyroptosis, a lytic form of programmed cell death mediated by gasdermin D, resulting in the formation of nonspecific pores in the plasma membrane and the release of intracellular components, which further exacerbates the inflammatory response (Broz and Dixit 2016). This form of programmed cell death affects not only cardiomyocytes but also other cardiac cell types, including fibroblasts, endothelial, and immune cells. Although pyroptosis in cardiomyocytes is recognized as a pivotal event in the pathogenesis of dilated cardiomyopathy (DCM) due to its direct impairment of cardiac contractile function, its occurrence in non-myocyte populations further exacerbates disease progression (Wang et al. 2023). Specifically, pyroptosis in cardiac fibroblasts or endothelial cells promotes adverse cardiac remodeling. Consequently, novel therapeutic strategies aimed at inhibiting pyroptosis within the myocardium are currently under development.

NLRP3 inflammasome activation has been strongly associated with metabolic diseases, including diabetes. Studies have demonstrated that NLRP3 is upregulated in both T1D and T2D, contributing to insulin resistance and β-cell dysfunction. Activation of NLRP3 in adipose tissue, liver, and pancreatic islets leads to increased secretion of pro-inflammatory cytokines, which exacerbate IR and promote β-cell apoptosis. Increased expression of NLRP3, ASC, and caspase-1 has been observed in pancreatic islets of type 2 diabetic patients, along with elevated serum levels of IL-1β and IL-18, correlating with poor glycemic control (Lee et al. 2013; Thorand et al. 2005) (Fig. 2).

In vivo studies using genetically modified mice lacking NLRP3, ASC, or caspase-1 have shown an improvement in glucose homeostasis as well as a reduction in inflammation, further highlighting the role of NLRP3 in diabetes pathophysiology (Sharma et al. 2021a). NLRP3 KO mice exhibit enhanced insulin sensitivity and reduced obesity-induced inflammation compared to WT mice, evidencing that NLRP3 activation is a key driver of metabolic inflammation and insulin resistance (Stienstra et al. 2011; Vandanmagsar et al. 2011).

DCM is a severe complication of long standing diabetes mellitus, characterized by myocardial cell death, fibrosis, left ventricular dysfunction, and metabolic deregulation (Westermeier et al. 2015). The NLRP3 inflammasome has been implicated in DCM pathogenesis through its role in promoting inflammation and fibrosis (Sun and Ding 2021). Chronic hyperglycemia and lipid accumulation in diabetic patients activate NLRP3 in cardiac cells, leading to the release of pro-inflammatory cytokines and the recruitment of inflammatory cells. This inflammatory response promotes fibrosis, hypertrophy, and apoptosis of cardiomyocytes, ultimately leading to cardiac dysfunction (Cosentino et al. 2022). Increased expression of NLRP3 and IL-1β has been observed in myocardial tissue of diabetic patients with heart failure, further supporting its role in DCM progression. In addition, clinical trials targeting the

NLRP3 inflammasome in diabetic patients have shown promising results, reducing cardiac inflammation and improving cardiac function (Sun and Ding 2021) (Fig. 2).

Among the various factors capable of activating the NLRP3 inflammasome, glucose has been identified as an effective activator (Shi et al. 2015). Chronic hyperglycemia, a hallmark of diabetes, leads to metabolic stress and the accumulation of metabolic by-products. These conditions activate the NLRP3 inflammasome in multiple cell types, including macrophages and cardiomyocytes. The subsequent activation of NLRP3 results in the production of pro-inflammatory cytokines IL-1β and IL-18, contributing to systemic inflammation, insulin resistance, and the progression of diabetic complications, including DCM. The chronic inflammatory state driven by NLRP3 activation exacerbates myocardial tissue damage and fibrosis, further worsening cardiac dysfunction (Ding et al. 2022).

Increasing evidence suggests that the NLRP3 inflammasome is emerging as a valuable molecular target for the treatment of DCM and other cardiovascular complications associated with diabetes. In this context, Luo et al. (2014) demonstrated that rosuvastatin (RSV), an anti-inflammatory drug, inhibits NLRP3 inflammasome activation via thioredoxin-interacting protein (TXNIP), suppressing the phosphorylation of MAPK signaling pathways in DCM. Additionally, INF4E, a synthetic NLRP3 inflammasome inhibitor, has been shown to protect against the ischemia-reperfusion-induced myocardial injury by inhibiting NLRP3 inflammasome, leading to the activation of the pro-survival reperfusion injury salvage kinase (RISK) pathway and improvement in mitochondrial function (Mastrocola et al. 2016).

Another approach to modulating NLRP3 inflammasome activity involves the administration of oral hypoglycemic drugs, which have been found to exert anti-inflammatory effects by targeting and regulating NLRP3. For instance, sulfonylureas can inhibit NLRP3 activation and reduce inflammatory cytokine levels (Hill et al. 2017). Sodium-glucose cotransporter 2 inhibitors (SGLT2i) suppress inflammasome activity by reducing oxidative stress and modulating intracellular signaling pathways (Hu et al. 2023); or dipeptidyl peptidase-4 inhibitors (DPP-4i) can mitigate inflammasome activation, thereby protecting against renal and vascular complications (Saini et al. 2023).

Targeting the NLRP3 inflammasome presents a promising dual therapeutic strategy for diabetes and its associated cardiovascular complications. Modulating this inflammasome not only contributes to glycemic control but also attenuates inflammation, addressing two critical aspects of diabetes management. While hypoglycemic drugs primarily regulate blood glucose levels by stimulating insulin secretion, enhancing insulin sensitivity, and decreasing glucose absorption or reabsorption, recent studies suggest that they may also exert anti-inflammatory effects by modulating the NLRP3 inflammasome pathway. Consequently, therapeutic interventions aimed at NLRP3 inhibition or modulation hold significant potential for improving both metabolic and cardiovascular outcomes in diabetic patients.

4 Conclusions

Although the inhibition of pattern recognition receptors (PRRs) has emerged as a promising therapeutic strategy to alleviate chronic inflammation in various inflammatory diseases, it also raises significant concerns due to the essential role of PRRs in host defense. PRRs confer a frontline defense, which is vital for maintaining host integrity and initiating adaptive immune responses. In this chapter, we have addressed the role of innate immunity in the context of the so-called "sterile inflammation" associated with chronic diseases, such as diabetes. Suppressing their activity may reduce pathological inflammation and tissue damage associated with chronic immune activation; however, it also compromises the immune system's ability to recognize and respond effectively to microbial threats. Thus, while targeting PRRs may offer therapeutic benefits in chronic inflammatory diseases, such strategies must be carefully optimized to preserve their essential protective functions. Approaches that allow for context-specific modulation rather than complete inhibition of PRR signaling may represent a more effective and safer avenue for clinical intervention.

This chapter has highlighted the crucial role of immune receptors in both the initiation and progression of metabolic diseases, as well as in the associated comorbidities, such as cardiovascular complications. Immune receptors, including TLRs and NLRS, emerge as promising therapeutic targets for both metabolic disorders and their associated cardiovascular complications. Given their pivotal role in mediating inflammatory responses, these PRRs should be considered in the development of therapeutic strategies aimed at preventing or mitigating complications in patients with metabolic diseases.

References

Ahmed I, Chakraborty R, Faizy AF, Moin S (2024) Exploring the key role of DNA methylation as an epigenetic modulator in oxidative stress related islet cell injury in patients with type 2 diabetes mellitus: a review. J Diabetes Metab Disord 23(2). https://doi.org/10.1007/S40200-024-01496-2

Amar J, Chabo C, Waget A, Klopp P, Vachoux C, Bermúdez-Humarán LG, Smirnova N, Bergé M, Sulpice T, Lahtinen S, Ouwehand A, Langella P, Rautonen N, Sansonetti PJ, Burcelin R (2011) Intestinal mucosal adherence and translocation of commensal bacteria at the early onset of type 2 diabetes: molecular mechanisms and probiotic treatment. EMBO Mol Med 3(9):559–572. https://doi.org/10.1002/emmm.201100159

Belinda A, Humardani FM, Dwi Putra SE, Widyadhana B (2025) The potential of circulating free DNA of methylated IGFBP as a biomarker for type 2 diabetes Mellitus: a comprehensive review. Clin Chim Acta 567. https://doi.org/10.1016/j.cca.2024.120104

Bernal-Lopez MR, Llorente-Cortes V, Calleja F, Lopez-Carmona D, Mayas MD, Gomez-Huelgas-R, Badimon L, Tinahones FJ (2013) Effect of different degrees of impaired glucose metabolism on the expression of inflammatory markers in monocytes of patients with atherosclerosis. Acta Diabetol 50(4):553–562. https://doi.org/10.1007/s00592-011-0337-2

Botchlett R, Woo S-L, Liu M, Pei Y, Guo X, Li H, Wu C (2017) Nutritional approaches for managing obesity-associated metabolic diseases. J Endocrinol 233:R145

Broz P, Dixit VM (2016) Inflammasomes: mechanism of assembly, regulation and signalling. Nat Rev Immunol 16(7):407–420). Nature Publishing Group. https://doi.org/10.1038/nri.2016.58

Brubaker SW, Bonham KS, Zanoni I, Kagan JC (2015) Innate immune pattern recognition: a cell biological perspective. Ann Rev Immunol 33:257–290). Annual Reviews Inc. https://doi.org/10.1146/annurev-immunol-032414-112240

Caruso R, Warner N, Inohara N, Núñez G (2014) NOD1 and NOD2: signaling, host defense, and inflammatory disease. Immunity 41(6):898–908). Cell Press. https://doi.org/10.1016/j.immuni.2014.12.010

Chen J, Sun Z, Jin M, Tu Y, Wang S, Yang X, Chen Q, Zhang X, Han Y, Pi R (2017) Inhibition of AGEs/RAGE/Rho/ROCK pathway suppresses non-specific neuroinflammation by regulating BV2 microglial M1/M2 polarization through the NF-κB pathway. J Neuroimmunol 305. https://doi.org/10.1016/j.jneuroim.2017.02.010

Chen X, Qian J, Liang S, Qian J, Luo W, Shi Y, Zhu H, Hu X, Wu G, Li X, Liang G (2024) Hyperglycemia activates FGFR1 via TLR4/c-Src pathway to induce inflammatory cardiomyopathy in diabetes. Acta Pharm Sin B 14(4):1693–1710. https://doi.org/10.1016/j.apsb.2024.01.013

Colleselli K, Stierschneider A, Wiesner C (2023) An update on toll-like receptor 2, its function and dimerization in pro- and anti-inflammatory processes. Int J Mol Sci 24(15). Multidisciplinary Digital Publishing Institute (MDPI). https://doi.org/10.3390/ijms241512464

Cosentino N, Ashraf Z, Li F, Dong N, Zheng Y, Xu L (2022) NLRP3 inflammasome: the rising star in cardiovascular diseases. Front Cardiovasc Med. https://doi.org/10.3389/fcvm.2022.927061

Cross K, Vetter SW, Alam Y, Hasan MZ, Nath AD, Leclerc E (2024) Role of the receptor for advanced glycation end products (RAGE) and its ligands in inflammatory responses. Biomolecules 14(12). https://doi.org/10.3390/BIOM14121550

Deets KA, Vance RE (2021) Inflammasomes and adaptive immune responses. Nat Immunol 22(4): 412–422). Nature Research. https://doi.org/10.1038/s41590-021-00869-6

Deng C, Li X, Ren M, Ye Z, Jin F, Yao B, Peng Y, Lu L, Dong K (2024) Paquinimod attenuates retinal injuries by suppressing the S100A9/TLR4 signaling in an experimental model of diabetic retinopathy. Exp Eye Res 249. https://doi.org/10.1016/j.exer.2024.110131

Denou E, Lolmède K, Garidou L, Pomie C, Chabo C, Lau TC, Fullerton MD, Nigro G, Zakaroff-Girard A, Luche E, Garret C, Serino M, Amar J, Courtney M, Cavallari JF, Henriksbo BD, Barra NG, Foley KP, McPhee JB et al (2015) Defective NOD 2 peptidoglycan sensing promotes diet-induced inflammation, dysbiosis, and insulin resistance. EMBO Mol Med 7(3):259–274. https://doi.org/10.15252/emmm.201404169

Ding K, Song C, Hu H, Yin K, Huang H, Tang H (2022) The role of NLRP3 Inflammasome in diabetic cardiomyopathy and its therapeutic implications. Oxid Med Cell Longev 2022: 3790721. Hindawi Limited. https://doi.org/10.1155/2022/3790721

Dong B, Qi D, Yang L, Huang Y, Xiao X, Tai N, Wen L, Susan Wong F (2012) TLR4 regulates cardiac lipid accumulation and diabetic heart disease in the nonobese diabetic mouse model of type 1 diabetes. J Physiol Heart Circ Physiol 303:732–742. https://doi.org/10.1152/ajpheart.00948.2011

Dvorkin S, Cambier S, Volkman HE, Stetson DB (2024) New frontiers in the cGAS-STING intracellular DNA-sensing pathway. Immunity 57(4):718–730. https://doi.org/10.1016/j.immuni.2024.02.019

Edfeldt K, Swedenborg J, Hansson GK, Yan Z (2002) Expression of toll-like receptors in human atherosclerotic lesions a possible pathway for plaque activation. Circulation. https://doi.org/10.1161/01.CIR.0000012489.17433.31

Eleazu C, Omar N, Lim OZ, Yeoh BS, Hussain NHN, Mohamed M (2019) Obesity and comorbidity: could simultaneous targeting of Esrage and srage be the panacea? Front Physiol 10. https://doi.org/10.3389/fphys.2019.00787

Escartín-Gutiérrez JR, Ponce-Figueroa M, Torres-Vega MÁ, Aguilar-Faisal L, Figueroa-Arredondo P (2023) Transcriptional activation of a pro-inflammatory response (NF-κB, AP-1, IL-1β) by the vibrio cholerae Cytotoxin (VCC) monomer through the MAPK signaling pathway in the THP-1 human macrophage cell line. Int J Mol Sci 24(8). https://doi.org/10.3390/ijms24087272

Esmaeilzadeh A, Mohammadi V, Elahi R, Rezakhani N (2023) The role of heat shock proteins (HSPs) in type 2 diabetes mellitus pathophysiology. J Diabetes Complicat 37(11). https://doi.org/10.1016/j.jdiacomp.2023.108564

Fink LN, Costford SR, Lee YS, Jensen TE, Bilan PJ, Oberbach A, Blüher M, Olefsky JM, Sams A, Klip A (2014) Pro-inflammatory macrophages increase in skeletal muscle of high fat-Fed mice and correlate with metabolic risk markers in humans. Obesity 22(3):747–757. https://doi.org/10.1002/oby.20615

Fitzgerald KA, Kagan JC (2020) Toll-like receptors and the control of immunity. Cell 180(6): 1044–1066). Cell Press. https://doi.org/10.1016/j.cell.2020.02.041

Frieler RA, Mortensen RM (2015) Immune cell and other noncardiomyocyte regulation of cardiac hypertrophy and remodeling. Circulation 131(11):1019–1030. https://doi.org/10.1161/CIRCULATIONAHA.114.008788

Frieler RA, Ramnarayanan S, Mortensen RM (1917) Nuclear receptor control of opposing macrophage phenotypes in cardiovascular disease. Front Biosci 17. https://doi.org/10.2741/4028

Fuentes-Antrás J, Ioan AM, Tuñón J, Egido J, Lorenzo Ó (2014) Activation of toll-like receptors and inflammasome complexes in the diabetic cardiomyopathy-associated inflammation. Int J Endocrinol 2014. Hindawi Publishing Corporation. https://doi.org/10.1155/2014/847827

Fukata M, Vamadevan AS, Abreu MT (2009) Toll-like receptors (TLRs) and Nod-like receptors (NLRs) in inflammatory disorders. Semin Immunol 21(4):242–253. https://doi.org/10.1016/j.smim.2009.06.005

Goldin A, Beckman JA, Schmidt AM, Creager MA (2006) Advanced glycation end products: sparking the development of diabetic vascular injury. Circulation 114(6). https://doi.org/10.1161/CIRCULATIONAHA.106.621854

Gonzalez LL, Garrie K, Turner MD (2020) Role of S100 proteins in health and disease. Biochimica et Biophysica Acta (BBA) 1867(6). https://doi.org/10.1016/j.bbamcr.2020.118677

González-Ramos S, Paz-García M, Rius C, del Monte-Monge A, Rodríguez C, Fernández-García V, Andrés V, Martínez-González J, Lasunción MA, Martín-Sanz P, Soehnlein O, Boscá L (2019) Endothelial NOD1 directs myeloid cell recruitment in atherosclerosis through VCAM-1. FASEB J 33(3). https://doi.org/10.1096/fj.201801231RR

Habas A, Reddy Natala S, Bowden-Verhoek JK, Stocking EM, Price DL, Wrasidlo W, Bonhaus DW, Gill MB (2022) NPT1220-312, a TLR2/TLR9 small molecule antagonist, inhibits pro-inflammatory signaling, cytokine release, and NLRP3 Inflammasome activation. Int J Inflamm 2022. https://doi.org/10.1155/2022/2337363

Haffner SM, Lehto S, Rönnemaa T, Pyörälä K, Laakso M (1998) Mortality from coronary heart disease in subjects with type 2 diabetes and in nondiabetic subjects with and without prior myocardial infarction. N Engl J Med 339(4):229–234. https://doi.org/10.1056/NEJM199807233390404

Harati MD, King J, Langer S, Binder F, Heilker R (2024) Recapitulation of NOD/RIPK2 signaling in iPSC-derived macrophages. SLAS Discov 29(7). https://doi.org/10.1016/J.SLASD.2024.100185

Hashemi N, Karimpour Reyhan S, Qahremani R, Seifouri K, Tavakoli M, Seyedi SA, Ghaemi F, Abbaszadeh M, Esteghamati A, Nakhjavani M, Mirmiranpour H, Rabizadeh S (2024) Vitamin D in type 2 diabetes and its correlation with heat shock protein 70, ferric reducing ability of plasma, advanced oxidation protein products and advanced glycation end products. Endocrinol Diabetes Metab 7(4). https://doi.org/10.1002/EDM2.508

He Y, Hara H, Núñez G (2016) Mechanism and regulation of NLRP3 Inflammasome activation. Trends Biochem Sci 41(12):1012–1021). Elsevier Ltd. https://doi.org/10.1016/j.tibs.2016.09.002

Hill JR, Coll RC, Sue N, Reid JC, Dou J, Holley CL, Pelingon R, Dickinson JB, Biden TJ, Schroder K, Cooper MA, Robertson AAB (2017) Sulfonylureas as concomitant insulin

Secretagogues and NLRP3 Inflammasome inhibitors. ChemMedChem 12(17):1449–1457. https://doi.org/10.1002/cmdc.201700270
Hu J, Xu J, Tan X, Li D, Yao D, Xu B, Lei Y (2023) Dapagliflozin protects against dilated cardiomyopathy progression by targeting NLRP3 inflammasome activation. Naunyn Schmiedeberg's Arch Pharmacol 396(7):1461–1470. https://doi.org/10.1007/s00210-023-02409-5
Iheagwam FN, Joseph AJ, Adedoyin ED, Iheagwam OT, Ejoh SA (2025) Mitochondrial dysfunction in diabetes: shedding light on a widespread oversight. Pathophysiology 32(1):9. https://doi.org/10.3390/PATHOPHYSIOLOGY32010009
Inohara N, Koseki T, del Peso L, Hu Y, Yee C, Chen S, Carrio R, Merino J, Liu D, Ni J, Nú G (1999) Nod1, an Apaf-1-like activator of Caspase-9 and nuclear factor-kappaB. J Biol Chem 274(21):14560–14567. http://www.jbc.org/
Irfan M, Abid F, Azhar A, Farooqui MU, Fatima U, Subhan M (2024) The dichotomy between heat shock protein-27 and microalbumin: covariate of early diabetic nephropathy. J Ayub Med College 36(1):40–44. https://doi.org/10.55519/JAMC-01-12499
Jangde N, Ray R, Rai V (2020) RAGE and its ligands: from pathogenesis to therapeutics. Crit Rev Biochem Mol Biol 55(6). https://doi.org/10.1080/10409238.2020.1819194
Kanneganti TD, Lamkanfi M, Núñez G (2007) Intracellular NOD-like receptors in host defense and disease. Immunity 27(4):549–559. https://doi.org/10.1016/j.immuni.2007.10.002
Kawai T, Akira S (2010) The role of pattern-recognition receptors in innate immunity: update on toll-like receptors. Nat Immunol 11(5):373–384. https://doi.org/10.1038/ni.1863
Kim HJ, Kim H, Lee JH, Hwangbo C (2023) Toll-like receptor 4 (TLR4): new insight immune and aging. Immun Ageing 20(1). BioMed Central Ltd. https://doi.org/10.1186/s12979-023-00383-3
Lamkanfi M, Dixit VM (2012) Inflammasomes and their roles in health and disease. In: Ann Rev Cell Dev Biol, vol 28, pp 137–161). Annual Reviews Inc. https://doi.org/10.1146/annurev-cellbio-101011-155745
Le Bagge S, Fotheringham AK, Leung SS, Forbes JM (2020) Targeting the receptor for advanced glycation end products (RAGE) in type 1 diabetes. Med Res Rev 40(4):1200–1219. https://doi.org/10.1002/MED.21654
Lee HM, Kim JJ, Kim HJ, Shong M, Ku BJ, Jo EK (2013) Upregulated NLRP3 inflammasome activation in patients with type 2 diabetes. Diabetes 62(1):194–204. https://doi.org/10.2337/db12-0420
Lei L, Hu H, Lei Y, Feng J (2018) Leukocytic toll-like receptor 2 knockout protects against diabetes-induced cardiac dysfunction. Biochem Biophys Res Commun 506(3):668–673. https://doi.org/10.1016/j.bbrc.2018.10.082
Li Z, Shang D (2024) NOD1 and NOD2: essential monitoring partners in the innate immune system. Curr Issues Mol Biol 46(9):9463–9479. https://doi.org/10.3390/CIMB46090561
Li B, Yim MM, Jin YX, Tao BK, Xie JS, Balas M, Khan H, Lam WC, Yan P, Navajas EV (2025) Circulating cell-free DNA as an epigenetic biomarker for early diabetic retinopathy: a Narrative Review. Diagnostics (Basel) 15(9). https://doi.org/10.3390/DIAGNOSTICS15091161
Liang W, Qi Y, Yi H, Mao C, Meng Q, Wang H, Zheng C (2022) The roles of adipose tissue macrophages in human disease. Front Immunol 13. Frontiers Media S.A. https://doi.org/10.3389/fimmu.2022.908749
Lim RR, Thomas A, Ramasubramanian A, Chaurasia SS (2024) Retinal microglia-derived S100A9 incite NLRP3 inflammasome in a Western diet fed Ossabaw pig retina. BioRxiv. https://doi.org/10.1101/2024.10.30.621160
Liu H-J, Gui L-K, Wei H, Zhou X-Y, Liu Z-L, Jin L-J (2024) The role of NF-κB in diabetic cardiomyopathy. All Life 17(1). https://doi.org/10.1080/26895293.2024.2397402
Luo B, Li B, Wang W, Liu X, Liu X, Xia Y, Zhang C, Zhang Y, Zhang M, An F (2014) Rosuvastatin alleviates diabetic cardiomyopathy by inhibiting NLRP3 inflammasome and MAPK pathways in a type 2 diabetes rat model. Cardiovasc Drugs Ther 28(1):33–43. https://doi.org/10.1007/s10557-013-6498-1

Ma P, Zha S, Shen X, Zhao Y, Li L, Yang L, Lei M, Liu W (2019) NFAT5 mediates hypertonic stress-induced atherosclerosis via activating NLRP3 inflammasome in endothelium. Cell Commun Signal 17(1). https://doi.org/10.1186/s12964-019-0406-7

Mao L, Kitani A, Strober W, Fuss IJ (2018) The role of NLRP3 and IL-1β in the pathogenesis of inflammatory bowel disease. Front Immunol 9. Frontiers Media S.A. https://doi.org/10.3389/fimmu.2018.02566

Mastrocola R, Penna C, Tullio F, Femminò S, Nigro D, Chiazza F, Serpe L, Collotta D, Alloatti G, Cocco M, Bertinaria M, Pagliaro P, Aragno M, Collino M (2016) Pharmacological inhibition of NLRP3 inflammasome attenuates myocardial ischemia/reperfusion injury by activation of RISK and mitochondrial pathways. Oxidative Med Cell Longev 2016. https://doi.org/10.1155/2016/5271251

Maya L, Villarreal FJ (2010) Diagnostic approaches for diabetic cardiomyopathy and myocardial fibrosis. J Mol Cell Cardiol 48(3):524–529. https://doi.org/10.1016/j.yjmcc.2009.06.021

McGettrick AF, O'Neill LAJ (2007) Toll-like receptors: key activators of leucocytes and regulator of haematopoiesis. Br J Haematol 139(2):185–193. https://doi.org/10.1111/j.1365-2141.2007.06802.x

Michetti F, Di Sante G, Clementi ME, Valeriani F, Mandarano M, Ria F, Di Liddo R, Rende M, Romano Spica V (2024) The multifaceted S100B protein: a role in obesity and diabetes? Int J Mol Sci 25(2). https://doi.org/10.3390/IJMS25020776

Midwood KS, Piccinini AM (2010) DAMPening inflammation by modulating TLR signalling. Mediators Inflamm 2010. https://doi.org/10.1155/2010/672395

Nackiewicz D, Dan M, He W, Kim R, Salmi A, Rütti S, Westwell-Roper C, Cunningham A, Speck M, Schuster-Klein C, Guardiola B, Maedler K, Ehses JA (2014) TLR2/6 and TLR4-activated macrophages contribute to islet inflammation and impair beta cell insulin gene expression via IL-1 and IL-6. Diabetologia 57(8):1645–1654. https://doi.org/10.1007/s00125-014-3249-1

Nakamura N, Lill JR, Phung Q, Jiang Z, Bakalarski C, De Mazière A, Klumperman J, Schlatter M, Delamarre L, Mellman I (2014) Endosomes are specialized platforms for bacterial sensing and NOD2 signalling. Nature 509(7499):240–244. https://doi.org/10.1038/nature13133

Nogueira-Machado JA, Volpe CMDO, Veloso CA, Chaves MM (2011) HMGB1, TLR and RAGE: A functional tripod that leads to diabetic inflammation. Expert Opin Ther Targets 15(8): 1023–1035. https://doi.org/10.1517/14728222.2011.575360

Oliveira-Nascimento L, Massari P, Wetzler LM (2012) The role of TLR2 ininfection and immunity. Front Immunol 3. https://doi.org/10.3389/fimmu.2012.00079

Oshitari T (2023) Advanced glycation end-products and diabetic neuropathy of the retina. Int J Mol Sci 24(3). https://doi.org/10.3390/ijms24032927

Pagliassotti MJ, Kim PY, Estrada AL, Stewart CM, Gentile CL (2016) Endoplasmic reticulum stress in obesity and obesity-related disorders: an expanded view. Metab Clin Exp 65(9): 1238–1246). W.B. Saunders. https://doi.org/10.1016/j.metabol.2016.05.002

Pickup JC, Mattock MB, Chusney GD, Butt D (1997) NIDDM as a disease of the innate immune system: association of acute-phase reactants and interleukin-6 with metabolic syndrome X. Diabetologia 40:1286

Pollastri A, Kovacs P, Keller M (2025) Circulating cell-free DNA in metabolic diseases. J Endocr Soc 9(2). https://doi.org/10.1210/JENDSO/BVAF006

Prajapati B, Jena K, Rajput P, Purandhar K, Seshadri S (2014) Send orders for reprints to reprints@benthamscience.net understanding and modulating the toll like receptors (TLRs) and NOD like receptors (NLRs) Cross talk in type 2 diabetes. Curr Diabetes Rev 10:190

Praveen PK, Jyothi MN, Prashant A (2025) Mitochondrial DNA variants in the pathogenesis and metabolic alterations of diabetes mellitus. Mol Genet Metab Rep 42. https://doi.org/10.1016/j.ymgmr.2024.101183

Prieto P, Vallejo-Cremades MT, Benito G, González-Peramato P, Francés D, Agra N, Terrón V, Gónzalez-Ramos S, Delgado C, Ruiz-Gayo M, Pacheco I, Velasco-Martín JP, Regadera J, Martín-Sanz P, López-Collazo E, Boscá L, Fernández-Velasco M (2014) NOD1 receptor is up-regulated in diabetic human and murine myocardium. Clin Sci 127(12):665–677. https://doi.org/10.1042/CS20140180

Rando MM, Biscetti F, Cecchini AL, Nardella E, Nicolazzi MA, Angelini F, Iezzi R, Eraso LH, Dimuzio PJ, Pitocco D, Gasbarrini A, Massetti M, Flex A (2022) Serum high mobility group box-1 levels associated with cardiovascular events after lower extremity revascularization: a prospective study of a diabetic population. Cardiovasc Diabetol 21(1). https://doi.org/10.1186/S12933-022-01650-1

Rathinam VAK, Fitzgerald KA (2016) Inflammasome complexes: emerging mechanisms and effector functions. Cell 165(4):792–800). Cell Press. https://doi.org/10.1016/j.cell.2016.03.046

Rosa B-LM, Vicenta L-C, Victor G-C, Dolores L-C, Fernando C, Ricardo G-H, Lina B, Francisco TJ (2012) Alterations of specific biomarkers of metabolic pathways in vascular tree from patients with Type 2 diabetes. Cardiovasc Diabetol. http://www.cardiab.com/content/11/1/86

Saini K, Sharma S, Khan Y (2023) DPP-4 inhibitors for treating T2DM – hype or hope? An analysis based on the current literature. Front Mol Biosci 10. Frontiers Media S.A. https://doi.org/10.3389/fmolb.2023.1130625

Saltiel AR, Olefsky JM (2017) Inflammatory mechanisms linking obesity and metabolic disease. J Clin Invest 127(1):1–4). American Society for Clinical Investigation. https://doi.org/10.1172/JCI92035

Santos-García I, Bascuñana P, Brackhan M, Villa M, Eiriz I, Brüning T, Pahnke J (2025) The ABC transporter A7 modulates neuroinflammation via NLRP3 inflammasome in Alzheimer's disease mice. Alzheimer's Res Ther 17(1):30. https://doi.org/10.1186/s13195-025-01673-2

Schertzer JD, Tamrakar AK, Magalhães JG, Pereira S, Bilan PJ, Fullerton MD, Liu Z, Steinberg GR, Giacca A, Philpott DJ, Klip A (2011) NOD1 activators link innate immunity to insulin resistance. Diabetes 60(9):2206–2215. https://doi.org/10.2337/db11-0004

Sharma A, Maurya CK, Arha D, Rai AK, Singh S, Varshney S, Schertzer JD, Tamrakar AK (2019) Nod1-mediated lipolysis promotes diacylglycerol accumulation and successive inflammation via PKCδ-IRAK axis in adipocytes. Biochim Biophys Acta Mol basis Dis 1865(1):136–146. https://doi.org/10.1016/j.bbadis.2018.10.036

Sharma A, Choi JSY, Stefanovic N, Al-Sharea A, Simpson DS, Mukhamedova N, Jandeleit-Dahm K, Murphy AJ, Sviridov D, Vince JE, Ritchie RH, de Haan JB (2021a) Specific NLRP3 inhibition protects against diabetes-associated atherosclerosis. Diabetes 70(3):772–787. https://doi.org/10.2337/DB20-0357

Sharma A, Singh S, Ahmad S, Gulzar F, Schertzer JD, Tamrakar AK (2021b) NOD1 activation induces oxidative stress via NOX1/4 in adipocytes. Free Radic Biol Med 162. https://doi.org/10.1016/j.freeradbiomed.2020.11.036

Shen J, Dai Z, Li Y, Zhu H, Zhao L (2022) TLR9 regulates NLRP3 inflammasome activation via the NF-kB signaling pathway in diabetic nephropathy. Diabetol Metab Syndr 14(1). https://doi.org/10.1186/s13098-021-00780-y

Shi H, Zhang Z, Wang X, Li R, Hou W, Bi W, Zhang X (2015) Inhibition of autophagy induces IL-1β release from ARPE-19 cells via ROS mediated NLRP3 inflammasome activation under high glucose stress. Biochem Biophys Res Commun 463(4):1071–1076. https://doi.org/10.1016/j.bbrc.2015.06.060

Srivastava SP, Kopasz-Gemmen O, Thurman A, Rajendran BK, Selvam MM, Kumar S, Srivastava R, Suresh MX, Kumari R, Goodwin JE, Inoki K (2025) The molecular determinants regulating redox signaling in diabetic endothelial cells. Front Pharmacol 16. https://doi.org/10.3389/FPHAR.2025.1563047/PDF

Stienstra R, Van Diepen JA, Tack CJ, Zaki MH, Van De Veerdonk FL, Perera D, Neale GA, Hooiveld GJ, Hijmans A, Vroegrijk I, Van Den Berg S, Romijn J, Rensen PCN, Joosten LAB, Netea MG, Kanneganti TD (2011) Inflammasome is a central player in the induction of obesity and insulin resistance. Proc Natl Acad Sci USA 108(37):15324–15329. https://doi.org/10.1073/pnas.1100255108

Sun Y, Ding S (2021) Nlrp3 inflammasome in diabetic cardiomyopathy and exercise intervention. Int J Mol Sci 22(24). MDPI. https://doi.org/10.3390/ijms222413228

Takeuchi O, Akira S (2010) Pattern recognition receptors and inflammation. Cell 140(6):805–820). Elsevier B.V. https://doi.org/10.1016/j.cell.2010.01.022

Teissier T, Boulanger É (2019) The receptor for advanced glycation end-products (RAGE) is an important pattern recognition receptor (PRR) for inflammaging. Biogerontology 20(3). https://doi.org/10.1007/s10522-019-09808-3

Thinschmidt JS, Colon Perez LM, Febo M, Caballero S, King MA, White FA, Grant MB (2016) Depressed basal hypothalamic neuronal activity in type-1 diabetic mice is correlated with proinflammatory secretion of HMBG1. Neurosci Lett 615:21–27. https://doi.org/10.1016/j.neulet.2016.01.014

Thorand B, Kolb H, Baumert J, Koenig W, Chambless L, Meisinger C, Illig T, Martin S, Herder C (2005) Elevated levels of Interleukin-18 predict the development of type 2 diabetes results from the MONICA/KORA Augsburg study, 1984–2002. Diabetes 54:2932

Timofeev YS, Kiselev AR, Dzhioeva ON, Drapkina OM (2023) Heat Shock Proteins (HSPs) and cardiovascular complications of obesity: searching for potential biomarkers. Curr Issues Mol Biol 45(12):9378–9389. https://doi.org/10.3390/CIMB45120588

Tuttle HA, Davis-Gorman G, Goldman S, Copeland JG, McDonagh PF (2004) Proinflammatory cytokines are increased in type 2 diabetic women with cardiovascular disease. J Diabetes Complicat 18(6):343–351. https://doi.org/10.1016/S1056-8727(03)00088-6

Val-Blasco A, Prieto P, Gonzalez-Ramos S, Benito G, Vallejo-Cremades MT, Pacheco I, González-Peramato P, Agra N, Terrón V, Delgado C, Martín-Sanz P, Boscá L, Fernández-Velasco M (2017) NOD1 activation in cardiac fibroblasts induces myocardial fibrosis in a murine model of type 2 diabetes. Biochem J 474(3):399–410. https://doi.org/10.1042/BCJ20160556

Vandanmagsar B, Youm YH, Ravussin A, Galgani JE, Stadler K, Mynatt RL, Ravussin E, Stephens JM, Dixit VD (2011) The NLRP3 inflammasome instigates obesity-induced inflammation and insulin resistance. Nat Med 17(2):179–189. https://doi.org/10.1038/nm.2279

Villafan-Bernal JR, Barajas-Olmos F, Guzmán-Guzmán IP, Martínez-Hernández A, Contreras-Cubas C, García-Ortiz H, Morales-Rivera MI, Martínez-Portilla RJ, Orozco L (2024) Relevant serum endoplasmic reticulum stress biomarkers in type 2 diabetes and its complications: a systematic review and meta-analysis. Antioxidants 13(12). https://doi.org/10.3390/ANTIOX13121564

Walle LV, Van Opdenbosch N, Jacques P, Fossoul A, Verheugen E, Vogel P, Beyaert R, Elewaut D, Kanneganti TD, Van Loo G, Lamkanfi M (2014) Negative regulation of the NLRP3 inflammasome by A20 protects against arthritis. Nature 512(1):69–73. https://doi.org/10.1038/nature13322

Wan R, Fang S, Zhang X, Zhou W, Bi X, Yuan L, Lv Q, Song Y, Tang W, Shi Y, Li T (2025) S100A9 as a promising therapeutic target for diabetic foot ulcers. Chin Med J 138(8). https://doi.org/10.1097/CM9.0000000000003543

Wang G, Wang G (2025) Effects of antidiabetic drugs on the level of serum uric acid in patients who have type 2 diabetes. Saudi Med J 46(3):213–225. https://doi.org/10.15537/SMJ.2025.46.3.20240920

Wang Y, Luo W, Han J, Khan ZA, Fang Q, Jin Y, Chen X, Zhang Y, Wang M, Qian J, Huang W, Lum H, Wu G, Liang G (2020a) MD2 activation by direct AGE interaction drives inflammatory diabetic cardiomyopathy. Nat Commun 11(1). https://doi.org/10.1038/s41467-020-15978-3

Wang D, Wang H, Gao H, Zhang H, Zhang H, Wang Q, Sun Z (2020b) P2X7 receptor mediates NLRP3 inflammasome activation in depression and diabetes. Cell Biosci 10(1). BioMed Central Ltd. https://doi.org/10.1186/s13578-020-00388-1

Wang G, Ma TY, Huang K, Zhong JH, Lu SJ, Li JJ (2023) Role of pyroptosis in diabetic cardiomyopathy: an updated review. Front Endocrinol 14. https://doi.org/10.3389/fendo.2023.1322907

Wei H, Sun M, Wang R, Zeng H, Zhao B, Jin S (2024) Puerarin mitigated LPS-ATP or HG-primed endothelial cells damage and diabetes-associated cardiovascular disease via ROS-NLRP3 signalling. J Cell Mol Med 28(10). https://doi.org/10.1111/JCMM.18239

Wentworth JM, Naselli G, Brown WA, Doyle L, Phipson B, Smyth GK, Wabitsch M, O'Brien PE, Harrison LC (2010) Pro-inflammatory CD11c+CD206+ adipose tissue macrophages are associated with insulin resistance in human obesity. Diabetes 59(7):1648–1656. https://doi.org/10.2337/db09-0287

Westermeier F, Navarro-Marquez M, López-Crisosto C, Bravo-Sagua R, Quiroga C, Bustamante M, Verdejo HE, Zalaquett R, Ibacache M, Parra V, Castro PF, Rothermel BA, Hill JA, Lavandero S (2015) Defective insulin signaling and mitochondrial dynamics in diabetic cardiomyopathy. Biochimica et Biophysica Acta (BBA) 1853(5):1113–1118. Elsevier B.V. https://doi.org/10.1016/j.bbamcr.2015.02.005

Wu RN, Yu TY, Zhou JC, Li M, Gao HK, Zhao C, Dong RQ, Peng D, Hu ZW, Zhang XW, Wu YQ (2018) Targeting HMGB1 ameliorates cardiac fibrosis through restoring TLR2-mediated autophagy suppression in myocardial fibroblasts. Int J Cardiol 267:156–162. https://doi.org/10.1016/j.ijcard.2018.04.103

Yang T, Luo L, Luo X, Liu X (2025) Metabolic crosstalk and therapeutic interplay between diabetes and hyperuricemia. Diabetes Res Clin Pract 224. https://doi.org/10.1016/j.diabres.2025.112204

Ye S, Lin K, Wu G, Xu MJ, Shan P, Huang W, Wang Y, Liang G (2021) Toll-like receptor 2 signaling deficiency in cardiac cells ameliorates Ang II-induced cardiac inflammation and remodeling. Transl Res 233:62–76. https://doi.org/10.1016/j.trsl.2021.02.011

Yuk JM, Jo EK (2011) Toll-like receptors and innate immunity. J Bacteriol Virol 41(4):225–235). The Korean Society for Mocrobiology/The Korean Society of Virology. https://doi.org/10.4167/jbv.2011.41.4.225

Zcan, U. O. ¨, Cao, Q., Yilmaz, E., Lee, A.-H., Iwakoshi, N. N., Zdelen, E. O. ¨, Tuncman, G., Görgün, C., Glimcher, L. H., & Hotamisligil, G. S. (2004). Endoplasmic reticulum stress links obesity, insulin action, and type 2 diabetes. www.sciencemag.org, Science, 306, 457

Zhang Y, Yang W, Li W, Zhao Y (2021) NLRP3 Inflammasome: checkpoint connecting innate and adaptive immunity in autoimmune diseases. Front Immunol 12. Frontiers Media S.A. https://doi.org/10.3389/fimmu.2021.732933

Zhang D, Li Y, Wang W, Lang X, Zhang Y, Zhao Q, Yan J, Zhang Y (2022) NOX1 promotes myocardial fibrosis and cardiac dysfunction via activating the TLR2/NF-κB pathway in diabetic cardiomyopathy. Front Pharmacol 13. https://doi.org/10.3389/fphar.2022.928762

Zhang Q, Guo S, Wang H (2024) The protective role of Baicalin in the regulation of NLRP3 Inflammasome in different diseases. Cell Biochem Biophys 83(2). https://doi.org/10.1007/S12013-024-01597-Y

Zhao H, Qi C, Zhang Y, Ren L, Chen S (2025a) Correlation between uric acid levels and bone mineral density in patients with type 2 diabetes mellitus: a systematic review and meta-analysis. Front Endocrinol 16. https://doi.org/10.3389/FENDO.2025.1415550/PDF

Zhao Y, Xu T, Wu Z, Li N, Liang Q (2025b) Rebalancing redox homeostasis: a pivotal regulator of the cGAS-STING pathway in autoimmune diseases. Autoimmun Rev 24(6). https://doi.org/10.1016/j.autrev.2025.103823

Zimbone S, Di Rosa MC, Chiechio S, Giuffrida ML (2023) Exploring the role of Hsp60 in Alzheimer's disease and type 2 diabetes: suggestion for common drug targeting. Int J Mol Sci 24(15). https://doi.org/10.3390/IJMS241512456

Cardiovascular Dysfunction in Type 2 Diabetes: The Role of MicroRNAs

Gizem Kayki-Mutlu and Ebru Arioglu-Inan

Contents

Abstract

Type 2 diabetes (T2D) is a major health concern that leads to multiple chronic complications. Among these, cardiovascular dysfunction is a prominent contributor to the morbidity and mortality associated with T2D. MicroRNAs (miRNAs) are non-coding RNAs that regulate protein synthesis by activating or suppressing target genes. Recently, their role in the cardiovascular complications of T2D has attracted significant attention. Several miRNAs have emerged as key regulators. In diabetic hearts, miRNAs such as miR-133, miR-1, miR-34a, and miR-21

G. Kayki-Mutlu · E. Arioglu-Inan (✉)
Department of Pharmacology, Faculty of Pharmacy, Ankara University, Ankara, Türkiye
e-mail: arioglu@ankara.edu.tr

A. Rueda, M. Nieves-Cintrón (eds.), *Cardiovascular Alterations in Metabolic Diseases*, Handbook of Experimental Pharmacology 293,
https://doi.org/10.1007/164_2026_799

influence critical processes, including hypertrophy, fibrosis, oxidative stress, and cell death. miR-126, in particular, is one of the most studied miRNAs in the context of vascular function in T2D, playing a crucial role in endothelial function, vascular integrity, and angiogenesis. Evidence to date suggests that altered levels of specific miRNAs contribute to cardiovascular dysfunction in T2D, making them potential therapeutic targets for preventing or treating these complications. In this chapter, we aim to discuss the impact of miRNAs on the cardiovascular system in T2D.

Keywords

Endothelial dysfunction · Heart · MicroRNAs · Type 2 diabetes · Vessels

1 Overview of the Effects of Type 2 Diabetes on the Cardiovascular System

Type 2 diabetes (T2D) is a chronic endocrine disorder characterized by impaired insulin secretion and/or insulin resistance in target tissues. The prevalence of T2D is estimated to reach 7,079 cases per 100,000 by 2030 (Khan et al. 2020). In its chronic stage, T2D is associated with severe health complications, among which cardiovascular dysfunction is particularly significant.

According to a systematic review by Einarson et al. (2018), the overall prevalence of cardiovascular disease (CVD) among 4,549,481 individuals with T2D was estimated at 32.2%. Moreover, CVD accounted for 50.3% of all deaths in people with T2D, with coronary heart disease (CHD) and stroke/cerebrovascular disease being the leading causes (Einarson et al. 2018). An incidence-based study of 29,863 patients also demonstrated that individuals with T2D had a significantly higher risk of developing coronary artery disease (CAD), myocardial infarction (MI), stroke and heart failure (HF) compared with non-diabetic patients (Straka et al. 2009). The coexistence of diabetes and hypertension further amplifies cardiovascular risk (Ormazabal et al. 2018). Consistently, a long-term longitudinal study reported higher cardiovascular mortality in T2D patients with hypertension than in hypertensive individuals without diabetes (Safar et al. 2017).

One of the most important cardiac complications of T2D is diabetic cardiomyopathy (DCM), defined as ventricular dysfunction in diabetic patients in the absence of CAD or hypertension (Rydén et al. 2013). Diastolic dysfunction, marked by increased ventricular stiffness, left atrial enlargement, and elevated left ventricular end diastolic pressure, represents the earliest stage of DCM (Battiprolu et al. 2010). This is followed by cardiac remodeling, left ventricular hypertrophy, and the clinical manifestations of HF (Ozasa et al. 2008). While some evidence suggests an association between chronic diabetes and impaired systolic function (Mbanya et al. 2001), left ventricular systolic function – measured by ejection fraction – remains normal in most T2D patients, keeping this issue under debate (Westermeier et al. 2016). More recently, DCM has been described as having two distinct phenotypes: one characterized by diastolic dysfunction, progressing to heart failure with preserved ejection fraction (HFpEF), and another characterized by systolic dysfunction, progressing to heart failure with reduced ejection fraction (HFrEF) (Zhao et al. 2022).

Oxidative stress is a major contributor to the development of cardiovascular complications in T2D. Chronic hyperglycemia enhances the production of reactive oxygen species (ROS) through multiple pathways, including the polyol and hexosamine pathways, protein kinase C (PKC) activation, and the formation of advanced glycation end products (AGEs) (Brownlee 2005). Mitochondria, the primary sites of cellular energy production, are also the major source of ROS in the cardiovascular system (Murphy and Steenbergen 2007). In T2D, mitochondrial dysfunction is characterized by excessive ROS generation and reduced ATP production (Rovira-Llopis et al. 2017). Myocardial contractile dysfunction has been linked to impaired mitochondrial function and dynamics in T2D patients (Montaigne et al. 2014). Additionally, mitochondrial respiratory dysfunction and increased H_2O_2 emission were reported in left atrial appendage tissue from T2D patients, contributing to impaired cardiac electromechanical function (Anderson et al. 2009).

AGEs are formed through non-enzymatic glycation of proteins, lipids, and nucleic acids (Caturano et al. 2025). Their hyperglycemia-driven overproduction plays a crucial role in the progression of diabetic complications (Pal and Bhadada 2023). Binding of AGEs to their receptor RAGE accelerates oxidative stress and inflammation, enhances vascular cell adhesion molecules (VCAM-1) and vascular endothelial growth factor (VEGF) expression, and impairs endothelial function, thereby promoting atherosclerosis (Pal and Bhadada 2023; Zhou et al. 2024). Several studies have confirmed the link between AGEs and macrovascular complications in T2D (Tanaka et al. 2012; Saremi et al. 2017; Yozgatli et al. 2018).

Endothelial dysfunction is another hallmark of T2D (McVeigh et al. 1992; Henry et al. 2004; Prior et al. 2005) and is recognized as an independent predictor of cardiovascular events (Nitenberg et al. 2004; Nitenberg et al. 2005). Endothelium-dependent vascular smooth muscle relaxation is impaired by 13–94% in T2D patients (Bahadoran et al. 2023). A meta-analysis further showed that vascular smooth muscle, alongside the endothelium, significantly contributes to vascular dysfunction in T2D (Montero et al. 2013). Vascular nitric oxide (NO) resistance, defined as impaired vasorelaxation in response to NO, has also been strongly associated with cardiovascular events in T2D (Bahadoran et al. 2023). The duration of T2D appears to be a major determinant of vascular NO resistance, with progressive deterioration observed in advanced disease stages (Bahadoran et al. 2023).

Several pathophysiological mechanisms underlie endothelial dysfunction in T2D, including oxidative stress, mitochondrial dysfunction, and inflammation. Excess ROS disrupt the balance between NO bioavailability and oxidative stress, further impairing endothelial function (Creager et al. 2003). ROS directly scavenge NO, reducing its bioavailability (Cubbon et al. 2007). In addition, PKC activation in the context of oxidative stress inhibits endothelial nitric oxide synthase (eNOS), further diminishing NO production (Naruse et al. 2006). Consistently, Kizhakekuttu et al. reported reduced eNOS-mediated vasodilation in arterioles from T2D patients, which was linked to mitochondrial hyperpolarization, reduced mitochondrial mass, and excessive mitochondrial superoxide generation (Kizhakekuttu et al. 2012).

Inflammation also plays a central role in regulating endothelial function in T2D, with strong interplay between oxidative stress and inflammation. Oxidative stress has been shown to activate inflammatory signaling through transcription factors such as NFκB (Caturano et al. 2025). NFκB modulates multiple pro-inflammatory and pro-atherosclerotic genes in endothelial cells (EC), vascular smooth muscle cells (VSMC), and macrophages (Sena et al. 2013). It also upregulates adhesion molecules such as E-selectin, VCAM-1, and intercellular adhesion molecule 1 (ICAM-1) (Chen et al. 1995).

Under the physiological conditions, insulin activates the phosphatidylinositol 3-kinase (PI3K) pathway in ECs, leading to eNOS phosphorylation and NO production (Dimmeler et al. 1999). However, in insulin resistance, PI3K pathway is disrupted, and the balance between PI3K/Akt pathway and mitogen-activated-protein kinase (MAPK)/extracellular signal-regulated kinases (ERK) pathway shifts toward MAPK/ERK. This shift promotes inflammation, vasoconstriction, and VSMC proliferation (Hsueh and Law 1999). Consequently, pro-inflammatory mediators such as plasminogen activator inhibitor-1 (PAI-1), ICAM-1, VCAM-1, and E-selectin are upregulated, further contributing to endothelial dysfunction (Montagnani et al. 2002).

2 MicroRNAs

MicroRNAs (miRNAs) are small, noncoding RNA molecules approximately 22 nucleotides long (Shantikumar et al. 2012). They are initially transcribed by RNA polymerase II and processed in the nucleus by the enzyme Drosha and its cofactor DiGeorge Critical Region 8 (DGCR8) to form precursor miRNAs. Exportin 5 then transports these precursors to the cytoplasm where the enzyme Dicer further processes them into mature miRNA duplexes. One strand of the duplex is then loaded onto an Argonaute (Ago) protein to form the RNA-induced silencing complex (RISC), which binds to 3′ untranslated region (UTR) of target mRNAs, leading to translational repression or mRNA degradation and ultimately silencing gene expression (Macvanin et al. 2023).

miRNAs are estimated to regulate up to 60% of human mRNAs, and more than 2000 miRNAs have been identified (Pérez-Cremades et al. 2023). These molecules play vital roles in gene regulation across a wide range of physiological and pathological processes. Dysregulation of miRNAs is associated with the development and progression of various diseases. In addition to exerting their gene regulatory functions within cells, miRNAs are also secreted into extracellular fluids – such as serum, plasma, and saliva – where they are transported by carriers including nucleophosmin, exosomes, and microvesicles. These extracellular miRNAs hold significant potential as biomarkers and therapeutic targets (Palihaderu et al. 2022).

Given their critical roles in gene regulation, they have been implicated in various physiological processes, including metabolic regulation. Notably, a large number of miRNAs act as crucial players in the control of glucose homeostasis and insulin signaling. They have important direct roles in the pathogenesis of type 2 diabetes (T2D) also contribute to its secondary complications, including cardiovascular disease (Tang, Tang et al. 2008). Hyperglycemia directly affects miRNA production, probably by altering the activity of the endonucleases DROSHA and DICER. High glucose lowers DROSHA levels, while DICER expression and pro-inflammatory markers are increased in diabetic mouse hearts, accompanied by widespread miRNA downregulation (Chavali et al. 2014; Lam et al. 2021). Besides, despite glucose normalization, dysregulated miRNAs persist – a phenomenon called "metabolic memory," contributing to ongoing cardiac issues in diabetes (Ceriello 2009).

3 The Effect of MicroRNAs on the Heart in Type 2 Diabetes

Diabetic complications are linked to altered miRNA levels in multiple organs, including the brain, heart, liver, and kidneys (Tang et al. 2008). Among these tissues, the heart is particularly vulnerable. A growing body of evidence supports central role for miRNAs in the development of DCM (Guo and Nair 2017). In the diabetic heart, miRNAs act as critical regulators of gene expression, contributing to complications such as cardiac hypertrophy, ventricular remodeling, and ultimately progression to HF.

In the diabetic heart, dysregulated miRNAs influence diverse pathological pathways, including oxidative stress, inflammation, apoptosis, fibrosis, mitochondrial dysfunction, and fetal gene reprogramming (Guo and Nair 2017). Rather than acting in isolation, many miRNAs converge on common signaling networks such as PI3K/Akt, transforming growth factor-beta (TGF-β), nuclear factor of activated T cells (NFAT), and MAPK pathways, underscoring their integrated role in diabetic cardiac remodeling.

3.1 Cardiac Hypertrophy and Remodeling

Several cardiomyocyte-enriched miRNAs are consistently linked to hypertrophic remodeling in diabetic models. Notably, miR-133 was the first miRNA reported to be dysregulated in diabetic hearts (Tang et al. 2008). In neonatal rat cardiomyocytes exposed to high glucose, hypertrophic growth is accompanied by a marked reduction in miR-133a (Feng et al. 2010). Importantly, restoration of miR-133a using miRNA mimics prevents glucose-induced hypertrophy by suppressing insulin-like growth factor 1 receptor *(IGF-1R)* and serum and glucocorticoid-regulated kinase 1 (*SGK1)* signaling, thereby limiting activation of the pro-hypertrophic transcription factor *myocyte-specific enhancer factor 2C (MEF2C)* (Feng et al. 2010). A similar anti-hypertrophic effect has been reported for miR-373; transfection of neonatal cardiomyocytes with a miR-373 mimic reduces cell size following glucose exposure and is associated with decreased *MEF2C* expression (Shen et al. 2011).

Beyond these early findings, additional miRNAs have emerged as key regulators of hypertrophic remodeling in type 2 diabetes. Reduced miR-30c levels have been shown to promote hyperglycemia-induced hypertrophy by increasing the expression of *CDC42* and p21-activated kinase *(PAK1)* (Raut et al. 2015). In contrast, miR-208a has been identified as a central early regulator of cardiac remodeling, acting downstream of α- myosin heavy chain (α-MHC) induction. This contributes to the pathological α-/β-MHC isoform switch and subsequent structural remodeling of the heart (Rawal et al. 2019). The senescence-associated miRNA, miR-34a is also upregulated in human type 2 diabetic hearts (Fomison-Nurse et al. 2018). Its expression correlates positively with HbA1c levels and promotes downregulation of Sirtuin 1 (*SIRT1*), a key modulator of metabolism homeostasis and cellular aging. Consistent with a causal role, inhibition of miR-34a in aged or diabetic models attenuates cardiac hypertrophy and improves ventricular remodeling (Boon et al. 2013; Fomison-Nurse et al. 2018). Interestingly, miR-34 expression was reduced in T2D rats following empagliflozin treatment, suggesting that cardioprotective therapies may partially act through normalization of this pathway (Kiyak-Kirmaci et al. 2025). Metabolic stress–responsive miRNAs also contribute to hypertrophic signaling in diabetes. Genetic deletion of miR-451, which targets calcium binding protein 39 *(CAB39)*, improves hypertrophy and contractile dysfunction in type 2 diabetic mice by enhancing AMP-activated protein kinase (AMPK) signaling (Kuwabara et al. 2015).

Collectively, these data indicate that multiple miRNAs converge on shared hypertrophic signaling hubs in the diabetic heart, including MEF2 signaling and AMPK-related pathways, which may account for similar remodeling phenotypes across different miRNA changes.

3.2 Cardiac Fibrosis

Fibrotic remodeling is a hallmark of DCM, and multiple miRNAs regulate fibroblast activation. miR-21 is a central regulator with highly context-dependent effects. In cardiac fibroblasts, high glucose increases miR-21 expression, enhancing collagen synthesis through targeting dual-specificity phosphatase 8 (*DUSP8*) and activating p38 MAPK signaling (Liu et al. 2014). miR-410-5p is another pro-fibrotic miRNA implicated in cardiac fibrosis. In high-fat-diet-fed rats, miR-410-5p was shown to suppress *SMAD7* – a negative regulator of TGFβ/SMAD signaling – thereby promoting fibrosis. Overexpression of miR-410-5p induced fibrotic changes even in healthy rats, whereas its inhibition reduced fibrosis in obese rats. Evidence suggest that miR-410-5p may originate from adipose or kidney tissue and exert endocrine-like effects on the heart, highlighting its potential as a therapeutic target in fibrotic remodeling (Zou et al. 2018).

In contrast, anti-fibrotic miR-29b is downregulated in Zucker diabetic fatty (ZDF) rat hearts, resulting in disrupted myofibrillar structure (Arnold et al. 2014). miR-1 has also been linked to anti-fibrotic and functional benefits in metabolic disease settings. Its expression increases following treatment with the phosphodiesterase 4D

(PDE4D) inhibitor, roflumilast. Restoring miR-1 improves cardiac function in high fat-induced hyperglycemia via activation of the cAMP–CREB–SIRT1 axis and enhanced SERCA2a expression (Xu et al. 2022). Cardiomyocyte-derived miR-194-3p similarly acts as an internal brake on cardiac fibrosis by inhibiting TGFβ-induced fibroblast-to-myofibroblast transformation. In T2D, reduced miR-194-3p contributes to increased fibrosis and diastolic dysfunction (Li et al. 2024). Overall, these findings place miRNAs at key control points of fibroblast activation.

3.3 Oxidative Stress and Energy Metabolism

Oxidative stress is a major driver of DCM and strongly influences miRNA expression. miR-30c, which normally exerts cardioprotective effects via peroxisome proliferator-activated receptor α (PPARα) signaling, is downregulated in T2D. This reduction is associated with increased peroxisome proliferator-activated receptor-gamma coactivator 1 β (PGC-1β) expression, promoting lipid accumulation, increased ROS, and metabolic dysfunction. Conversely, miR-30c overexpression reduces oxidative stress, improves metabolic balance, and mitigates cardiac damage (Yin et al. 2019). Functional benefits have been reported at the organ level, including improved left ventricular ejection fraction and reduced left ventricular mass in diabetic models with miR-30c augmentation (Chen et al. 2017).

miR-21 plays a multifaceted role in the regulation of cardiac remodeling and oxidative stress. In one setting, reduced LAZ3 expression is linked to elevated miR-21 levels, which suppress PPARα and nuclear factor erythroid 2-related factor 2 (Nrf2) signaling, thereby impairing antioxidant and anti-inflammatory responses (Gao et al. 2018). Consistently, miR-21 is upregulated in T2D patients and is associated with increased ROS (La Sala et al. 2019). In contrast, miR-21 levels were reduced in the hearts of diabetic db/db mice. Restoring miR-21 improved diastolic function, decreased oxidative stress markers, and increased phospho-Akt and phospho-eNOS levels (Dai et al. 2018a). These apparently conflicting observations support the idea that miR-21 regulation may be tissue-, model-, and disease stage–dependent rather than uniformly directional across diabetic settings.

Several additional miRNAs modulate oxidative stress responses. In high-fat-diet-fed rats subjected to multiple low-dose streptozotocin (STZ), increased miR-503 expression was accompanied by enhanced oxidative stress, reduced Nrf2 expression, and worsened cardiac function. However, its inhibition – particularly in combination with the antioxidant inducer CPDT – restored Nrf2 activity and alleviated DCM features (Miao et al. 2017). Conversely, miR-22 is downregulated in diabetic rat hearts; its overexpression increases SIRT1 levels and reduces oxidative damage (Tang et al. 2018). Similarly, miR-92a-2-5p is significantly downregulated in T2D rat models and high-glucose-stimulated cardiomyocytes. Overexpression of miR-92a-2-5p via agomiRs or adenoviral vectors reduces oxidative damage, apoptosis, and myocardial remodeling, at least partly by targeting MKNK2 and decreasing p38-MAPK phosphorylation (Yu et al. 2022).

Beyond redox control, miRNAs also govern cardiac bioenergetics and substrate handling. miR-301b regulates translation of AMP deaminase 3 (AMPD3); its downregulation increases AMPD3 levels and contributes to ATP depletion, impaired energy metabolism, and reduced cardiac contractility in T2D rat hearts (Tatekoshi et al. 2018). Conversely, miR-223 is upregulated in diabetic human hearts and may represent an adaptive response, promoting glucose uptake through increased GLUT4 expression in cardiomyocytes (Lu et al. 2010). Increased mitochondrial miR-378a in DCM is associated with reduced mt-ATP6 levels, a critical ATP synthase subunit. Genetic deletion of miR-378a preserves mt-ATP6 expression, sustains ATP synthase activity, and improves cardiac function in diabetic mice (Durr et al. 2022). Collectively, these studies support a unifying model in which multiple miRNAs shape diabetic cardiac remodeling by regulating antioxidant capacity and by tuning cellular energetics.

3.4 Lipotoxicity and Adipose Crosstalk

Myocardial lipotoxicity is another key pathological mechanism contributing to DCM and is driven by excess free fatty acid (FFAs) accumulation in cardiac tissue. Lipid overload impairs mitochondrial function, increases ROS, and disrupts cellular homeostasis. Several miRNAs regulate these lipotoxic responses (Pérez-Cremades et al. 2023). For example, miR-451 is upregulated in insulin-resistant hearts and in cardiomyocytes treated with palmitic acid, a saturated fatty acid that induces lipotoxicity. Deletion of miR-451 attenuates high-fat-diet-induced hypertrophy by targeting *CAB39* (a scaffold protein for liver kinase B1), enhancing AMPK activation and reducing mTOR signaling, (Kuwabara et al. 2015). Similarly, miR-320 contributes to diabetes-induced lipotoxicity by functioning as a nuclear activating RNA and directly upregulating fatty acid metabolism genes such as *CD36*, a key FFA transporter in db/db mice (Li et al. 2019). In contrast, miR-30c is protective; its overexpression improves glucose utilization, reduces oxidative stress and lipid accumulation, and enhances overall cardiac function in db/db mice. These benefits are mediated, in part, through inhibition of PGC-1β, a central regulator of mitochondrial lipid metabolism (Yin et al. 2019).

Adiposity, particularly epicardial adipose tissue (EAT), is increasingly implicated in DCM progression. EAT not only provides metabolic and thermogenic support but also releases bioactive molecules that influence myocardial function. In patients with T2D, 42 miRNAs were differentially expressed in EAT compared to healthy individuals, with hsa-miR-4,687-3p emerging as a key regulatory candidate (Liu et al. 2016). In addition, miR-22-3p has been implicated in adipose tissue remodeling and SIRT1 regulation, both critical for fat distribution and metabolic homeostasis. Suppression of miR-22-3p appears to increase SIRT1 expression, and prolonged PDE5 inhibitor treatment has been reported to downregulate miR-22-3p, thereby promoting beneficial metabolic effects (Fiore et al. 2016).

Moreover, secretory products from EAT in T2D can induce mitochondrial dysfunction via activation of renin-angiotensin system and upregulation of miR-208a

(Blumensatt et al. 2017). Exposure to angiotensin II impairs mitochondrial function, and this effect can be reversed by miR-208a inhibition, suggesting a mechanistic link between adipose-derived miRNAs and cardiac mitochondrial health (Blumensatt et al. 2017). Taken together, these studies emphasize that miRNAs integrate lipid handling, mitochondrial stress, and endocrine-like adipose–heart crosstalk, providing a plausible route by which systemic metabolic dysfunction is translated into cardiac remodeling.

3.5 Cell Death Pathways

miRNAs also play crucial roles in regulating cell death mechanisms in diabetic heart. Hyperglycemia promotes cardiomyocyte apoptosis, in part through disruption of pro-survival signaling. For example, insulin-like growth factor 1 (IGF-1), which normally limits apoptosis, is suppressed by upregulated miR-1 in cardiomyocytes under diabetic conditions (Yu et al. 2008). Another survival factor, Pim-1 (proviral integration site for Moloney murine leukemia virus-1), is also diminished due to increased miR-1. Restoring Pim-1 levels – either by Pim-1 overexpression or miR-1 inhibition – reduces glucose-induced cell death (Katare et al. 2011). In addition, miR-206 is upregulated in high glucose-treated cardiomyocytes and reduces heat shock protein 60 (Hsp-60), a mitochondrial chaperone with anti-apoptotic roles (Shan et al. 2003).

Among the miRNAs involved in diabetes-related apoptosis, miR-340-5p aggravates DCM by targeting the antiapoptotic MCL-1, promoting mitochondrial dysfunction, oxidative stress, apoptosis, and myocardial fibrosis; inhibition of miR-340-5p is protective in db/db mice (Zhu et al. 2022). miR-34a upregulation in human diabetic hearts is associated with reduced SIRT1 and increased caspase activity (Fomison-Nurse et al. 2018). miR-207 promotes type 2 DCM in mice by targeting the lysosomal-associated membrane protein LAMP2, reducing autophagy and increasing cardiomyocyte apoptosis (Xing et al. 2019). A long non-coding RNA (lncRNA), FENDRR, were upregulated in type 2 diabetic patients, promoting cardiomyocyte injury through the miR-296-5p/*HMGA1* axis. Silencing FENDRR reduces apoptosis, inflammation, and oxidative stress. (Gu and Zhou 2025). miR 320 promotes apoptosis in myocardial microvascular EC of type 2 diabetic rats by targeting multiple pro-survival genes, including VEGF, fibroblast growth factor (FGF), and IGF-1 (Wang et al. 2009). Similarly, miR-483-3p enhances cardiomyocyte apoptosis by suppressing *IGF-1* expression under high glucose conditions (Qiao et al. 2016), and elevated miR-195 levels promotes EC death, while its inhibition protects against non-esterified fatty acid (NEFA)-induced apoptosis in db/db mice (Zheng et al. 2015).

Conversely, several protective miRNAs are reduced in diabetic settings. miR-181a and miR-30c are downregulated and regulate p53/p21-associated apoptotic signaling, contributing to pro-apoptotic activation in DCM (Raut et al. 2016). miR-675 is downregulated under high glucose and targets *VDAC1*, linking miRNA changes to mitochondrial permeability and apoptosis (Li et al. 2016b). miR-22 prevents apoptosis by downregulating ATP-binding cassette transporter A1 (ABCA1) in db/db mice and high-glucose-exposed cardiomyocytes (Wang et al. 2021), and miR-29a targets *BAK1* and regulates apoptosis (Wang et al. 2022). Diabetic mice lacking cardiac miR-17-92 display a larger infarct size after ischemia reperfusion (I/R) injury, attributed to the loss of STAT3-induced miR-17-92 and derepression of the pro-apoptotic target *EGLN3/PHD3* (Samidurai et al. 2020). miR-186-5p is downregulated under high glucose and promotes apoptosis via Toll-like receptor 3 (Liu et al. 2019), whereas its mimic reduces apoptosis (Jiang et al. 2018). miR-133 is also downregulated in diabetic mice hearts and is accompanied by reduced anti-apoptotic signaling and increased apoptotic markers (Habibi et al. 2020).

In parallel, miRNAs regulate autophagy and other cell death pathways. miR-494 has been reported to increase under diabetic conditions and modulate autophagy through PI3K/AKT/mTOR signaling (Ning et al. 2023). However, miR-24, an insulin-sensitive miRNA downregulated in patients with T2D exerts cardioprotective effects (Pérez-Cremades et al. 2023). Its overexpression reduces infarct size after ischemia/reperfusion in diabetic mice by targeting regulators of apoptosis and autophagy, including O-GlcNAc transferase (*OGT*), the autophagy-related protein (*ATG4A*), and the apoptosis-associated protein *BIM* (Wang et al. 2018). In contrast, elevated miR-30d promotes pyroptosis under high glucose conditions by increasing pro-inflammatory mediators, including IL-1β, IL-18, and caspase-1 (Li et al. 2014). miR-34b-3p also promotes pyroptosis in DCM by targeting aryl hydrocarbon receptor; lncRNA GAS5 (growth arrest-specific transcript) inhibits miR-34b-3p, suppressing NLRP3 inflammasome activation and protecting the heart (Xu et al. 2020). miR-9 is downregulated in diabetic human heart and is associated with increased pyroptosis and upregulation of *ELAVL1*, a pro-inflammatory RNA-binding protein (Jeyabal et al. 2016). miR-214-3p is also downregulated in the serum of type 2 diabetic patients in association with increased pyroptosis-related markers (Yang et al. 2018). Overall, these data indicate that miRNAs influence cardiomyocyte survival by targeting mitochondrial checkpoints (e.g., VDAC1, MCL-1), growth factor/pro-survival pathways, and autophagy–pyroptosis balance.

3.6 Inflammation and Immune Regulation

Inflammation contributes substantially to DCM progression, and multiple miRNAs modulate inflammatory signaling after myocardial injury and metabolic stress. The anti-inflammatory miR-146a is downregulated in diabetic models, and miR-146 mimic approaches have shown promise in alleviating diabetic inflammatory phenotypes, supporting its therapeutic potential in diabetes-related organ damage (Ghaffari et al. 2023). Sodium-glucose cotransporter 2 (SGLT2) inhibitors such as empagliflozin and dapagliflozin have also been reported to increase miR-146a levels in T2D rats, alongside histopathological and biochemical improvement (Kiyak-Kirmaci et al. 2025). Mechanistically, miR-146a suppresses IRAK1 and TRAF6 signaling to reduce pro-inflammatory cytokine production in T2D (Alipoor et al. 2017). Interestingly, its expression may depend on exercise modality and intensity. High-intensity training decreases miR-146a (Cirilli et al. 2019), whereas resistance training has been reported to increase it (Morais Junior et al. 2017), suggesting differential regulation by distinct training programs.

In contrast, miR-155 functions as a pro-inflammatory miRNA and is elevated in db/db mouse hearts following myocardial infarction (Kishore et al. 2013). Intramyocardial delivery of bone marrow-derived progenitor cells lowered miR-155 and improved cardiac repair in diabetic mice (Kishore et al. 2013). Inhibition of miR-150-5p also reduces inflammation by dampening both NF-kB and TGF-β1 pathways, supporting its candidacy as a therapeutic target for diabetic cardiac complications (Che et al. 2020). Collectively, inflammatory miRNAs link metabolic stress to cytokine signaling and remodeling pathways.

3.7 Circulating miRNAs and Biomarkers

In addition to tissue-specific changes, circulating miRNAs can reflect early and progressive alterations associated with diabetic cardiac injury (Zhu and Leung 2015). In a serum profiling study evaluating 798 miRNAs, six miRNAs (miR-615-3p, miR-3147, miR-1224-5p, miR-5196-3p, miR-6732-3p, and miR-548b-3p) were significantly upregulated in T2D patients with ischemic heart disease. These changes were linked to pathways including endothelin-1, glucocorticoid and apelin pathways – axes relevant to vascular tone, inflammation, and cardiac remodeling (Bielska et al. 2022). Importantly, miR-221 and miR-34a have been proposed to sustain disease progression even after blood glucose normalization, suggesting that miRNA-mediated dysfunction may persist independently of glycemic control and thus require targeted therapeutic strategies (Macvanin et al. 2023).

Given their stability in circulation and sensitivity to pathological changes, miRNAs have emerged as promising diagnostic and prognostic biomarkers. In healthy individuals, miRNAs transferred between cells and tissues maintain stable expression patterns, but in disease states, their levels become dysregulated. This fluctuation offers opportunities for using circulating miRNAs as non-invasive indicators of disease onset, progression or response to therapy (Guo and Nair 2017). Consistent with this concept, multiple studies have identified circulating miRNAs as reliable biomarkers in both diabetes and cardiovascular disease (Shantikumar et al. 2012; Saini et al. 2022).

For example, plasma levels of miR-1 and miR-133a have been proposed as biomarkers for early cardiac complications in T2D (Pérez-Cremades et al. 2023). Both miRNAs were significantly increased in T2D patients and in high-fat-diet-fed mice exhibiting increased myocardial lipid accumulation. These changes were also reflected in exosomes released from lipid-loaded cardiomyocytes, suggesting their role in intercellular communication and pathogenesis. Notably, miR-1 and miR-133a independently predicted myocardial steatosis, emphasizing their potential as diagnostic biomarkers for early-stage DCM (de Gonzalo-Calvo et al. 2017).

Beyond environmental and metabolic influences, genetic variation can also affect miRNA function and contribute to the pathophysiology of diabetic complications. Polymorphisms in miRNA genes such as miR-133a-1-rs8089787 and let-7f-rs10877887 have been linked to altered diastolic function in patients with T2D, suggesting their potential as genetic markers and therapeutic targets for diastolic dysfunction (Sun et al. 2022). Collectively, circulating miRNAs reflect key pathological features of diabetic cardiac injury – including hypertrophy, metabolic stress, and inflammation – and may provide a noninvasive tool for early diagnosis and risk assessment.

3.8 Clinical Relevance and Therapeutic Perspectives

Given their ability to regulate multiple genes simultaneously, RNA-based therapies offer a promising alternative to traditional treatments. In the context of miRNA modulation, two major strategies have been developed: (1) restoring downregulated miRNAs with miRNA mimics or viral vectors and (2) inhibiting overactive miRNAs using antisense oligonucleotides (ASOs, antimiRs), or competitive inhibitors (Macvanin et al. 2023). miRNA mimics, synthetic double-stranded RNAs, restore the function of downregulated miRNAs by targeting multiple mRNAs. In contrast, ASOs are single-stranded DNAs that block mRNA function, while antimiRs directly target miRNAs; their cholesterol-conjugated forms are known as antagomiRs (Macvanin et al. 2023).

In experimental diabetes models, antagomiR-155 was shown to reduce inflammation and improve cardiac damage and function (Corsten et al. 2012). Viral vectors such as adeno-associated virus (AAV) can also deliver miRNA modulators in a tissue-targeted manner. For example, an adenoviral approach was used to inhibit miR-503 in diabetic limb ischemia (Caporali et al. 2011). However, because adenoviruses mediate only short-term gene expression, they may be less suitable for chronic diseases such as diabetes (Shantikumar et al. 2012).

Beyond DCM specifically, anti-miR therapies are being investigated for broader metabolic disorders. Anti-miR-103/107 is under development for NAFLD (non-alcoholic fatty liver disease) and NASH (non-alcoholic steatohepatitis) in patients with T2D or prediabetes (La Sala et al. 2024). This agent has successfully completed phase I clinical trials and entered phase II trials, with proposed insulin-sensitizing effects linked to improved insulin signaling, reduced hepatic triglyceride accumulation, improved adipose features, and decreased adipocyte size and steatosis (Pal and Bhadada 2023; Trajkovski et al. 2011). Ongoing studies should clarify efficacy, safety, tissue specificity, and whether combining miRNA therapies with established cardiometabolic drugs yields additive benefits. In summary, miRNA-based interventions are attractive because they can modulate entire disease-relevant networks. At the same time, the convergence of many miRNAs on shared pathways underscores the need for careful targeting to maximize cardioprotection while minimizing off-target effects – particularly in a systemic disease such as type 2 diabetes (see Fig. 1 for a summary of cardiac miRNA targets in T2D).

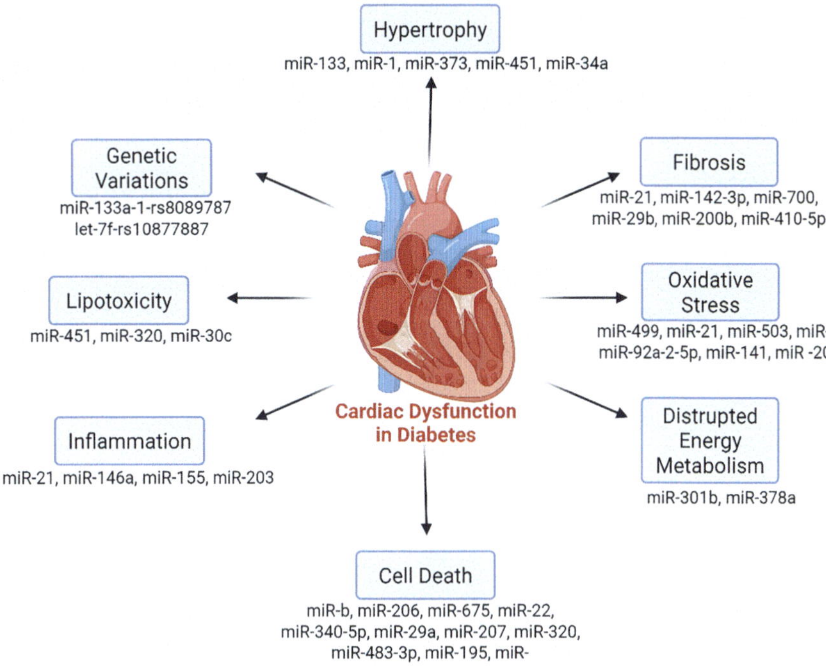

Fig. 1 miRNAs involved in the cardiac function in T2D. (This figure is created in https://BioRender.com)

4 The Effect of MicroRNAs on the Vascular System in Type 2 Diabetes

Current preclinical and clinical findings demonstrate that several miRNAs play essential roles in vascular function. It has also been reported that the alteration of miRNAs in the vessels contributes to vascular dysfunction seen in T2D (Fig. 2). In this regard, most of the studies have focused on the role of miRNAs in angiogenesis and endothelial dysfunction in T2D.

4.1 The Role of miRNAs in Endothelial Dysfunction and Angiogenesis

miR-126 is one of the most extensively studied miRNAs in the context of angiogenesis (Table 1). Highly expressed in ECs, miR-126 is crucial for maintaining endothelial homeostasis, vascular integrity, and angiogenesis (Wang et al. 2008; Arunachalam et al. 2015). Mechanistically, it promotes VEGF signaling by inhibiting *Sprouty-related protein (SPRED1)* and *phosphoinositol-3 kinase*

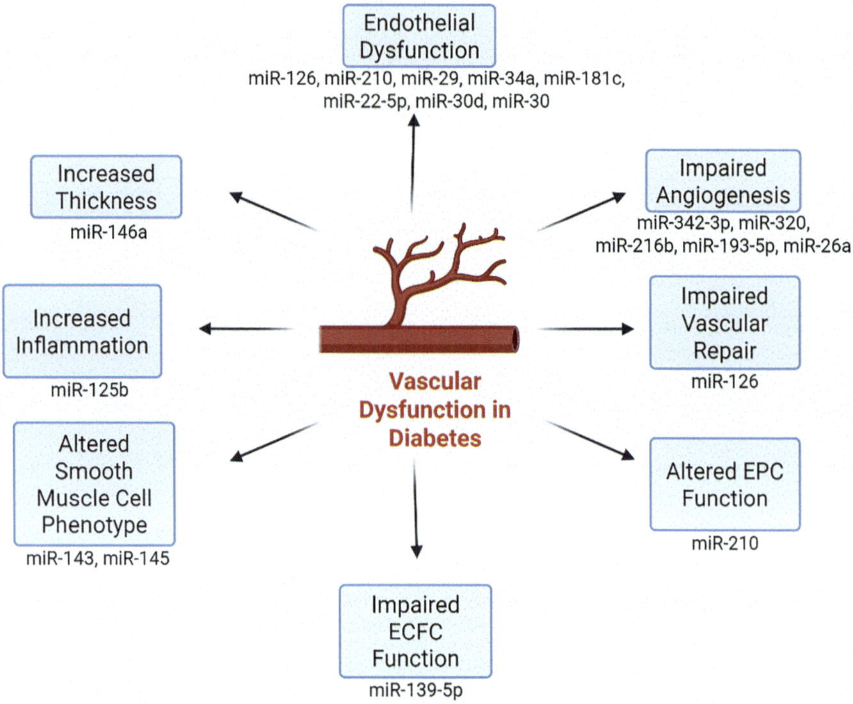

Fig. 2 miRNAs related to vascular function in T2D. (This figure is created in https://BioRender.com)

regulatory subunit 2 (PIK3R2/p85-beta) (Fish et al. 2008). In human umbilical vein endothelial cells (HUVEC), miR-126 levels were found to be reduced in apoptotic bodies under hyperglycemic conditions (Zampetaki et al. 2010). Furthermore, the same study reported diminished expression of miR-126 in the plasma of hyperglycemic leptin-obese mice. Consistently, lower plasma levels of miR-126 have been observed in T2D patients (Zampetaki et al. 2010; Al-Kafaji et al. 2017). It has been suggested that this reduction may impair miR-126 delivery to monocytes, contributing to *VEGF* resistance and endothelial dysfunction (Zampetaki et al. 2010) (Fig. 2).

Endothelial progenitor cells (EPCs) are essential for angiogenesis and endothelial regeneration following vascular injury, as they can differentiate into mature ECs (Rabelink et al. 2004; Hristov and Weber 2008). The number and function of EPCs are inversely correlated with cardiovascular risk factors (Hristov and Weber 2008). EPC dysfunction – characterized by reduced cell number, impaired damaged proliferation, adhesion, and angiogenesis – is a common feature in T2D (Prattichizzo et al. 2015; De Pascale et al. 2016; Li et al. 2020). Notably, reduced expression of miR-126 has been demonstrated in EPCs of patients with T2D and has been proposed to contribute to impaired vascular repair in these patients (Meng et al.

Table 1 Key miRNAs that play a role in the cardiovascular dysfunction in T2D

miRNA	Effect	Alteration in T2D	Potential target/ pathway	Source	Reference
miR-133a	Anti-hypertrophic, anti-apoptotic	↓, heart	*IGF1R*, *SGK1* → *MEF2C* signaling	Cardiomyocytes	Tang et al. (2008), Feng et al. (2010)
miR-1	Pro-apoptotic (when ↑); anti-fibrotic (context-dependent)	↑ in diabetic cardiomyocytes; ↓ in some models	*IGF-1, PIM-1*	Cardiomyocytes	Yu et al. (2008), Katare et al. (2011)
miR-34a	Promotes hypertrophy, apoptosis	↑, heart	*SIRT1*	Diabetic heart	Boon et al. (2013), Fomison-Nurse et al. (2018)
miR-30c	Anti-hypertrophic, anti-lipotoxic, antioxidant	↓, heart	*CDC42/PAK1; PGC-1β; PPARα* signaling	Diabetic heart	Raut et al. (2015), Yin et al. (2019)
miR-21	Pro-fibrotic, redox regulator (context-dependent)	↑ in fibroblasts; variable in heart	*DUSP8* → *p38 MAPK; PPARα/Nrf2*	Cardiac fibroblasts / heart	Liu et al. (2014), Dai et al. (2018a)
miR-126	Angiogenesis, endothelial regeneration	↓, plasma		Hyperglycemic leptin-obese mice	Zampetaki et al. (2010)
		↓, plasma		T2D patients	Zampetaki et al. (2010), Al-Kafaji et al. (2017)
		↓, EPCs	*SPRED1*: *Ras/ERK/VEGF* and *PI3K/Akt/eNOS*	T2D patients	Meng et al. (2012)
		↓, circulating micro particles		T2D patients	Jansen et al. (2016)
		↓, circulating micro particles (including those derived from EPCs)		T2D patients	Wu et al. (2016)
miR-210	EPC number/function	↑, peripheral blood		T2D patients	Li et al. (2020)
	Endothelial dysfunction	↓, RBCs; ↓, plasma	*PTP1B*	T2D patients	Zhou et al. (2022)

(continued)

Table 1 (continued)

miRNA	Effect	Alteration in T2D	Potential target/ pathway	Source	Reference
	Endothelial dysfunction	↓, aorta	*PTP1B/GPD2*	Db/db mice	Collado et al. (2025)

T2D type 2 diabetes, *IGF1R* Insulin-like growth factor 1 receptor, *SGK1* Serum and glucocorticoid-regulated kinase 1, *MEF2C Myocyte-specific enhancer factor 2C*, *PIM-1* provirus integration site for Moloney murine leukemia virus 1, *SIRT1* Sirtuin 1, *PAK1* p21-activated kinase, *PGC-1β* Peroxisome proliferator-activated receptor-gamma coactivator 1 *β*, *PPARα* Peroxisome proliferator-activated receptor *α*, *DUSP8* Dual-specificity phosphatase 8, *p38 MAPK* P38 Mitogen-Activated Protein Kinase, *Nrf2* Nuclear factor erythroid 2-related factor 2, *EPC* endothelial progenitor cells, *RBC* red blood cell, *PI3K* phosphoinositol-3-kinase, *eNOS* endothelial nitric oxide synthase, *SPRED1* Sprouty-related protein 1, *ERK* extracellular signal-regulated kinase, *VEGF* vascular growth factor, *PTP1B* vascular tyrosine phosphatase 1B, *GPD2* mitochondrial glycerol-3-phosphate dehydrogenase 2

2012) (Fig. 2). Restoration of miR-126 expression in EPCs improved colony formation, proliferation, migration, and reduced apoptosis, although it did not affect cell differentiation. These beneficial effects were mediated through miR-126 targeting *SPRED1*, activating *Ras/ERK/VEGF* and *PI3K/Akt/eNOS* signaling pathways. In addition to miR-126, other miRNAs, including miR-21, miR-27a, miR-27b, and miR-130, were also found to be downregulated in EPCs derived from the patients with T2D (Meng et al. 2012).

Jansen et al. demonstrated that endothelial microparticles derived from hyperglycemia-impaired ECs contain reduced levels of miR-126 and consequently lose their regenerative capacity (Jansen et al. 2013). The same group later reported that both miR-126 and miR-26a were markedly downregulated in circulating micro particles in T2D patients (Jansen et al. 2016). Clinically, patients with reduced levels of these miRNAs were found to have a higher risk for concomitant CAD. Furthermore, in vitro hyperglycemic conditions diminished the packaging of these miRNAs into endothelial microparticles.

Additional studies further support the impact of miR-126 level on vascular function in T2D. Wu et al. (2016) reported that circulating microvesicles, including those derived from EPCs, exhibited reduced levels of both miR-126 and *VEGF receptor 2 (VEGFR2)* in patients with uncontrolled T2D (Wu et al. 2016). Functional studies using miR-126 mimics and inhibitors confirmed its regulatory role in EPC-derived microvesicle function, suggesting that downregulation of miR-126 impairs the protective effects of circulating and EPC-derived microvesicles in T2D. In db/db mice, the vascular protective effect of exercise was attributed to the expression level of miR-126 (Lew et al. 2020). The same study also suggested that EC integrity and small arteriole density were closely associated with plasma and cardiac miR-126 levels. Collectively, these findings highlight the central role of miRNA-126 in the pathogenesis of T2D-related vascular disease (Fig. 2, Table 1).

Another miRNA which plays role in angiogenesis in T2D is miR-26a. miR-26a, in particular, has an antiapoptotic effect in vascular ECs and is dysregulated in atherosclerosis (Zhang et al. 2015). It regulates both physiological and pathological angiogenesis via *BMP/SMAD-1* signaling (Icli et al. 2013). As mentioned above, miR-26a was found to be downregulated in circulating micro particles in T2D patients (Jansen et al. 2016). Thus, its reduction has been proposed as a compensatory proangiogenic mechanism that may slow the progression of angiogenesis impairment in this pathology (Jansen et al. 2016).

Cai et al. (2025) investigated EPC dysfunction in T2D within the framework of the *TGF-β1*/miR-130a/IL-18 axis (Cai et al. 2025). In EPCs isolated from patients with T2D, miR-130a expression was negatively correlated with *TGF-β1* and positively correlated with IL-18. Functionally, overexpression of miR-130a inhibited tube formation, cell adhesion, and migration in EPCs. This finding was linked to the inverse relationship between miR-130a and IL-18, as IL-18 exerted a favorable effect on EPC function (Cai et al. 2025). In addition to miR-126 and miR-130a, miR-210 has also been implicated in number and function of EPCs in T2D (Fig. 2, Table 1). Li et al. reported that EPC counts in the peripheral blood were significantly lower in newly diagnosed T2D patients, whereas miR-210 levels were increased

(Li et al. 2020). These EPCs exhibited impaired proliferation, adhesion, migration, and tube formation, along with enhanced apoptosis. Upregulation of miR-210 was identified as an independent risk factor for the reduced EPC numbers. Importantly, transfection of EPCs with a miR-210 inhibitor restored their biological function, suggesting that downregulation of miR-210 may promote EPC mobilization, differentiation, and angiogenesis (Li et al. 2020). Conversely, Zhou et al. (2022) demonstrated that miR-210 expression was reduced in red blood cells (RBC) and plasma of T2D patients (Zhou et al. 2022) (Table 1). Rat aortas incubated with RBCs isolated from T2D patients displayed endothelial dysfunction, and a similar impairment of endothelium-dependent relaxation in rats transfused with RBCs from diabetic Goto-Kakizaki rats. This effect was referred to the downregulation of miR-210, linked to *vascular tyrosine phosphatase 1B (PTP1B)* – a regulator of insulin signaling – and increased ROS. Of note, endothelial dysfunction was improved by restoring miR-210 expression using a mimic. Further supporting these findings, Collado et al. showed that miR-210 was downregulated in the aorta of db/db mice. Its suppression contributed to endothelial dysfunction through the downstream targets including *PTP1B, mitochondrial glycerol-3-phosphate dehydrogenase 2 (GPD2)*, and mitochondrial oxidative stress (Collado et al. 2025) (Table 1). The conflicting findings regarding miR-210 expression in patients with T2D may reflect differences in disease duration and comorbid cardiovascular conditions. Li et al. (2020) studied newly diagnosed T2D patients without evident cardiac disease, whereas Zhou et al. (2022) analyzed samples from individuals with established diabetes who were receiving oral antidiabetic drugs or insulin. In addition, participants in the Zhou et al. (2022) cohort had hypertension and were treated with antihypertensive medications, factors that may further influence miR-210 expression.

miR-29 was found to be dysregulated in resistance arteriole biopsies from T2D patients (Widlansky et al. 2018). Remarkably, intraluminal transfection with miR-29a-3p or miR-29b-3p mimics restored impaired endothelium-dependent vasodilation in these arterioles. Consistent with this, administration of anti-miR-29b-3p in arterioles of nondiabetic human subjects impaired endothelium-dependent vasodilatation, an effect also observed in rats. Moreover, in a miR-29a-3p and miR-29b-3p knockdown rat model (Mir29b-1/a$^{-/-}$), endothelium-dependent vasodilatation was impaired and mean arterial pressure was elevated (Widlansky et al. 2018). The same study further showed that the beneficial effect of miR-29 on endothelial vasodilatation partly involves modulation of *lysophospholipase I (Lypla1)* expression. Collectively, these findings indicate that miR-29 is essential for normal endothelial function and may represent a therapeutic target in cardiometabolic disorders.

Elevated levels of miR-320 were detected in myocardial microvascular endothelial cells (MMEC) of diabetic Goto-Kakizaki rats (Wang et al. 2009). This upregulation was linked to reduced cell proliferation, impaired migration, and downregulation of *IGF-1*. Notably, transfection with a miR-320 inhibitor reversed these effects, suggesting that inhibition of miR-320 may have therapeutic potential for restoring angiogenesis in T2D (Wang et al. 2009) (Fig. 2). Similarly, miR-193-5p (Yi et al. 2017) and miR-216b (Dai et al. 2018b) were significantly upregulated in

MMECs isolated from diabetic Goto-Kakizaki (GK) rats. Downregulation of miR-193-5 using its antagomiR promoted angiogenesis by enhancing cell migration and proliferation (Yi et al. 2017). This effect was accompanied by upregulation of *insulin-like growth factor 2 (IGF2)* gene, a key regulator of angiogenesis (Alders et al. 2025). Thus, the angiogenic improvement was attributed to suppression of miR-193-5p and subsequent *IGF2* induction. In parallel, inhibition of miR-216b stimulated angiogenesis through increased cell invasion and proliferation (Dai et al. 2018b). This effect was linked to enhanced expression of *frizzled class receptor 5 (FDZ5)*, a component of *Wnt* signaling pathway, which plays an essential role in angiogenesis and vascular remodeling (Goodwin and D'Amore 2002; Muley et al. 2010). Taken together, these findings support that miR-193-5p and miR-216b regulate angiogenesis in diabetes via targeting *IGF2* and *FDZ5*, respectively (Yi et al. 2017; Dai et al. 2018a) (Fig. 2).

Luo et al. (2021) further implicated miR-139-5p in diabetic endothelial dysfunction through *c-Jun*-initiated pathways (Luo et al. 2020). They reported that miR-139-5p was upregulated in endothelial colony-forming cells (ECFCs) from patients with T2D, in ECs isolated from diabetic rodents' aortas, and in HUVECs exposed to hyperglycemia. Furthermore, miR-139-5p regulated ECFC function via the *c-Jun-VEGF/PDGF-B* pathway. Elevated miR-139-5p expression suppressed this pathway, resulting in reduced migration, tube formation, and proliferation of ECFCs, as well as impaired EC survival (Luo et al. 2020). These findings suggest that targeting miR-139-5p may represent a potential therapeutic strategy for diabetic vascular dysfunction.

In the study by Li et al. (2016a), impaired endothelium-dependent vasodilatation in db/db mice was attributed to *P66Shc*-induced upregulation of miR-34a in both endothelium and media of aortas (Li et al. 2016a). *P66Shc*, a pro-apoptotic protein, has been implicated in the pathogenesis of diabetic complications (Mousavi et al. 2022). Inhibition of miR-34a suppressed its elevated expression and preserved endothelial vasodilatation. Mechanistically, miR-34a was shown to target *Sirt1*, a critical regulator of vascular endothelial function. *Sirt1* activates *endothelial nitric oxide synthase (eNOS)* through deacetylation, thereby increasing NO levels (Mattagajasingh et al. 2007). Thus, the authors concluded that *P66Shc*-driven upregulation of miR-34a contributes to endothelial dysfunction in db/db mice via downregulation of *Sirt1* (Li et al. 2016a) (Fig. 2). In the context of *eNOS* and NO, miR-4521 has also been implicated in diabetes-induced EC dysfunction. Zhang et al. (2024) reported that inhibition of miR-4521 further aggravated vascular endothelial dysfunction in high fat-high sucrose (HFHG) diet induced diabetic mice (Zhang et al. 2024). The study showed that circHMGCS1 functions as a miR-4521 sponge, leading to upregulation of *arginase I*, reduced vascular NO secretion and *eNOS* activity, increased adhesion molecule expression, and enhanced ROS formation. These alterations blunted vascular relaxation and accelerated endothelial dysfunction. Accordingly, inhibition of circHMGCS1 or overexpression of miR-4521 has been proposed as a therapeutic strategy to mitigate vascular endothelial dysfunction in diabetes (Zhang et al. 2024). miRNAs have also been reported to be associated with nitrative stress in diabetes. In a study by Yang et al. (2017), miR-181c expression was reduced, whereas *forkhead protein FoxO1* was upregulated in primary mouse aortic ECs isolated from db/db mice and in a mouse EC line exposed to high glucose (Yang et al. 2017) (Fig. 2). Transfection with a miR-181c mimic reversed high glucose-induced nitration stress in mouse aortic ECs, while this effect was abolished by *FoxO1* overexpression. Moreover, systemic delivery of a miR-181c mimic attenuated nitration stress in db/db mice. These findings indicate that miR-181c alleviates diabetes-associated nitration stress by suppressing *FoxO1* expression (Yang et al. 2017).

As discussed in the first section, AGEs are major contributors to endothelial dysfunction in T2D. Ji et al. (2025) demonstrated a link between AGEs, miR-22-5p, and EC function (Ji et al. 2025). miR-22-5p is upregulated in exosomes exposed to AGEs and subsequently transferred to ECs (Ji et al. 2025) (Fig. 2). Both AGE-derived exosomes and overexpression of miR-22-5p resulted in downregulation of *FOXP1* and impaired EC function. Consistent with this, unfavorable effects of AGE-exosomes on EC proliferation, migration, *FOXP1* expression, and the levels of *VCAM-1*, *ICAM-1*, and *MCP-1* were alleviated when a miR-22-5p inhibitor was used. In addition, the authors reported a link between *Rab27a* and EC function in AGE-exosomes. This was confirmed by using *Rab27a*-knockout type 2 diabetic mice, in which exosome release was reduced and EC inflammation was attenuated. Thus, the authors concluded that targeting miR-22-5p or *Rab27a* may represent a therapeutic strategy for preventing and treating diabetic vascular lesions (Pal and Bhadada 2023).

In addition to miRNAs discussed above, many others have been investigated in the context of angiogenesis and EC function in T2D. Stepien et al. (2018) screened miRNAs in ectosomes obtained from patients with T2D and identified altered expression of miR-193b-3p, miR-199a-3p, miR-20a-3p, miR-26b-5p, miR-30b-5p, miR-30c-5p, miR-374a-5p, miR-409-3p, and miR-95-3p (Stępień et al. 2018). Importantly both pro-angiogenic and anti-angiogenic miRNAs were found to be dysregulated in T2D. For example, ectosome-specific miRNAs – including hsa-miR-26a-5p, hsa-miR-26b-5p, hsa-miR-30b-5p, and hsa-miR-30c-5p – were shown to target the mRNAs of *MTDH* and *PDCD10*, two genes involved in angiogenesis. Notably, both the pro-angiogenic hsa-miR-30 family miRNAs and the anti-angiogenic 26 hsa-miR-26 family targeted these transcripts, suggesting that their dysregulation contributes to impaired angiogenesis and, consequently, the development of diabetic vascular complications (Stępień et al. 2018). Increased expression of miR-30d and miR-30e in cardiac endothelium is thought to contribute to microvascular and consequently diastolic dysfunction in diabetes (Veitch et al. 2022). In rodents with T2D, miR-30d and miR-30e were found to be upregulated in circulating plasma endothelial vesicles (Veitch et al. 2022). The upregulation of miR-30e was associated with coronary microvascular dysfunction and rarefaction during the early stages of diabetes. Mechanistically, miR-30 promoted oxidative stress, lipid peroxidation, and endothelial dysfunction in cultured ECs by regulating the β-oxidation of exogenous fatty acids (Fig. 2). Collectively, these findings indicate that miRNAs play a crucial role in regulating angiogenesis and endothelial dysfunction in T2D, thereby contributing to the vascular complications associated with this condition.

4.2 The Role of miRNAs in Vascular Smooth Muscle and Remodeling

There are few studies examining the relationship between vascular smooth muscle and miRNAs in T2D. In db/db mice, miR-125b expression was increased in aortic VSMCs, concomitant with downregulation of *Suv39h1*, a histone lysine N methyltransferase (Villeneuve et al. 2010). Similarly, upregulation of miR-125b was associated with enhanced expression of inflammatory proteins, including *monocyte chemoattractant protein-1 (MCP-1)*, interleukin-6 (IL-6), as well as increased monocyte-VSMCs binding (Cheng et al. 2018).

miR-146a has been proposed as both a biomarker for early diagnosis and a therapeutic target in atherosclerosis associated with T2D. In patients with newly diagnosed T2D, higher plasma levels of miR-146a were positively correlated with increased carotid intima-media thickness and brachial-ankle pulse wave velocity – the markers of subclinical atherosclerosis – independent of other cardiovascular risk factors (Guo et al. 2020). Moreover, in T2D patients, the expression levels of miR-146a, miR34a, miR-124a, miR-155, miR221, and miR-126 were positively correlated with markers of vascular endothelial changes, including VEGF, apolipoprotein A-I (ApoAI), apolipoprotein B (ApoB), and ApoB/ApoAI ratio (Al-Rawaf et al. 2025). Alterations in saphenous vein smooth muscle cell phenotype in T2D were found to be associated with increased expression of miR-143 and miR-145 (Riches et al. 2014). Suppression of these miRNAs using antimiR-143/145 ameliorated the phenotypic changes in saphenous vein smooth muscle cells. Therefore, it has been suggested that this distinct saphenous vein smooth muscle cell phenotype, along with the upregulation of miR-143 and miR-145, may contribute to vascular complications in T2D. Compared with the extensive evidence on angiogenesis and endothelial dysfunction, relatively limited data are available on the role of microRNAs in vascular smooth muscle function and remodeling. Further studies are therefore needed to better understand this area.

5 Conclusion

Current evidence indicates that dysregulated expression of specific miRNAs plays a significant role in cardiovascular dysfunction in T2D. Some of these miRNAs have demonstrated clear impact in preclinical and, in some cases, clinical studies. In the diabetic heart, it has been shown that miR-133, miR-1, and miR-144 influence major pathological abnormalities such as hypertrophy, fibrosis, oxidative stress, and cell death. On the other hand, in the vascular system, miR-126 appears to play a crucial role in diabetes-related alterations in endothelial function, vascular integrity, and angiogenesis. Together, these findings highlight that miRNA dysregulation contributes to both cardiac and vascular complications of T2D.

It is also evident that, beyond the most extensively studied miRNAs, many others linked to cardiovascular dysfunction in T2D have been investigated in single or limited studies. Therefore, it remains difficult to fully interpret the impact of all the miRNAs discussed in this chapter. Importantly, the concept of metabolic memory – where cardiovascular abnormalities persist despite glycemic normalization – suggests that sustained miRNA dysregulation may contribute to long-lasting cardiac and vascular damage in T2D.

Future studies are needed to better define the roles of these miRNAs and clarify how they contribute to cardiovascular complications in T2D. Further clinical trials of miRNA-based therapies and additional research on circulating miRNAs for early detection of DCM will be important for translating these findings into clinical practice. With continued progress, miRNA-targeted strategies may offer more precise approaches for managing cardiovascular complications in type 2 diabetes.

References

Alders L, Pirlet E, Gesquiere E, Bronckaers A (2025) The role of IGF-2 and its variants in enhancing endothelial migration and angiogenesis. Front Cell Dev Biol 13:1598705

Alipoor B, Ghaedi H, Meshkani R, Torkamandi S, Saffari S, Iranpour M, Omrani MD (2017) Association of MiR-146a expression and type 2 diabetes mellitus: a meta-analysis. Int J Mol Cell Med 6(3):156–163

Al-Kafaji G, Al-Mahroos G, Abdulla Al-Muhtaresh H, Sabry MA, Abdul Razzak R, Salem AH (2017) Circulating endothelium-enriched microRNA-126 as a potential biomarker for coronary artery disease in type 2 diabetes mellitus patients. Biomarkers 22(3–4):268–278

Al-Rawaf HA, Gabr SA, Alghadir T, Alghadir F, Iqbal A, Alghadir AH (2025) Correlation between circulating microRNAs and vascular biomarkers in type 2 diabetes based upon physical activity: a biochemical analytic study. BMC Endocr Disord 25(1):55

Anderson EJ, Kypson AP, Rodriguez E, Anderson CA, Lehr EJ, Neufer PD (2009) Substrate-specific derangements in mitochondrial metabolism and redox balance in the atrium of the type 2 diabetic human heart. J Am Coll Cardiol 54(20):1891–1898

Arnold N, Koppula PR, Gul R, Luck C, Pulakat L (2014) Regulation of cardiac expression of the diabetic marker microRNA miR-29. PLoS One 9(7):e103284

Arunachalam G, Upadhyay R, Ding H, Triggle CR (2015) MicroRNA signature and cardiovascular dysfunction. J Cardiovasc Pharmacol 65(5):419–429

Bahadoran Z, Mirmiran P, Kashfi K, Ghasemi A (2023) Vascular nitric oxide resistance in type 2 diabetes. Cell Death Dis 14(7):410

Battiprolu PK, Gillette TG, Wang ZV, Lavandero S, Hill JA (2010) Diabetic cardiomyopathy: mechanisms and therapeutic targets. Drug Discov Today Dis Mech 7(2):e135–e143

Bielska A, Niemira M, Bauer W, Sidorkiewicz I, Szałkowska A, Skwarska A, Raczkowska J, Ostrowski D, Gugała K, Dobrzycki S, Krętowski A (2022) Serum miRNA profile in diabetic patients with ischemic heart disease as a promising non-invasive biomarker. Front Endocrinol (Lausanne) 13:888948

Blumensatt M, Fahlbusch P, Hilgers R, Bekaert M, Herzfeld de Wiza D, Akhyari P, Ruige JB, Ouwens DM (2017) Secretory products from epicardial adipose tissue from patients with type 2 diabetes impair mitochondrial β-oxidation in cardiomyocytes via activation of the cardiac renin-angiotensin system and induction of miR-208a. Basic Res Cardiol 112(1):2

Boon RA, Iekushi K, Lechner S, Seeger T, Fischer A, Heydt S, Kaluza D, Tréguer K, Carmona G, Bonauer A, Horrevoets AJ, Didier N, Girmatsion Z, Biliczki P, Ehrlich JR, Katus HA, Müller OJ, Potente M, Zeiher AM, Hermeking H, Dimmeler S (2013) MicroRNA-34a regulates cardiac ageing and function. Nature 495(7439):107–110

Brownlee M (2005) The pathobiology of diabetic complications: a unifying mechanism. Diabetes 54(6):1615–1625

Cai Y, Zhu Y, Xu N, Chen T (2025) The study of miR-130a expression and its mechanism of action in peripheral blood endothelial progenitor cells (EPCs) in type 2 diabetes mellitus (T2DM). Sci Rep 15(1):11038

Caporali A, Meloni M, Völlenkle C, Bonci D, Sala-Newby GB, Addis R, Spinetti G, Losa S, Masson R, Baker AH, Agami R, le Sage C, Condorelli G, Madeddu P, Martelli F, Emanueli C (2011) Deregulation of microRNA-503 contributes to diabetes mellitus-induced impairment of endothelial function and reparative angiogenesis after limb ischemia. Circulation 123(3): 282–291

Caturano A, Rocco M, Tagliaferri G, Piacevole A, Nilo D, Di Lorenzo G, Iadicicco I, Donnarumma M, Galiero R, Acierno C, Sardu C, Russo V, Vetrano E, Conte C, Marfella R, Rinaldi L, Sasso FC (2025) Oxidative stress and cardiovascular complications in type 2 diabetes: from pathophysiology to lifestyle modifications. Antioxidants 14(1):72

Ceriello A (2009) Hypothesis: the "metabolic memory", the new challenge of diabetes. Diabetes Res Clin Pract 86(Suppl 1):S2–S6

Chavali V, Tyagi SC, Mishra PK (2014) Differential expression of dicer, miRNAs, and inflammatory markers in diabetic Ins2+/− Akita hearts. Cell Biochem Biophys 68(1):25–35

Che H, Wang Y, Li Y, Lv J, Li H, Liu Y, Dong R, Sun Y, Xu X, Zhao J, Wang L (2020) Inhibition of microRNA-150-5p alleviates cardiac inflammation and fibrosis via targeting Smad7 in high glucose-treated cardiac fibroblasts. J Cell Physiol 235(11):7769–7779

Chen CC, Rosenbloom CL, Anderson DC, Manning AM (1995) Selective inhibition of E-selectin, vascular cell adhesion molecule-1, and intercellular adhesion molecule-1 expression by inhibitors of I kappa B-alpha phosphorylation. J Immunol 155(7):3538–3545

Chen C, Yang S, Li H, Yin Z, Fan J, Zhao Y, Gong W, Yan M, Wang DW (2017) Mir30c is involved in diabetic cardiomyopathy through regulation of cardiac autophagy via BECN1. Mol Ther Nucleic Acids 7:127–139

Cheng S, Cui Y, Fan L, Mu X, Hua Y (2018) T2DM inhibition of endothelial miR-342-3p facilitates angiogenic dysfunction via repression of FGF11 signaling. Biochem Biophys Res Commun 503(1):71–78

Cirilli I, Silvestri S, Marcheggiani F, Olivieri F, Galeazzi R, Antonicelli R, Recchioni R, Marcheselli F, Bacchetti T, Tiano L, Orlando P (2019) Three months monitored metabolic fitness modulates cardiovascular risk factors in diabetic patients. Diabetes Metab J 43(6):893–897

Collado A, Jiao T, Kontidou E, Carvalho L, Chernogubova E, Yang J, Zaccagnini G, Zhao A, Tengbom J, Zheng X, Rethi B, Alvarsson M, Catrina SB, Mahdi A, Carlström M, Martelli F, Pernow J, Zhou Z (2025) miR-210 as a therapeutic target in diabetes-associated endothelial dysfunction. Br J Pharmacol 182(2):417–431

Corsten MF, Papageorgiou A, Verhesen W, Carai P, Lindow M, Obad S, Summer G, Coort SL, Hazebroek M, van Leeuwen R, Gijbels MJ, Wijnands E, Biessen EA, De Winther MP, Stassen FR, Carmeliet P, Kauppinen S, Schroen B, Heymans S (2012) MicroRNA profiling identifies microRNA-155 as an adverse mediator of cardiac injury and dysfunction during acute viral myocarditis. Circ Res 111(4):415–425

Creager MA, Lüscher TF, Cosentino F, Beckman JA (2003) Diabetes and vascular disease: pathophysiology, clinical consequences, and medical therapy: part I. Circulation 108(12): 1527–1532

Cubbon RM, Rajwani A, Wheatcroft SB (2007) The impact of insulin resistance on endothelial function, progenitor cells and repair. Diab Vasc Dis Res 4(2):103–111

Dai B, Li H, Fan J, Zhao Y, Yin Z, Nie X, Wang DW, Chen C (2018a) MiR-21 protected against diabetic cardiomyopathy induced diastolic dysfunction by targeting gelsolin. Cardiovasc Diabetol 17(1):123

Dai Y, Lu H, Wang S, Chang S, Li C, Huang Z, Zhang F, Yang H, Shen Y, Chen Z, Qian J, Ge J (2018b) MicroRNA-216b actively modulates diabetic angiopathy through inverse regulation on FZD5. Gene 658:129–135 de Gonzalo-Calvo D, van der Meer RW, Rijzewijk LJ, Smit JW, Revuelta-Lopez E, Nasarre L, Escola-Gil JC, Lamb HJ, Llorente-Cortes V (2017) Serum microRNA-1 and microRNA-133a levels reflect myocardial steatosis in uncomplicated type 2 diabetes. Sci Rep 7(1):47

De Pascale MR, Bruzzese G, Crimi E, Grimaldi V, Liguori A, Brongo S, Barbieri M, Picascia A, Schiano C, Sommese L, Ferrara N, Paolisso G, Napoli C (2016) Severe type 2 diabetes induces reversible modifications of endothelial progenitor cells which are ameliorate by glycemic control. Int J Stem Cells 9(1):137–144

Dimmeler S, Fleming I, Fisslthaler B, Hermann C, Busse R, Zeiher AM (1999) Activation of nitric oxide synthase in endothelial cells by Akt-dependent phosphorylation. Nature 399(6736): 601–605

Durr AJ, Hathaway QA, Kunovac A, Taylor AD, Pinti MV, Rizwan S, Shepherd DL, Cook CC, Fink GK, Hollander JM (2022) Manipulation of the miR-378a/mt-ATP6 regulatory axis rescues ATP synthase in the diabetic heart and offers a novel role for lncRNA Kcnq1ot1. Am J Physiol Cell Physiol 322(3):C482–c495

Einarson TR, Acs A, Ludwig C, Panton UH (2018) Prevalence of cardiovascular disease in type 2 diabetes: a systematic literature review of scientific evidence from across the world in 2007-2017. Cardiovasc Diabetol 17(1):83

Feng B, Chen S, George B, Feng Q, Chakrabarti S (2010) miR133a regulates cardiomyocyte hypertrophy in diabetes. Diabetes Metab Res Rev 26(1):40–49

Fiore D, Gianfrilli D, Giannetta E, Galea N, Panio G, di Dato C, Pofi R, Pozza C, Sbardella E, Carbone I, Naro F, Lenzi A, Venneri MA, Isidori AM (2016) PDE5 inhibition ameliorates visceral adiposity targeting the miR-22/SIRT1 pathway: evidence from the CECSID trial. J Clin Endocrinol Metab 101(4):1525–1534

Fish JE, Santoro MM, Morton SU, Yu S, Yeh RF, Wythe JD, Ivey KN, Bruneau BG, Stainier DY, Srivastava D (2008) miR-126 regulates angiogenic signaling and vascular integrity. Dev Cell 15(2):272–284

Fomison-Nurse I, Saw EEL, Gandhi S, Munasinghe PE, Van Hout I, Williams MJA, Galvin I, Bunton R, Davis P, Cameron V, Katare R (2018) Diabetes induces the activation of pro-ageing miR-34a in the heart, but has differential effects on cardiomyocytes and cardiac progenitor cells. Cell Death Differ 25(7):1336–1349

Gao L, Liu Y, Guo S, Xiao L, Wu L, Wang Z, Liang C, Yao R, Zhang Y (2018) LAZ3 protects cardiac remodeling in diabetic cardiomyopathy via regulating miR-21/PPARa signaling. Biochim Biophys Acta Mol basis Dis 1864(10):3322–3338

Ghaffari M, Razi S, Zalpoor H, Nabi-Afjadi M, Mohebichamkhorami F, Zali H (2023) Association of MicroRNA-146a with type 1 and 2 diabetes and their related complications. J Diabetes Res 2023:2587104

Goodwin AM, D'Amore PA (2002) Wnt signaling in the vasculature. Angiogenesis 5(1–2):1–9

Gu L, Zhou Z (2025) Unlocking the therapeutic potential of lncRNA FENDRR in DCM: novel targets and insights via the miR-296-5p/HMGA1 axis. J Cardiothorac Surg 20(1):254

Guo R, Nair S (2017) Role of microRNA in diabetic cardiomyopathy: from mechanism to intervention. Biochim Biophys Acta Mol basis Dis 1863(8):2070–2077

Guo W, Li XN, Li J, Lu J, Wu J, Zhu WF, Qin P, Xu NZ, Zhang Q (2020) Increased plasma miR-146a levels are associated with subclinical atherosclerosis in newly diagnosed type 2 diabetes mellitus. J Diabetes Complicat 34(12):107725

Habibi P, Alihemmati A, Ahmadiasl N, Fateh A, Anvari E (2020) Exercise training attenuates diabetes-induced cardiac injury through increasing miR-133a and improving pro-apoptosis/anti-apoptosis balance in ovariectomized rats. Iran J Basic Med Sci 23(1):79–85

Henry RM, Ferreira I, Kostense PJ, Dekker JM, Nijpels G, Heine RJ, Kamp O, Bouter LM, Stehouwer CD (2004) Type 2 diabetes is associated with impaired endothelium-dependent, flow-mediated dilation, but impaired glucose metabolism is not; the Hoorn study. Atherosclerosis 174(1):49–56

Hristov M, Weber C (2008) Endothelial progenitor cells in vascular repair and remodeling. Pharmacol Res 58(2):148–151

Hsueh WA, Law RE (1999) Insulin signaling in the arterial wall. Am J Cardiol 84(1a):21j–24j
Icli B, Wara AK, Moslehi J, Sun X, Plovie E, Cahill M, Marchini JF, Schissler A, Padera RF, Shi J, Cheng HW, Raghuram S, Arany Z, Liao R, Croce K, MacRae C, Feinberg MW (2013) MicroRNA-26a regulates pathological and physiological angiogenesis by targeting BMP/SMAD1 signaling. Circ Res 113(11):1231–1241
Jansen F, Yang X, Hoelscher M, Cattelan A, Schmitz T, Proebsting S, Wenzel D, Vosen S, Franklin BS, Fleischmann BK, Nickenig G, Werner N (2013) Endothelial Microparticle–Mediated Transfer of MicroRNA-126 Promotes Vascular Endothelial Cell Repair via SPRED1 and Is Abrogated in Glucose-Damaged Endothelial Microparticles. Circulation 128(18):2026–2038
Jansen F, Wang H, Przybilla D, Franklin BS, Dolf A, Pfeifer P, Schmitz T, Flender A, Endl E, Nickenig G, Werner N (2016) Vascular endothelial microparticles-incorporated microRNAs are altered in patients with diabetes mellitus. Cardiovasc Diabetol 15:49
Jeyabal P, Thandavarayan RA, Joladarashi D, Suresh Babu S, Krishnamurthy S, Bhimaraj A, Youker KA, Kishore R, Krishnamurthy P (2016) MicroRNA-9 inhibits hyperglycemia-induced pyroptosis in human ventricular cardiomyocytes by targeting ELAVL1. Biochem Biophys Res Commun 471(4):423–429
Ji Y, Chen H, Pang L, Chen C, Wang S, Chen J, Fang L, Liu B, Cheng Y, Liu S, Zhong Y (2025) AGE induced macrophage-derived exosomes induce endothelial dysfunction in diabetes via miR-22-5p/FOXP1. Cardiovasc Diabetol 24(1):158
Jiang J, Mo H, Liu C, Wu B, Wu Z, Li X, Li T, He S, Li S, You Q, Wu K, Guo R (2018) Inhibition of miR-186-5p contributes to high glucose-induced injury in AC16 cardiomyocytes. Exp Ther Med 15(1):627–632
Katare R, Caporali A, Zentilin L, Avolio E, Sala-Newby G, Oikawa A, Cesselli D, Beltrami AP, Giacca M, Emanueli C, Madeddu P (2011) Intravenous gene therapy with PIM-1 via a cardiotropic viral vector halts the progression of diabetic cardiomyopathy through promotion of prosurvival signaling. Circ Res 108(10):1238–1251
Khan MAB, Hashim MJ, King JK, Govender RD, Mustafa H, Al Kaabi J (2020) Epidemiology of type 2 diabetes - global burden of disease and forecasted trends. J Epidemiol Glob Health 10(1): 107–111
Kishore R, Verma SK, Mackie AR, Vaughan EE, Abramova TV, Aiko I, Krishnamurthy P (2013) Bone marrow progenitor cell therapy-mediated paracrine regulation of cardiac miRNA-155 modulates fibrotic response in diabetic hearts. PLoS One 8(4):e60161
Kiyak-Kirmaci H, Hazar-Yavuz AN, Polat EB, Alsaadoni H, Cilingir-Kaya OT, Aktas HS, Elcioglu HK (2025) Effects of empagliflozin and dapagliflozin, SGLT2 inhibitors, on miRNA expressions in diabetes-related cardiovascular damage in rats. J Diabetes Complicat 39(7): 109063
Kizhakekuttu TJ, Wang J, Dharmashankar K, Ying R, Gutterman DD, Vita JA, Widlansky ME (2012) Adverse alterations in mitochondrial function contribute to type 2 diabetes mellitus-related endothelial dysfunction in humans. Arterioscler Thromb Vasc Biol 32(10):2531–2539
Kuwabara Y, Horie T, Baba O, Watanabe S, Nishiga M, Usami S, Izuhara M, Nakao T, Nishino T, Otsu K, Kita T, Kimura T, Ono K (2015) MicroRNA-451 exacerbates lipotoxicity in cardiac myocytes and high-fat diet-induced cardiac hypertrophy in mice through suppression of the LKB1/AMPK pathway. Circ Res 116(2):279–288
La Sala L, Mrakic-Sposta S, Tagliabue E, Prattichizzo F, Micheloni S, Sangalli E, Specchia C, Uccellatore AC, Lupini S, Spinetti G, de Candia P, Ceriello A (2019) Circulating microRNA-21 is an early predictor of ROS-mediated damage in subjects with high risk of developing diabetes and in drug-naïve T2D. Cardiovasc Diabetol 18(1):18
La Sala L, Carlini V, Conte C, Macas-Granizo MB, Afzalpour E, Martin-Delgado J, D'Anzeo M, Pedretti RFE, Naselli A, Pontiroli AE, Cappato R (2024) Metabolic disorders affecting the liver and heart: therapeutic efficacy of miRNA-based therapies? Pharmacol Res 201:107083
Lam B, Nwadozi E, Haas TL, Birot O, Roudier E (2021) High glucose treatment limits drosha protein expression and alters AngiomiR maturation in microvascular primary endothelial cells via an Mdm2-dependent mechanism. Cells 10(4):742

Lew JK, Pearson JT, Saw E, Tsuchimochi H, Wei M, Ghosh N, Du CK, Zhan DY, Jin M, Umetani K, Shirai M, Katare R, Schwenke DO (2020) Exercise regulates microRNAs to preserve coronary and cardiac function in the diabetic heart. Circ Res 127(11):1384–1400
Li X, Du N, Zhang Q, Li J, Chen X, Liu X, Hu Y, Qin W, Shen N, Xu C, Fang Z, Wei Y, Wang R, Du Z, Zhang Y, Lu Y (2014) MicroRNA-30d regulates cardiomyocyte pyroptosis by directly targeting foxo3a in diabetic cardiomyopathy. Cell Death Dis 5(10):e1479
Li Q, Kim YR, Vikram A, Kumar S, Kassan M, Gabani M, Lee SK, Jacobs JS, Irani K (2016a) P66Shc-induced microRNA-34a causes diabetic endothelial dysfunction by downregulating Sirtuin1. Arterioscler Thromb Vasc Biol 36(12):2394–2403
Li X, Wang H, Yao B, Xu W, Chen J, Zhou X (2016b) lncRNA H19/miR-675 axis regulates cardiomyocyte apoptosis by targeting VDAC1 in diabetic cardiomyopathy. Sci Rep 6(1):36340
Li H, Fan J, Zhao Y, Zhang X, Dai B, Zhan J, Yin Z, Nie X, Fu XD, Chen C, Wang DW (2019) Nuclear miR-320 mediates diabetes-induced cardiac dysfunction by activating transcription of fatty acid metabolic genes to cause lipotoxicity in the heart. Circ Res 125(12):1106–1120
Li X, Jia Z, Zhao X, Xu M, Chen M (2020) Expression of miR-210 in the peripheral blood of patients with newly diagnosed type 2 diabetes mellitus and its effect on the number and function of endothelial progenitor cells. Microvasc Res 131:104032
Li Y, Du Y, Liu Y, Chen X, Li X, Duan Y, Qin Y, Liu H, Ma X, Nie S, Zhang H (2024) Cardiomyocyte-derived small extracellular vesicle: a new mechanism driving diabetic cardiac fibrosis and cardiomyopathy. Theranostics 14(15):5926–5944
Liu S, Li W, Xu M, Huang H, Wang J, Chen X (2014) Micro-RNA 21targets dual specific phosphatase 8 to promote collagen synthesis in high glucose–treated primary cardiac fibroblasts. Can J Cardiol 30(12):1689–1699
Liu Y, Fu W, Lu M, Huai S, Song Y, Wei Y (2016) Role of miRNAs in epicardial adipose tissue in CAD patients with T2DM. Biomed Res Int 2016:1629236
Liu Y, Zheng W, Pan Y, Hu J (2019) Low expression of miR-186-5p regulates cell apoptosis by targeting toll-like receptor 3 in high glucose-induced cardiomyocytes. J Cell Biochem 120(6): 9532–9538
Lu H, Buchan RJ, Cook SA (2010) MicroRNA-223 regulates Glut4 expression and cardiomyocyte glucose metabolism. Cardiovasc Res 86(3):410–420
Luo YF, Wan XX, Zhao LL, Guo Z, Shen RT, Zeng PY, Wang LH, Yuan JJ, Yang WJ, Yue C, Mo ZH (2020) MicroRNA-139-5p upregulation is associated with diabetic endothelial cell dysfunction by targeting c-jun. Aging (Albany NY) 13(1):1186–1211
Macvanin MT, Gluvic Z, Radovanovic J, Essack M, Gao X, Isenovic ER (2023) Diabetic cardiomyopathy: the role of microRNAs and long non-coding RNAs. Front Endocrinol (Lausanne) 14:1124613
Mattagajasingh I, Kim C-S, Naqvi A, Yamamori T, Hoffman TA, Jung S-B, DeRicco J, Kasuno K, Irani K (2007) SIRT1 promotes endothelium-dependent vascular relaxation by activating endothelial nitric oxide synthase. Proc Natl Acad Sci 104(37):14855–14860
Mbanya JC, Sobngwi E, Mbanya DS, Ngu KB (2001) Left ventricular mass and systolic function in African diabetic patients: association with microalbuminuria. Diabetes Metab 27(3):378–382
McVeigh GE, Brennan GM, Johnston GD, McDermott BJ, McGrath LT, Henry WR, Andrews JW, Hayes JR (1992) Impaired endothelium-dependent and independent vasodilation in patients with type 2 (non-insulin-dependent) diabetes mellitus. Diabetologia 35(8):771–776
Meng S, Cao JT, Zhang B, Zhou Q, Shen CX, Wang CQ (2012) Downregulation of microRNA-126 in endothelial progenitor cells from diabetes patients, impairs their functional properties, via target gene Spred-1. J Mol Cell Cardiol 53(1):64–72
Miao Y, Wan Q, Liu X, Wang Y, Luo Y, Liu D, Lin N, Zhou H, Zhong J (2017) miR-503 is involved in the protective effect of phase II enzyme inducer (CPDT) in diabetic cardiomyopathy via Nrf2/ARE signaling pathway. Biomed Res Int 2017:9167450
Montagnani M, Golovchenko I, Kim I, Koh GY, Goalstone ML, Mundhekar AN, Johansen M, Kucik DF, Quon MJ, Draznin B (2002) Inhibition of phosphatidylinositol 3-kinase enhances mitogenic actions of insulin in endothelial cells. J Biol Chem 277(3):1794–1799

Montaigne D, Marechal X, Coisne A, Debry N, Modine T, Fayad G, Potelle C, El Arid JM, Mouton S, Sebti Y, Duez H, Preau S, Remy-Jouet I, Zerimech F, Koussa M, Richard V, Neviere R, Edme JL, Lefebvre P, Staels B (2014) Myocardial contractile dysfunction is associated with impaired mitochondrial function and dynamics in type 2 diabetic but not in obese patients. Circulation 130(7):554–564

Montero D, Walther G, Pérez-Martin A, Vicente-Salar N, Roche E, Vinet A (2013) Vascular smooth muscle function in type 2 diabetes mellitus: a systematic review and meta-analysis. Diabetologia 56(10):2122–2133

Morais Junior GS, Souza VC, Machado-Silva W, Henriques AD, Melo Alves A, Barbosa Morais D, Nóbrega OT, Brito CJ, Dos Santos Silva RJ (2017) Acute strength training promotes responses in whole blood circulating levels of miR-146a among older adults with type 2 diabetes mellitus. Clin Interv Aging 12:1443–1450

Mousavi S, Khazeei Tabari MA, Bagheri A, Samieefar N, Shaterian N, Kelishadi R (2022) The role of p66Shc in diabetes: a comprehensive review from bench to bedside. J Diabetes Res 2022: 7703520

Muley A, Majumder S, Kolluru GK, Parkinson S, Viola H, Hool L, Arfuso F, Ganss R, Dharmarajan A, Chatterjee S (2010) Secreted frizzled-related protein 4: an angiogenesis inhibitor. Am J Pathol 176(3):1505–1516

Murphy E, Steenbergen C (2007) Preconditioning: the mitochondrial connection. Annu Rev Physiol 69:51–67

Naruse K, Rask-Madsen C, Takahara N, Ha SW, Suzuma K, Way KJ, Jacobs JR, Clermont AC, Ueki K, Ohshiro Y, Zhang J, Goldfine AB, King GL (2006) Activation of vascular protein kinase C-beta inhibits Akt-dependent endothelial nitric oxide synthase function in obesity-associated insulin resistance. Diabetes 55(3):691–698

Ning S, Zhang S, Guo Z (2023) MicroRNA-494 regulates high glucose-induced cardiomyocyte apoptosis and autophagy by PI3K/AKT/mTOR signalling pathway. ESC Heart Fail 10(2): 1401–1411

Nitenberg A, Valensi P, Sachs R, Cosson E, Attali JR, Antony I (2004) Prognostic value of epicardial coronary artery constriction to the cold pressor test in type 2 diabetic patients with angiographically normal coronary arteries and no other major coronary risk factors. Diabetes Care 27(1):208–215

Nitenberg A, Pham I, Antony I, Valensi P, Attali JR, Chemla D (2005) Cardiovascular outcome of patients with abnormal coronary vasomotion and normal coronary arteriography is worse in type 2 diabetes mellitus than in arterial hypertension: a 10 year follow-up study. Atherosclerosis 183(1):113–120

Ormazabal V, Nair S, Elfeky O, Aguayo C, Salomon C, Zuñiga FA (2018) Association between insulin resistance and the development of cardiovascular disease. Cardiovasc Diabetol 17(1): 122

Ozasa N, Furukawa Y, Morimoto T, Tadamura E, Kita T, Kimura T (2008) Relation among left ventricular mass, insulin resistance, and hemodynamic parameters in type 2 diabetes. Hypertens Res 31(3):425–432

Pal R, Bhadada SK (2023) AGEs accumulation with vascular complications, glycemic control and metabolic syndrome: a narrative review. Bone 176:116884

Palihaderu P, Mendis B, Premarathne J, Dias W, Yeap SK, Ho WY, Dissanayake AS, Rajapakse IH, Karunanayake P, Senarath U, Satharasinghe DA (2022) Therapeutic potential of miRNAs for type 2 diabetes mellitus: an overview. Epigenet Insights 15:25168657221130041

Pérez-Cremades D, Chen J, Assa C, Feinberg MW (2023) MicroRNA-mediated control of myocardial infarction in diabetes. Trends Cardiovasc Med 33(4):195–201

Prattichizzo F, Giuliani A, Ceka A, Rippo MR, Bonfigli AR, Testa R, Procopio AD, Olivieri F (2015) Epigenetic mechanisms of endothelial dysfunction in type 2 diabetes. Clin Epigenetics 7(1):56

Prior JO, Quiñones MJ, Hernandez-Pampaloni M, Facta AD, Schindler TH, Sayre JW, Hsueh WA, Schelbert HR (2005) Coronary circulatory dysfunction in insulin resistance, impaired glucose tolerance, and type 2 diabetes mellitus. Circulation 111(18):2291–2298

Qiao Y, Zhao Y, Liu Y, Ma N, Wang C, Zou J, Liu Z, Zhou Z, Han D, He J, Sun Q, Liu Y, Xu C, Du Z, Huang H (2016) miR-483-3p regulates hyperglycaemia-induced cardiomyocyte apoptosis in transgenic mice. Biochem Biophys Res Commun 477(4):541–547

Rabelink TJ, de Boer HC, de Koning EJ, van Zonneveld AJ (2004) Endothelial progenitor cells: more than an inflammatory response? Arterioscler Thromb Vasc Biol 24(5):834–838

Raut SK, Kumar A, Singh GB, Nahar U, Sharma V, Mittal A, Sharma R, Khullar M (2015) miR-30c mediates upregulation of Cdc42 and Pak1 in diabetic cardiomyopathy. Cardiovasc Ther 33(3):89–97

Raut SK, Singh GB, Rastogi B, Saikia UN, Mittal A, Dogra N, Singh S, Prasad R, Khullar M (2016) miR-30c and miR-181a synergistically modulate p53-p21 pathway in diabetes induced cardiac hypertrophy. Mol Cell Biochem 417(1–2):191–203

Rawal S, Nagesh PT, Coffey S, Van Hout I, Galvin IF, Bunton RW, Davis P, Williams MJA, Katare R (2019) Early dysregulation of cardiac-specific microRNA-208a is linked to maladaptive cardiac remodelling in diabetic myocardium. Cardiovasc Diabetol 18(1):13

Riches K, Alshanwani AR, Warburton P, O'Regan DJ, Ball SG, Wood IC, Turner NA, Porter KE (2014) Elevated expression levels of miR-143/5 in saphenous vein smooth muscle cells from patients with Type 2 diabetes drive persistent changes in phenotype and function. J Mol Cell Cardiol 74:240–250

Rovira-Llopis S, Bañuls C, Diaz-Morales N, Hernandez-Mijares A, Rocha M, Victor VM (2017) Mitochondrial dynamics in type 2 diabetes: pathophysiological implications. Redox Biol 11: 637–645

Rydén L, Grant PJ, Anker SD, Berne C, Cosentino F, Danchin N, Deaton C, Escaned J, Hammes HP, Huikuri H, Marre M, Marx N, Mellbin L, Ostergren J, Patrono C, Seferovic P, Uva MS, Taskinen MR, Tendera M, Tuomilehto J, Valensi P, Zamorano JL, Zamorano JL, Achenbach S, Baumgartner H, Bax JJ, Bueno H, Dean V, Deaton C, Erol C, Fagard R, Ferrari R, Hasdai D, Hoes AW, Kirchhof P, Knuuti J, Kolh P, Lancellotti P, Linhart A, Nihoyannopoulos P, Piepoli MF, Ponikowski P, Sirnes PA, Tamargo JL, Tendera M, Torbicki A, Wijns W, Windecker S, De Backer G, Sirnes PA, Ezquerra EA, Avogaro A, Badimon L, Baranova E, Baumgartner H, Betteridge J, Ceriello A, Fagard R, Funck-Brentano C, Gulba DC, Hasdai D, Hoes AW, Kjekshus JK, Knuuti J, Kolh P, Lev E, Mueller C, Neyses L, Nilsson PM, Perk J, Ponikowski P, Reiner Z, Sattar N, Schächinger V, Scheen A, Schirmer H, Strömberg A, Sudzhaeva S, Tamargo JL, Viigimaa M, Vlachopoulos C, Xuereb RG (2013) ESC guidelines on diabetes, pre-diabetes, and cardiovascular diseases developed in collaboration with the EASD: the task force on diabetes, pre-diabetes, and cardiovascular diseases of the European Society of Cardiology (ESC) and developed in collaboration with the European Association for the Study of Diabetes (EASD). Eur Heart J 34(39):3035–3087

Safar ME, Gnakaméné JB, Bahous SA, Yannoutsos A, Thomas F (2017) Longitudinal study of hypertensive subjects with type 2 diabetes mellitus: overall and cardiovascular risk. Hypertension 69(6):1029–1035

Saini VM, Liu KR, Surve AS, Gupta S, Gupta A (2022) MicroRNAs as biomarkers for monitoring cardiovascular changes in Type II Diabetes Mellitus (T2DM) and exercise. J Diabetes Metab Disord 21(2):1819–1832

Samidurai A, Roh SK, Prakash M, Durrant D, Salloum FN, Kukreja RC, Das A (2020) STAT3-miR-17/20 signalling axis plays a critical role in attenuating myocardial infarction following rapamycin treatment in diabetic mice. Cardiovasc Res 116(13):2103–2115

Saremi A, Howell S, Schwenke DC, Bahn G, Beisswenger PJ, Reaven PD (2017) Advanced glycation end products, oxidation products, and the extent of atherosclerosis during the VA diabetes trial and follow-up study. Diabetes Care 40(4):591–598

Sena CM, Pereira AM, Seiça R (2013) Endothelial dysfunction - a major mediator of diabetic vascular disease. Biochim Biophys Acta 1832(12):2216–2231

Shan YX, Liu TJ, Su HF, Samsamshariat A, Mestril R, Wang PH (2003) Hsp10 and Hsp60 modulate Bcl-2 family and mitochondria apoptosis signaling induced by doxorubicin in cardiac muscle cells. J Mol Cell Cardiol 35(9):1135–1143

Shantikumar S, Caporali A, Emanueli C (2012) Role of microRNAs in diabetes and its cardiovascular complications. Cardiovasc Res 93(4):583–593

Shen E, Diao X, Wang X, Chen R, Hu B (2011) MicroRNAs involved in the mitogen-activated protein kinase cascades pathway during glucose-induced cardiomyocyte hypertrophy. Am J Pathol 179(2):639–650

Stępień E, Durak-Kozica M, Kamińska A, Targosz-Korecka M, Libera M, Tylko G, Opalińska A, Kapusta M, Solnica B, Georgescu A, Costa MC, Czyżewska-Buczyńska A, Witkiewicz W, Małecki MT, Enguita FJ (2018) Circulating ectosomes: determination of angiogenic microRNAs in type 2 diabetes. Theranostics 8(14):3874–3890

Straka RJ, Liu LZ, Girase PS, DeLorenzo A, Chapman RH (2009) Incremental cardiovascular costs and resource use associated with diabetes: an assessment of 29,863 patients in the US managed-care setting. Cardiovasc Diabetol 8:53

Sun D, Zhu Z, Zhang Y, Bai R, Zhu F, Shan Z, Ma C, Yang J (2022) Relation of genetic polymorphisms in microRNAs with diastolic and systolic function in type 2 diabetes mellitus. Nutr Metab Cardiovasc Dis 32(12):2877–2882

Tanaka K, Tani Y, Asai J, Nemoto F, Kusano Y, Suzuki H, Hayashi Y, Asahi K, Nakayama M, Miyata T, Watanabe T (2012) Skin autofluorescence is associated with severity of vascular complications in Japanese patients with Type 2 diabetes. Diabet Med 29(4):492–500

Tang X, Tang G, Ozcan S (2008) Role of microRNAs in diabetes. Biochim Biophys Acta 1779(11): 697–701

Tang Q, Len Q, Liu Z, Wang W (2018) Overexpression of miR-22 attenuates oxidative stress injury in diabetic cardiomyopathy via Sirt 1. Cardiovasc Ther 36(2):e12318

Tatekoshi Y, Tanno M, Kouzu H, Abe K, Miki T, Kuno A, Yano T, Ishikawa S, Ohwada W, Sato T, Niinuma T, Suzuki H, Miura T (2018) Translational regulation by miR-301b upregulates AMP deaminase in diabetic hearts. J Mol Cell Cardiol 119:138–146

Trajkovski M, Hausser J, Soutschek J, Bhat B, Akin A, Zavolan M, Heim MH, Stoffel M (2011) MicroRNAs 103 and 107 regulate insulin sensitivity. Nature 474(7353):649–653

Veitch S, Njock MS, Chandy M, Siraj MA, Chi L, Mak H, Yu K, Rathnakumar K, Perez-Romero CA, Chen Z, Alibhai FJ, Gustafson D, Raju S, Wu R, Zarrin Khat D, Wang Y, Caballero A, Meagher P, Lau E, Pepic L, Cheng HS, Galant NJ, Howe KL, Li RK, Connelly KA, Husain M, Delgado-Olguin P, Fish JE (2022) MiR-30 promotes fatty acid beta-oxidation and endothelial cell dysfunction and is a circulating biomarker of coronary microvascular dysfunction in pre-clinical models of diabetes. Cardiovasc Diabetol 21(1):31

Villeneuve LM, Kato M, Reddy MA, Wang M, Lanting L, Natarajan R (2010) Enhanced levels of microRNA-125b in vascular smooth muscle cells of diabetic db/db mice lead to increased inflammatory gene expression by targeting the histone methyltransferase Suv39h1. Diabetes 59(11):2904–2915

Wang S, Aurora AB, Johnson BA, Qi X, McAnally J, Hill JA, Richardson JA, Bassel-Duby R, Olson EN (2008) The endothelial specific microRNA miR-126 governs vascular integrity and angiogenesis. Dev Cell 15(2):261–271

Wang XH, Qian RZ, Zhang W, Chen SF, Jin HM, Hu RM (2009) MicroRNA-320 expression in myocardial microvascular endothelial cells and its relationship with insulin-like growth factor-1 in type 2 diabetic rats. Clin Exp Pharmacol Physiol 36(2):181–188

Wang D, Hu X, Lee SH, Chen F, Jiang K, Tu Z, Liu Z, Du J, Wang L, Yin C, Liao Y, Shang H, Martin KA, Herzog RI, Young LH, Qian L, Hwa J, Xiang Y (2018) Diabetes exacerbates myocardial ischemia/reperfusion injury by down-regulation of microRNA and up-regulation of O-GlcNAcylation. JACC Basic Transl Sci 3(3):350–362

Wang C, Liu G, Yang H, Guo S, Wang H, Dong Z, Li X, Bai Y, Cheng Y (2021) MALAT1-mediated recruitment of the histone methyltransferase EZH2 to the microRNA-22 promoter leads to cardiomyocyte apoptosis in diabetic cardiomyopathy. Sci Total Environ 766:142191

Wang X, Zhang Z, Wang M (2022) MiR-29a regulates cardiomyocyte apoptosis by targeting Bak1 in diabetic cardiomyopathy. J Biochem 171(6):663–671

Westermeier F, Riquelme JA, Pavez M, Garrido V, Díaz A, Verdejo HE, Castro PF, García L, Lavandero S (2016) New molecular insights of insulin in diabetic cardiomyopathy. Front Physiol 7:125

Widlansky ME, Jensen DM, Wang J, Liu Y, Geurts AM, Kriegel AJ, Liu P, Ying R, Zhang G, Casati M, Chu C, Malik M, Branum A, Tanner MJ, Tyagi S, Usa K, Liang M (2018) miR-29 contributes to normal endothelial function and can restore it in cardiometabolic disorders. EMBO Mol Med 10(3)

Wu K, Yang Y, Zhong Y, Ammar HM, Zhang P, Guo R, Liu H, Cheng C, Koroscil TM, Chen Y, Liu S, Bihl JC (2016) The effects of microvesicles on endothelial progenitor cells are compromised in type 2 diabetic patients via downregulation of the miR-126/VEGFR2 pathway. Am J Physiol Endocrinol Metab 310(10):E828–E837

Xing R, Liu D, Cheng X, Tian X, Yan C, Han Y (2019) MiR-207 inhibits autophagy and promotes apoptosis of cardiomyocytes by directly targeting LAMP2 in type 2 diabetic cardiomyopathy. Biochem Biophys Res Commun 520(1):27–34

Xu Y, Fang H, Xu Q, Xu C, Yang L, Huang C (2020) LncRNA GAS5 inhibits NLRP3 inflammasome activation-mediated pyroptosis in diabetic cardiomyopathy by targeting miR-34b-3p/AHR. Cell Cycle 19(22):3054–3065

Xu R, Fu J, Hu Y, Yang X, Tao X, Chen L, Huang K, Fu Q (2022) Roflumilast-mediated phosphodiesterase 4D inhibition reverses diabetes-associated cardiac dysfunction and remodeling: effects beyond glucose lowering. Diabetes 71(8):1660–1678

Yang G, Wu Y, Ye S (2017) MiR-181c restrains nitration stress of endothelial cells in diabetic db/db mice through inhibiting the expression of FoxO1. Biochem Biophys Res Commun 486(1):29–35

Yang F, Qin Y, Lv J, Wang Y, Che H, Chen X, Jiang Y, Li A, Sun X, Yue E, Ren L, Li Y, Bai Y, Wang L (2018) Silencing long non-coding RNA Kcnq1ot1 alleviates pyroptosis and fibrosis in diabetic cardiomyopathy. Cell Death Dis 9(10):1000

Yi F, Shang Y, Li B, Dai S, Wu W, Cheng L, Wang X (2017) MicroRNA-193-5p modulates angiogenesis through IGF2 in type 2 diabetic cardiomyopathy. Biochem Biophys Res Commun 491(4):876–882

Yin Z, Zhao Y, He M, Li H, Fan J, Nie X, Yan M, Chen C, Wang DW (2019) MiR-30c/PGC-1β protects against diabetic cardiomyopathy via PPARα. Cardiovasc Diabetol 18(1):7

Yozgatli K, Lefrandt JD, Noordzij MJ, Oomen PHN, Brouwer T, Jager J, Castro Cabezas M, Smit AJ (2018) Accumulation of advanced glycation end products is associated with macrovascular events and glycaemic control with microvascular complications in type 2 diabetes mellitus. Diabet Med 35:1242

Yu XY, Song YH, Geng YJ, Lin QX, Shan ZX, Lin SG, Li Y (2008) Glucose induces apoptosis of cardiomyocytes via microRNA-1 and IGF-1. Biochem Biophys Res Commun 376(3):548–552

Yu M, Sun Y, Shan X, Yang F, Chu G, Chen Q, Han L, Guo Z, Wang G (2022) Therapeutic overexpression of miR-92a-2-5p ameliorated cardiomyocyte oxidative stress injury in the development of diabetic cardiomyopathy. Cell Mol Biol Lett 27(1):85

Zampetaki A, Kiechl S, Drozdov I, Willeit P, Mayr U, Prokopi M, Mayr A, Weger S, Oberhollenzer F, Bonora E, Shah A, Willeit J, Mayr M (2010) Plasma microRNA profiling reveals loss of endothelial miR-126 and other microRNAs in type 2 diabetes. Circ Res 107(6): 810–817

Zhang Y, Qin W, Zhang L, Wu X, Du N, Hu Y, Li X, Shen N, Xiao D, Zhang H, Li Z, Zhang Y, Yang H, Gao F, Du Z, Xu C, Yang B (2015) MicroRNA-26a prevents endothelial cell apoptosis by directly targeting TRPC6 in the setting of atherosclerosis. Sci Rep 5:9401

Zhang M, Du G, Xie L, Xu Y, Chen W (2024) Circular RNA HMGCS1 sponges MIR4521 to aggravate type 2 diabetes-induced vascular endothelial dysfunction. elife 13

Zhao X, Liu S, Wang X, Chen Y, Pang P, Yang Q, Lin J, Deng S, Wu S, Fan G, Wang B (2022) Diabetic cardiomyopathy: clinical phenotype and practice. Front Endocrinol (Lausanne) 13: 1032268

Zheng D, Ma J, Yu Y, Li M, Ni R, Wang G, Chen R, Li J, Fan GC, Lacefield JC, Peng T (2015) Silencing of miR-195 reduces diabetic cardiomyopathy in C57BL/6 mice. Diabetologia 58(8): 1949–1958

Zhou Z, Collado A, Sun C, Tratsiakovich Y, Mahdi A, Winter H, Chernogubova E, Seime T, Narayanan S, Jiao T, Jin H, Alvarsson M, Zheng X, Yang J, Hedin U, Catrina SB, Maegdefessel L, Pernow J (2022) Downregulation of erythrocyte miR-210 induces endothelial dysfunction in type 2 diabetes. Diabetes 71(2):285–297

Zhou M, Zhang Y, Shi L, Li L, Zhang D, Gong Z, Wu Q (2024) Activation and modulation of the AGEs-RAGE axis: implications for inflammatory pathologies and therapeutic interventions - a review. Pharmacol Res 206:107282

Zhu H, Leung SW (2015) Identification of microRNA biomarkers in type 2 diabetes: a meta-analysis of controlled profiling studies. Diabetologia 58(5):900–911

Zhu Y, Yang X, Zhou J, Chen L, Zuo P, Chen L, Jiang L, Li T, Wang D, Xu Y, Li Q, Yan Y (2022) miR-340-5p mediates cardiomyocyte oxidative stress in diabetes-induced cardiac dysfunction by targeting Mcl-1. Oxidative Med Cell Longev 2022:3182931

Zou T, Zhu M, Ma Y-C, Xiao F, Yu X, Xu L, Ma L-Q, Yang J, Dong J-Z (2018) MicroRNA-410-5p exacerbates high-fat diet-induced cardiac remodeling in mice in an endocrine fashion. Sci Rep 8(1):8780

In Search of a Biomarker for Vasculopathy Associated with Metabolic Syndrome

Donjuán-Loredo Guadalupe, Saavedra-Serrato Luis, Chávez-Morales Tómas, and Espinosa-Tanguma Ricardo

Contents

D.-L. Guadalupe · E.-T. Ricardo (✉)
Departamento de Fisiología y Biofísica, Facultad de Medicina, Universidad Autónoma de San Luis Potosí, San Luis Potosí, Mexico
e-mail: espinosr@uaslp.mx

S.-S. Luis · C.-M. Tómas
Facultad de Ciencias Químicas, Universidad Autónoma de San Luis Potosí, San Luis Potosí, Mexico
e-mail: A316019@alumnos.uaslp.mx; A298828@alumnos.uaslp.mx

A. Rueda, M. Nieves-Cintrón (eds.), *Cardiovascular Alterations in Metabolic Diseases*, Handbook of Experimental Pharmacology 293,
https://doi.org/10.1007/164_2026_791

Abstract

Central obesity is associated with a group of metabolic and cardiovascular alterations known as metabolic syndrome (MetS). MetS affects an estimated 20–25% of the global population. The clinical diagnosis of MetS is made using different methodologies, depending on the parameter being measured; however, no established molecule or biomarker unifies these alterations and allows MetS to be identified from its inception. Fatty acid-binding proteins (FABPs) have been studied as molecules that accompany MetS abnormalities, from their role in intracellular lipid transport to their release into the circulation under pathological conditions and their elevation in various biofluids, which may be indicative of MetS. In this chapter, we will focus on adipocyte, epidermal, and intestinal FABPs as metabolic biomarkers of the early stages of MetS since they are associated with alterations such as inflammation of the tissues containing them, which allows them to be identified even in the early stages of the disease. The ability to have a molecule that combines all the parameters of MetS remains and important goal, given the existence of possible candidates. This would allow the early identification of MetS, which would represent a new approach to its clinical diagnosis.

Keywords

Biomarkers · Diabetes · Fatty acid · Hypertension · Metabolic syndrome · Obesity

1 Introduction

The Metabolic Syndrome (MetS) is a cluster of metabolic defects that includes central obesity, hypertension (HT), insulin resistance, hyperglycemia, and atherogenic dyslipidemia, characterized by hypertriglyceridemia and low high-density lipoprotein cholesterol (HDL-c); three of these are required for clinical diagnosis. The presence of MetS increases the risk of developing type 2 diabetes (T2D) and cardiovascular disease (CVD) (Mohamed et al. 2023). It is important to detect it in its early stages to implement lifestyle changes and prevent its progression and complications.

Prevalence estimates vary depending on the criteria used to define MetS and often coincide with the prevalence of obesity and T2D, with MetS affecting nearly 25% of the global adult population (Mohamed et al. 2023). In some projections, the prevalence of MetS is expected to reach up to 53% by 2035 (Saklayen 2018). The age at which MetS is diagnosed has been decreasing in recent years. More than 25 years ago, the highest risk of developing MetS was in people over 50 years of age; currently, increasing rates are observed among individuals between 30 and 35 years of age, although risk continues to increase with age. Of all the changes, central obesity has been identified as the leading risk factor for its development (Lemieux and Després 2020). Interestingly, MetS could be the general indicator of adipose tissue disease, with an aggregation of activated macrophages causing low-grade inflammation and an increase in the number of adipokines released by the abnormal activity of the inflamed adipocyte (Oda 2018). Adipose tissue and lipids, as biological molecules, are involved in fundamental processes that are critical for proper cellular function and in the pathogenesis of many metabolic disorders. Cells with active lipid metabolism, such as adipocytes and keratinocytes, contain fatty acid binding proteins (FABPs) that coordinate the intracellular transport of lipids to different cell compartments (Furuhashi et al. 2014).

The gut microbiota is directly related to host metabolism; changes in the balance of the microbiota influence the development of inflammation, abnormalities in glucose metabolism, and regulation of blood pressure. Together with the microbiota associated with host aging, these factors influence the development of MetS (Pelsers et al. 2003). Evidence suggests that alterations in the gut microbiota contribute to insulin resistance, T2D, HT, and CVD. The microbial population of the human intestine comprises approximately 10^{13}–10^{14} bacteria of around 1000 different species, which modulate normal metabolic activities and physiological functions. For example, cecal bacteria of the phylum Bacteroidetes are reduced in obesity, and this reduction is accompanied by a proportional increase of phylum Firmicutes associated with obesity. Oral administration of good bacteria has been shown to ameliorate intestinal barrier dysfunction and metabolic disorders in obese mice, suggesting that the transmissibility of gut microbes and metabolic phenotypes is closely linked and that it is possible to influence the context of MetS (Lau et al. 2016).

Because the development of MetS involves alterations across multiple tissues and functions, early diagnosis is complex. Early therapeutic intervention, monitoring response to treatment, reducing morbidity and mortality, and establishing the prognosis of associated diseases are goals to be achieved when a biomarker is available (Ellis and Goodacre 2006). Most of the current routine biochemical studies (fasting serum glucose, oral glucose tolerance curve, lipid profile) to detect any of the disorders associated with MetS are based on the measurement of specific markers to obtain results and establish the alteration, anthropometric tests (body mass index), or taking blood pressure, making it difficult to detect early pathologies that occur simultaneously, such as MetS. The idea is to have a biomarker that helps detect this spectrum of alterations in a single molecule from some of the tissues that pathologically intervene in its development (Ellis and Goodacre 2006).

Adipose tissue, the epidermis, and the gastrointestinal tract are tissues that show inflammation and other metabolic abnormalities related to the pathogenesis of MetS; it is crucial to find an associated molecule that allows the identification of a population at risk. It has become of great interest to search for and investigate new biomarkers to detect MetS at an early stage. However, no single biomarker is currently available, which is a challenge (Haka et al. 2016).

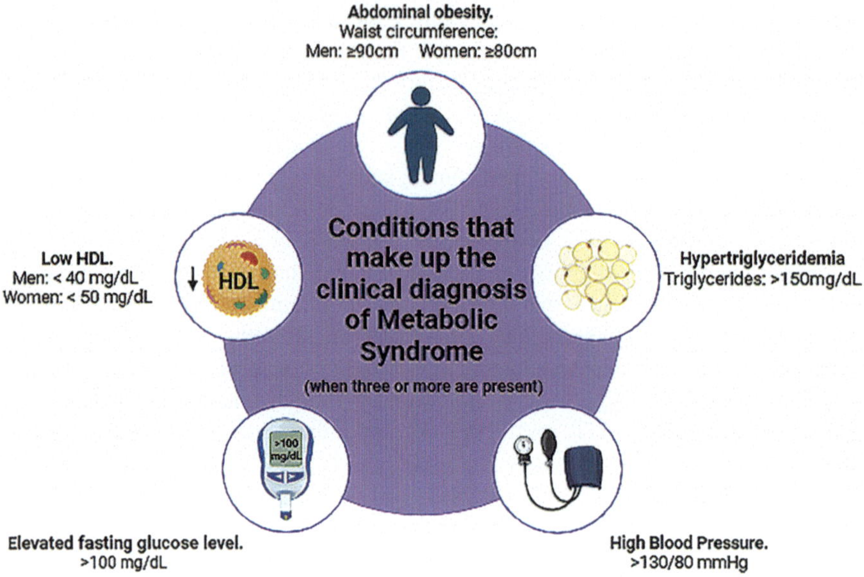

Fig. 1 Conditions that make up the clinical diagnosis of metabolic syndrome. The American Heart Association defines the clinical diagnosis of MetS as the presence of three or more of these conditions. Central obesity is regarded as the primary risk factor and an important driver of the development of other metabolic diseases. (Created with BioRender)

2 Metabolic Syndrome

Central obesity is excess abdominal fat and is considered the major risk factor for the development of metabolic diseases such as insulin resistance, hyperinsulinemia, oral glucose intolerance, hyperglycemia, and dyslipidemia, characterized by high triglycerides and cholesterol. Low HDL-c, HT, and inflammation, which predispose to the development of T2D and a wide variety of CVD, including acute myocardial infarction and cerebrovascular events; this entire spectrum of alterations is clinically known as MetS (Katsiki et al. 2014). Different health organizations worldwide have defined MetS, with the American Heart Association noting that clinical diagnosis is made when three or more of the following conditions are present (Fig. 1) (Hernández et al. 2018).

3 Description of the Components Associated with Metabolic Syndrome

3.1 Central Obesity

The main risk factor for MetS is obesity. In particular, the accumulation of visceral fat, also known as central obesity, is closely linked to a wide range of metabolic changes. Excessive adipose tissue accumulation in the abdomen and trunk is promoted by a high caloric intake and reduced physical activity (Bovolini et al. 2021). The World Health Organization (WHO), as part of World Obesity Day 2022, reported that there are more than 800 million adults aged 18 years and above with obesity (World Health Organization 2024a, b).

The adipocytes of people with central obesity are hypertrophied due to the excessive accumulation of lipids inside, which causes dysfunction of these cells, altering, on the one hand, adipogenesis and lipolysis, leading to an increase in free fatty acids, allowing the accumulation of ectopic lipids and causing lipotoxicity (Unger et al. 2010). Furthermore, this adipocyte dysfunction favors a greater release of adipokines, which is why adipose tissue is considered an important endocrine organ. In addition to the adipokines mentioned above, new molecules have recently been identified that have very different effects and important implications in the development of MetS (Kumari et al. 2019). Obesity induces metabolic stress and inflammatory responses in adipose tissue, which are important mediators of obesity-related metabolic and cardiovascular pathologies.

3.2 Hypertension

According to the American Heart Association (AHA) criteria, HT is diagnosed when blood pressure values are ≥130 and/or ≥80 mmHg (Espinosa Brito 2018; Flack and Adekola 2020).

With these new criteria for its diagnosis (Table 1), the prevalence of HT in the United States alone suddenly increased to 103 million, or about 46% of adults in that country. Uncontrolled chronic HT is associated with cardiovascular, cerebrovascular, and renal damage, making early diagnosis and treatment very important (Flack and Adekola 2020).

Up to now, the way of diagnosis in clinical practice is to use a sphygmomanometer. However, it is necessary to develop new tools or detect biomarkers that are present in the early stages of this pathology. For example, in HT, there is dysfunction in the vascular endothelium with a different biochemical profile than the healthy endothelium, so the detection of this biochemical change could help to make an early diagnosis of the disease, even before the blood pressure levels rise. Similarly, this could be done with perivascular adipose tissue, which has a specific secretory profile in HT associated with obesity (Pacia et al. 2016). Similarly, platelets from patients with HT could be studied since they show abnormal behavior in the release of

Table 1 AHA criteria for the diagnosis of HT

Blood pressure category	Systolic (mmHg)	Diastolic (mmHg)
Normal	<120	<80
Elevated	120–129	≤80
Hypertension stage 1	130–139	80–89
Hypertension stage 2	≥140	≥90
Hypertensive crisis	>180	>120

proteins, lipids, and receptors from their cell membrane, which can lead to thrombus formation and, consequently, stroke (García-Rubio et al. 2019).

At the biochemical level, an increase in the concentration of renin is also observed, an enzyme secreted by the juxtaglomerular cells of the kidney in response to hypovolemia and hypotension, which catalyzes the conversion of angiotensinogen to angiotensin I. This increase in renin has been considered a possible biomarker for monitoring the response to treatment since many of the antihypertensive drugs used are directed at some point in the regulation of the renin-angiotensin-aldosterone system (Zheng et al. 2019).

3.3 Type 2 Diabetes Mellitus (T2D)

T2D is a chronic disease characterized by hyperglycemia, which is associated with resistance to the action of the hormone insulin or a deficiency in its production. T2D is associated with multiple complications affecting organs such as the heart, blood vessels, eyes, kidneys, and nerves (Eizirik et al. 2020). Approximately 422 million people worldwide have T2D, and approximately 1.6 million deaths each year are directly related to T2D and its complications (World Health Organization 2024a, b). Its complications can be prevented, so early diagnosis and timely treatment play a crucial role. Routine biochemical tests for blood glucose analysis include fasting serum glucose, oral glucose tolerance test (OGTT), and glycated hemoglobin (HbA1c) (World Health Organization 2024a, b). In addition, there is a method widely used by patients for ambulatory monitoring at home: capillary blood glucose measured by a glucometer.

3.4 Dyslipidemia

Hypertriglyceridemia, along with low levels of the lipoprotein HDL-c, with an important cardioprotective function, and elevated levels of low-density and very-low-density lipoproteins (LDL-c and VLDL-c, respectively), are the primary alterations in lipid metabolism observed in MetS. It is well established that these factors significantly increase cardiovascular morbidity and mortality (Bovolini et al. 2021; Vekic et al. 2019). Consumption of foods containing excess calories predisposes to the storage of triglycerides in adipocytes. There are multiple factors that determine the capacity of this storage, and when this limit is exceeded, ectopic lipid deposition begins in organs and tissues such as skeletal muscle, liver, heart, and pancreas, which can impair their function and cause lipotoxicity (Vekic et al. 2019). Currently, serum lipid levels are obtained with biochemical analyses using specific reagents for the detection of each of these in venous blood. Inflammatory biomarkers have been used for the early detection of pathologies associated with dyslipidemia, such as atherosclerosis and acute myocardial infarction, among others.

3.5 Inflammation

Inflammation is of great pathophysiological importance in the development of MetS; certain markers of inflammation, such as C-reactive protein (CRP) and interleukin-6 (IL-6), have been repeatedly associated with this pathology, particularly in the context of insulin resistance. The association between systemic inflammation and MetS may reflect a cytokine-mediated acute phase response of the innate immune system. IL-6 is a key regulator of the inflammatory process, which is secreted in part from visceral and subcutaneous fat, and plays an important role in regulating glucose and lipid metabolism (Ingelsson et al. 2008). Inflammation also contributes to the pathogenesis of atherosclerosis and coronary heart disease in MetS. Recent evidence suggests that abnormalities between inflammatory and insulin signaling pathways cause insulin resistance and endothelial dysfunction, which together predispose to cardiovascular disease in MetS. Routine complementary studies linking levels of proinflammatory cytokines to these pathologies are rare, and even the use of anti-inflammatory drugs is not part of routine therapy for MetS (Koh et al. 2005).

4 Metabolic Biomarkers

A biological marker or biomarker is a physiological, biochemical, or morphological change that can be objectively measured at the molecular, biochemical, or cellular level; these markers identify normal or abnormal biological processes or, in some cases, responses to a drug used. In many pathologies, biomarkers are usually proteins whose appearance or increase in plasma or other biofluid levels is associated with the predisposition, onset, or progression of the disease (Griffiths et al. 2002). The main purpose of using metabolic biomarkers is to detect the early and intermediate stages of a pathological process and to identify individuals who are sensitive or predisposed to the pathology.

Both in animal models of MetS and obesity and in clinical studies performed in metabolically ill and obese humans (Ishimura et al. 2013), the presence of elevated serum levels of A-FABP (adipocytic) and E-FABP (epidermal) has been directly associated with dyslipidemia, insulin resistance, T2D, atherosclerosis, HT, renal dysfunction, fatty liver disease, cardiac dysfunction, among other cardiovascular events, showing a strong involvement of these and other FABPs, such as intestinal FABP (I-FABP), associated with changes in the gut microbiota as a consequence of high-fat food intake (Furuhashi et al. 2020). On the other hand, it has been shown in these models that genetic deficiency, antibody neutralization (Uysal et al. 2000; Makowski et al. 2001; Chung et al. 2019), or pharmacological inhibition of these FABPs (Yao et al. 2020) attenuates the metabolic, cardiovascular, and inflammatory dysfunctions present in MetS and obesity. Because of their relevance, they have been considered biomarkers of metabolic and cardiovascular diseases.

5 Fatty Acid Binding Proteins (FABPs)

In lipid metabolism, a series of molecules are involved at some point in its regulation, some to transport them in the plasma, others in the transmembrane transport, or at the intracellular level. One of these molecules is the fatty acid binding protein (FABP), which belongs to a family of cytosolic proteins that can bind with high affinity and reversibly to hydrophobic ligands, such as long-chain saturated and unsaturated fatty acids and other lipids, facilitating their intracellular transport to specific organelles in the cell (Furuhashi and Hotamisligil 2008). This group includes several members, all with the same function, but named according to the tissue to which they belong (heart fatty acid binding protein, H-FABP or FABP3; adipocyte fatty acid binding protein, A-FABP or FABP4, intestinal fatty acid binding protein, I-FABP or FABP2, liver fatty acid binding protein, L-FABP or FABP1, epidermal fatty acid binding protein, E-FABP or FABP5), etc. (Gillilan et al. 2007). Although there is a specific or predominant FABP in a tissue, more than one type of FABP can be found in it, even showing expression patterns that vary depending on the pathological state of the individual.

The primary structure of FABPs is characterized by having 126–137 amino acids, with a molecular weight of approximately 14–15 kDa, and up to 70% similarity in amino acid sequence can be found among its members. Its tertiary structure is of the beta-barrel type, with ten antiparallel chains organized in two beta sheets facing each other and two small alpha helices located between the first and second beta sheets. The ligand binding site is in the center of the beta-barrel; all family members bind a single ligand except hepatic FABP, which binds two (Li and Ishibashi 1992). FABPs have been shown to undergo specific conformational changes during ligand binding, which depend on the type of fatty acid to which they bind. These changes also indicate the intracellular site to which they are targeted (Ishimura et al. 2013).

The main functions attributed to FABPs include the following (Ishimura et al. 2013):

1. Facilitate the entry of fatty acids into cells.
2. Facilitate the transport of fatty acids within the cytosol of cells.
3. Transport fatty acids to the various organelles and metabolic pathways where they are needed.
4. Regulate the activity of enzymes involved in lipid metabolism.
5. Mitigate the adverse effects of fatty acids on cell membranes and enzymes.
6. Regulate the expression of certain genes, particularly those involved in pathways such as lipid and carbohydrate metabolism.

Numerous functions have been proposed for FABPs. As lipid chaperones, FABPs may actively facilitate the transport of lipids to specific compartments in the cell, such as the lipid droplet for storage, the endoplasmic reticulum for signaling, trafficking, and membrane synthesis, the mitochondria or peroxisome for oxidation, cytosolic or other enzymes to regulate their activity, the nucleus for lipid-mediated transcriptional regulation, or even outside the cell to signal in an autocrine or paracrine manner. FABP content in most cells is generally proportional to the rates of fatty-acid metabolism (Furuhashi and Hotamisligil 2008).

6 Adipocyte Fatty Acid Binding Protein (A-FABP, FABP4, ap2)

A-FABP is one of the most abundant cytosolic proteins in adipocytes and is also expressed in macrophages and endothelial cells. In adipocytes, it carries out intracellular physiological functions, but in obesity, where it is known that there is a dysfunction of adipose tissue, there is an overexpression and release of adipokines (leptin, adiponectin, proinflammatory cytokines, among others); this is the case of A-FABP, which has been detected in the bloodstream in the presence of adiposity and which reaches other organs such as the liver and is involved in the regulation of proteins that control both lipid metabolism and insulin sensitivity (Rodríguez-Calvo et al. 2019).

Expression of A-FABP is induced during adipocyte differentiation from progenitor cells and is transcriptionally controlled by PPAR-gamma agonists, circulating free fatty acids, dexamethasone, and insulin. Functionally, A-FABP regulates lipolysis by activating hormone-sensitive lipase (HSL) and by transporting HSL-derived fatty acids in adipocytes. A-FABP is also elevated during the differentiation of monocytes into macrophages. In macrophages, its expression can be induced by fatty acids, lipopolysaccharide (LPS), toll-like receptor (TLR) agonists, oxidized low-density lipoprotein (oxLDL), and advanced glycation end products (AGEs). A-FABP also promotes cholesterol ester accumulation, foam cell formation, and inflammatory responses by activating the IKK-NF-κB and JNK-AP-1 pathways (Rodriguez-Calvo et al. 2017). In endothelial cells, increased A-FABP induces endothelial dysfunction by modulating endothelial NO synthase (eNOS) nitric oxide (NO) signaling. In addition to its intracellular effects, A-FABP is also recognized as a hormone that is released into circulation and exerts effects on target tissues, such as adipose tissue and endothelium (Li et al. 2021). In general, these cytosolic proteins do not have a typical secretory signal peptide in their sequence; therefore, they are released into the blood by a non-classical route and due to the presence of tissue damage, such as in the case of adipose tissue, which represents a dysfunctional process due to the hypertrophy and hyperplasia present in obesity (Ertunc et al. 2015; Kralisch et al. 2014). The release of A-FABP from adipocytes is also favored by increased lipolysis and activation of the sympathetic nervous system, so it is considered an adipokine that is directed to the circulation in pathological conditions affecting target organs (Mita et al. 2015). A-FABP has been proposed as a very useful biomarker in the context of MetS (Xu et al. 2007) and CVD (Saito et al. 2021), since it promotes the development of insulin resistance (Uysal et al. 2000), promotes the formation of foam cells and atherosclerosis, inhibits endothelial nitric oxide synthase (Furuhashi et al. 2018), in addition to increasing serum A-FABP levels promoting the onset of T2D, HT and obesity-related CV events (Tso et al. 2007; Chow et al. 2013; Li et al. 2016) (Fig. 2).

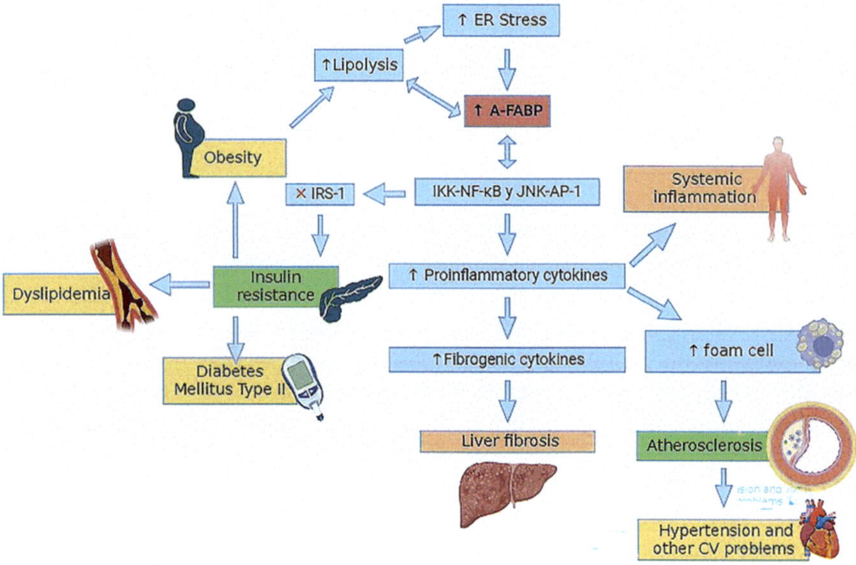

Fig. 2 Cycle of A-FABP elevation and progression of metabolic syndrome. The development of obesity is associated with an increase in basal lipolysis, leading to a higher concentration of A-FABP, which in turn induces further lipolysis, favoring increased secretion of A-FABP in a continuous cycle. In macrophages, A-FABP triggers inflammatory responses through activation of the IKK-NF-κB and JNK-AP-1 pathways, causing both systemic inflammation and the formation of foam cells that accumulate and initiate atherosclerotic lesions that can eventually lead to hypertension and other cardiovascular diseases. The release of pro-inflammatory cytokines resulting from the activation of these pathways also affects other organs, such as the liver, where it promotes the development of hepatic fibrosis. In addition, activation of protein kinases such as IKK and JNK inhibits IRS-1 and reduces insulin signaling, which ultimately promotes the onset of type 2 diabetes mellitus, dyslipidemias, hypertension, and obesity, thereby perpetuating the cycle of A-FABP elevation and progression of the metabolic syndrome (Rodriguez-Calvo et al. 2017). (Created with BioRender)

7 Epidermal Fatty Acid Binding Protein (E-FABP, FABP5, mal1)

E-FABP is mainly expressed in the epidermis but can also be found at lower levels in adipocytes and macrophages. Macrophages have been shown to primarily express A-FABP and E-FABP, providing a unique perspective to analyze how they regulate fatty acid (FA) metabolism and inflammatory pathways, thus shaping macrophage function (Jin et al. 2021). Fatty acids are shown to be critical in the maintenance of the water permeability barrier that is ascribed to the lipids in the intracellular milieu of the cornified cell layer in the epidermis. The cytosolic proteins lack secretory signal peptides in their sequence; therefore, they are released into the blood by a non-classical route. The overexpression and secretion of A-FABP into the circulation are associated with obesity, MetS, and CVD (Furuhashi et al. 2017).

The amount of E-FABP found in the blood is approximately 100 times less than that of A-FABP. Both have a similarity in amino acid sequence of 52% and bind to several fatty acids with the same affinity and selectivity (Uysal et al. 2000; Lin and Khnykin 2014). The skin is a very extensive tissue and has a very complex lipid metabolism. The presence of lipids is critical for the epidermis in four ways: (1) Fatty acids and ceramides are essential for the formation of the stratum corneum. (2) Serve as basic components of the sebum produced by the sebaceous glands. (3) Play an important role in keratinocyte signaling to regulate epidermal homeostasis. (4) Contribute to the acidification of the stratum corneum, promoting its structural integrity and barrier function (Makowski et al. 2001).

Skin involvement in metabolic pathologies is evident by the presence of inflammatory processes triggered by cytokines from the nearby subcutaneous adipose tissue that are deposited in the skin (Lin and Khnykin 2014); some are damage to the integrity of the barrier, alterations in the structure and function of collagen, changes in micro- and macrocirculation, damage to lymphatic vessels causing lymphedema, difficulty in wound healing, and increased production of sebum and sweat by the sebaceous and sweat glands (Makowski et al. 2001). Dietary fatty acids are directed to nearby tissues for deposition, such as subcutaneous adipose tissue and skin. Once they enter keratinocytes by passive diffusion or through membrane proteins, they are transported in the cytosol attached to the E- FABP to carry out a rather complex metabolism; in MetS, where the skin is also affected by inflammatory processes, we can identify skin biomarkers related to abnormal lipid metabolism (Nakamizo et al. 2019) (Table 2). In an obese mouse model with a high-fat diet, skin lesions were associated with CD11c + macrophage accumulation. Further analysis of the skin indicated that IL-1β signaling was significantly upregulated in CD11c + macrophages. Interestingly, saturated, but not unsaturated, FAs promote CD11c expression and induce IL-1β secretion in an E-FABP-dependent manner, suggesting that E-FABP enhances saturated FAs-mediated CD11c + macrophage differentiation and IL-1β signaling pathways. Recent studies demonstrate that saturated FAs are transported to lysosomes to form crystals for inflammasome activation and IL-1β release, suggesting that E-FABP may deliver saturated FAs to lysosomes in macrophages (Jin et al. 2021).

Table 2 Fatty acid binding proteins function in health and disease (Li et al. 2020)

Type of FABP	Function in health	Function in disease
Adipose-FABP (A-FABP, FABP4)	Lipid storage, lipolysis, and metabolism	Metabolic diseases (e.g. atherosclerosis, insulin resistance, type 2 diabetes), cardiovascular diseases, asthma, cancer
Epidermal-FABP (E-FABP, FABP5)	FA binding and oxidation, transportation of other signaling molecules	Inflammatory skin diseases (e.g. psoriasis, dermatitis), cancer, atherosclerosis, autoimmune diseases
Intestine-FABP (I-FABP, FABP2)	Dietary lipid absorption	Metabolic syndrome

8 Intestinal Fatty Acid Binding Protein (I-FABP, FABP2)

I-FABP is expressed in the epithelial cells of the intestinal mucosa and is responsible for the intracellular transport of fatty acids in the small intestine after their absorption into the epithelial cells of the enterocytes (Pelsers et al. 2003). The intestinal mucosa plays an important role not only in the absorption of fats and nutrients but also in defense, preventing the passage of harmful substances and promoting the development of the intestinal immune system. A high-fat diet alters the composition of the intestinal microbiota by increasing intestinal permeability. Obesity and insulin resistance have been described as the major metabolic changes mediated by the gut microbiota (Lau et al. 2016). Recent studies have shown that intestinal expression of I-FABP appears to positively correlate with ingested energy, with increased expression resulting in what could be considered an adaptive response to increasing dietary fat content. As a result, basal plasma levels of I-FABP reflect the physiological turnover rate of enterocytes, whereas elevated levels may indicate damage to intestinal epithelial cells (Lau et al. 2016; Weiss et al. 2002).

In metabolic diseases such as MS, the inflammation and loss of integrity of the intestinal wall observed during the consumption of high-fat diets seem to compromise its function by increasing the levels of I-FABP. This loss of the wall allows a displacement of this protein from the interior of the wall cells into the bloodstream and the intestinal lumen. This has enabled it to emerge as a potential non-invasive fecal biomarker for evaluating the loss of intestinal wall integrity, inflammation, and dysbiosis associated with these metabolic diseases (Thuijls et al. 2011; Wells et al. 2017) (Table 2).

There are two polymorphic variants of I-FABP at codon 54 of exon 2, replacing alanine (Ala) with threonine (Thr) in the small helical region of the protein. Several studies have shown that, although this mutation is functional, its binding and transport capacity for fatty acids differ, as it has a greater capacity to transport long-chain fatty acids (Turkovic et al. 2012). In addition, the Thr54 allele of I-FABP has been shown to be significantly associated with higher total cholesterol, dyslipidemia, stroke incidence, and obesity, and weakly associated with insulin resistance in different ethnic groups (Gomez et al. 2007).

A high-fat diet promotes the development of metabolic disorders such as obesity and insulin resistance but also alters the composition of the gut microbiota, ultimately causing inflammation, damage, and increased intestinal wall permeability (Fig. 3). In this context, the translocation of I-FABP from the gut to the bloodstream and into the intestinal lumen has emerged as a potential non-invasive fecal biomarker to assess intestinal wall integrity loss, inflammation, and dysbiosis in these metabolic diseases. Serum I-FABP concentration is designated to be 2.0 ng/mL or less in the circulation of normal healthy individuals (Funaoka et al. 2010). I-FABP mRNA levels increase from the duodenum to reach the highest levels in the proximal ileum. It has been shown that I-FABP is released into the circulation following small intestinal mucosal injury, and its plasma concentration has been associated with small intestinal diseases—necrotizing enterocolitis and celiac disease. Basal I-FABP plasma levels may reflect the physiological turnover rate of enterocytes, whereas

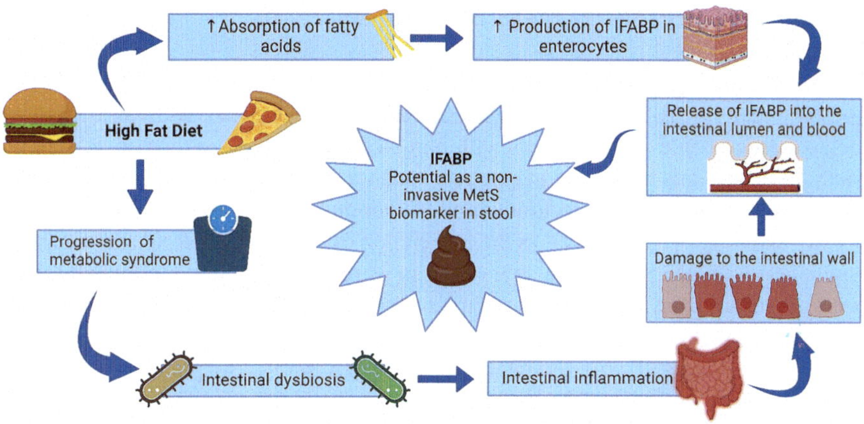

Fig. 3 Potential of I-FABP as a biomarker for MetS. Intestinal expression of I-FABP appears to be positively correlated with energy intake, with increased expression as an adaptive response to higher dietary fat content. (Created with BioRender)

elevated levels might indicate intestinal epithelial cell damage. Nevertheless, in the case of obesity-associated metabolic diseases, the existing data about I-FABP and intestinal barrier dysfunction is limited (Lau et al. 2016).

9 Inflammation in MetS and Its Association with FABPs

A-FABP is expressed in endothelial cells and macrophages in addition to adipocytes. E-FABP has a more widespread expression profile, including skin, adipose tissue, and immune system cellular populations. In studies focused on lipid metabolism in immune cells and their function, it has been found that in obesity and MetS, A-FABP and E-FABP show unique expression patterns in macrophages that regulate their metabolic and inflammatory pathways, particularly in the development of atherosclerosis, HT, and other MetS-associated CV diseases (Jin et al. 2021).

A-FABP4, one of the most abundant cytoplasmic proteins in adipocytes, acts at the interface of metabolic and inflammatory pathways. A positive correlation has been found between pro-inflammatory factors such as CRP, IL-6, TNF receptors, and leptin with A-FABP in obese individuals, suggesting that it plays a role in systemic inflammation and is involved in the development of key pathologies associated with MetS (Terra et al. 2011). Chronic consumption of high-fat diets damages the intestinal barrier, leading to dysbiosis and the subsequent migration of bacteria or their by-products, such as LPS. Together with I-FABP, these are recognized as key factors in the development of intestinal inflammation characteristic of metabolic disorders (Lau et al. 2016).

10 Other Potential MetS Biomarkers

Concentrations of pro-inflammatory markers in adolescents and young people with obesity, such as IL-6, have been associated with MetS, as well as a certain metabolomic profile in individuals with non-alcoholic fatty liver disease present in MetS. Other studies have used magnetic resonance imaging to investigate its potential use as a marker for the accumulation of liver and pancreatic fat associated with obesity and overweight, as well as the association of certain microRNAs in the adult population with MetS. Resistin, one of the most recently identified adipokines, has been proposed as an inflammatory marker involved in the regulation of obesity in humans (Terra et al. 2011). There is evidence for an association between GLP2, gut growth, and increased energy intake. It has been shown to play a role in the inflammatory state induced by changes in the microbiota after feeding a high-fat diet, as its production is increased to improve the integrity of the intestinal barrier. This amino acid has been postulated as a biomarker of metabolic changes (Baldassano et al. 2013).

11 Vasculopathy and Its Relationship with FABPs

A-FABP was identified as a key mediator in these pathophysiological pathways involved in the development of hypertension, including being associated with endothelial dysfunction through mediating endothelial NO pathways and activation of the sympathetic nervous system. Circulating levels of A-FABP are closely associated with carotid intima-media thickness (CIMT), a well-established marker of atherosclerosis. Moreover, the expression of AFABP was elevated in carotid plaques in patients with CVD and was associated with plaque vulnerability. Animal studies showed that A-FABP mediates the pathogenesis of atherosclerosis by inducing endothelial dysfunction, vascular smooth muscle cell invasion, and foam cell formation (Li et al. 2021).

A-FABP has long been implicated in the progression and severity of ischemic stroke; circulating A-FABP levels are elevated after acute ischemic stroke and are positively correlated with early death and poor functional outcome, myocardial perfusion abnormalities, and left ventricular mass and hypertrophy (Li et al. 2021). Endothelial cell FABP4 expression is strongly induced by pro-angiogenic mediators, vascular endothelial growth factor (VEGF), and basic fibroblast growth factor (bFGF), and FABP4 significantly promotes the angiogenic responses of endothelial cells. Interestingly, although FABP4 is not expressed in normal brain blood vessels, it demonstrates an upregulation of FABP4 in both arteriovenous malformations (AVMs) and cavernous malformations (CMs), which are the most common cerebral vascular malformations (Cataltepe et al. 2015). Cholesterol efflux capacity (CEC) from lipid-loaded cells is a key athero-protective event that counteracts cholesterol uptake. The imbalance between CEC and uptake determines whether atherosclerosis is prevented or developed. Many proteins and factors participate in the CEC. FABP5 is independently associated with both carotid atherosclerosis and decreased CEC, suggesting that FABP5 level is a novel regulatory factor of CEC and a potential biomarker for residual risk of atherosclerosis in relation to cholesterol efflux from macrophages (Furuhashi et al. 2017).

12 FABPs as a Therapeutic Target

As the functions of this protein's family have been further elucidated, it has become evident that they are critical mediators of metabolism, CV and inflammatory processes, both locally and systemically, and therefore are potential therapeutic targets for cardioimmunometabolic diseases. Genetic deficiency and small molecule-mediated inhibition of FABP4 and FABP5 can potently improve glucose homeostasis and reduce atherosclerosis in mouse models (Hotamisligil and Bernlohr 2015).

As FABPs are involved in various metabolic and CV diseases and represent a therapeutic target, multiple small molecule inhibitors, including BMS309403, HTS01037, and other triazolopyrimidine derivatives, which inhibit by various modes of binding, and polyclonal and monoclonal neutralizing antibodies, such as CA33 and 2E4, have been developed, aiming to inhibit FABP activity. A fluoroquinolone antibiotic (levofloxacin) and a uricosuric agent (benzbromarone) were also found to exhibit anti-A-FABP properties (Hotamisligil and Bernlohr 2015).

Recent studies reported on the development of an isoform-specific and biologically active synthetic A-FABP inhibitor and demonstrated that chemical inhibition of A-FABP could be a potential therapeutic strategy against IR, diabetes, fatty liver disease, and atherosclerosis in independent experimental models. Previous studies suggest that the expression, regulation, and metabolic function of human A-FABP may be like that of mice; studies are needed to determine whether FABP inhibitors could be used safely in humans and show efficacy against metabolic diseases. If successful, the inhibition of FABPs in humans may become a promising new class of therapies against a wide range of metabolic, CV diseases, and possibly other inflammatory diseases (Furuhashi and Hotamisligil 2008).

13 Conclusions

MetS is the subject of numerous studies that have provided new insights into its pathophysiology, the search for biomarkers, and the development of new drugs, among other areas of research. Being a disease with high prevalence and in which there are different mechanisms involved in its presentation, one of them related to FABPs, we can conclude that these cytosolic proteins are candidates that have unique characteristics and are involved in basic functions of the organism but that in pathological conditions offer us an open window for the early detection of MetS and CV complications.

References

Baldassano S, Amato A, Cappello F, Rappa F, Mulè F (2013) Glucagon-like peptide-2 and mouse intestinal adaptation to a high-fat diet. J Endocrinol 217(1):11–20. https://doi.org/10.1530/JOE-12-0500. PMID: 23308022

Bovolini A, Garcia J, Andrade MA, Duarte JA (2021) Metabolic syndrome pathophysiology and predisposing factors. Int J Sports Med 42(03):199–214

Cataltepe S, Arikan MC, Liang X, Smith TW, Cataltepe O (2015) Fatty acid binding protein 4 expression in cerebral vascular malformations: implications for vascular remodelling. Neuropathol Appl Neurobiol 41(5):646-656

Chow WS, Tso AWK, Xu A, Yuen MMA, Fong CHY, Lam TH et al (2013) Elevated circulating adipocyte-fatty acid binding protein levels predict incident cardiovascular events in a community-based cohort: a 12-year prospective study. J Am Heart Assoc 2(1):e004176

Chung JY, Ain QU, Song Y, Yong SB, Kim YH (2019) Targeted delivery of CRISPR interference system against Fabp4 to white adipocytes ameliorates obesity, inflammation, hepatic steatosis, and insulin resistance. Genome Res 29(9):1442–1452

Eizirik DL, Pasquali L, Cnop M (2020) Pancreatic β-cells in type 1 and type 2 diabetes mellitus: different pathways to failure. Nat Rev Endocrinol 16(7):349–362

Ellis DI, Goodacre R (2006) Metabolic fingerprinting in disease diagnosis: biomedical applications of infrared and Raman spectroscopy. Analyst 131(8):875–885

Ertunc ME, Sikkeland J, Fenaroli F, Griffiths G, Daniels MP, Cao H et al (2015) Secretion of fatty acid binding protein aP2 from adipocytes through a nonclassical pathway in response to adipocyte lipase activity. J Lipid Res 56(2):423–434

Espinosa Brito A (2018) Hipertensión arterial: cifras para definirla al comenzar 2018. Revista Finlay 8(1):66–74

Flack JM, Adekola B (2020) Blood pressure and the new ACC/AHA hypertension guidelines. Trends Cardiovasc Med 30(3):160–164

Funaoka H, Kanda T, Fujii H (2010) Intestinal fatty acid-binding protein (I-FABP) as a new biomarker for intestinal diseases. Rinsho Byori Jpn J Clin Pathol 58(2):162–168

Furuhashi M, Hotamisligil GS (2008) Fatty acid-binding proteins: role in metabolic diseases and potential as drug targets. Nat Rev Drug Discov 7(6):489–503

Furuhashi M, Saitoh S, Shimamoto K, Miura T (2014) Fatty acid-binding protein 4 (FABP4): pathophysiological insights and potent clinical biomarker of metabolic and cardiovascular diseases. Clin Med Insights Cardiol 8:CMC-S17067

Furuhashi M, Ogura M, Matsumoto M, Yuda S, Muranaka A, Kawamukai M et al (2017) Serum FABP5 concentration is a potential biomarker for residual risk of atherosclerosis in relation to cholesterol efflux from macrophages. Sci Rep 7(1):1–10

Furuhashi M, Yuda S, Muranaka A, Kawamukai M, Matsumoto M, Tanaka M et al (2018) Circulating fatty acid-binding protein 4 concentration predicts the progression of carotid atherosclerosis in a general population without medication. Circ J 82(4):1121–1129

Furuhashi M, Sakuma I, Morimoto T, Higashiura Y, Sakai A, Matsumoto M et al (2020) Independent and distinct associations of FABP4 and FABP5 with metabolic parameters in type 2 diabetes mellitus. Front Endocrinol 11:575557

García-Rubio DL, de la Mora MB, Badillo-Ramírez I, Cerecedo D, Saniger JM, Benítez-Benítez JL, Villagrán-Muniz M (2019) Analysis of platelets in hypertensive and normotensive individuals using Raman and Fourier transform infrared-attenuated total reflectance spectroscopies. J Raman Spectrosc 50(4):509–521

Gillilan RE, Ayers SD, Noy N (2007) Structural basis for activation of fatty acid-binding protein 4. J Mol Biol 372(5):1246–1260

Gomez LC, Real SM, Ojeda MS, Gimenez S, Mayorga LS, Roqué M (2007) Polymorphism of the FABP2 gene: a population frequency analysis and an association study with cardiovascular risk markers in Argentina. BMC Med Genet 8:39. https://doi.org/10.1186/1471-2350-8-39

Griffiths HR, Møller L, Bartosz G, Bast A, Bertoni-Freddari C, Collins A et al (2002) Biomarkers. Mol Aspects Med 23(1–3):101–208

Haka AS, Sue E, Zhang C, Bhardwaj P, Sterling J, Carpenter C et al (2016) Non-invasive detection of inflammatory changes in white adipose tissue by label-free Raman spectroscopy. Anal Chem 88(4):2140–2148

Hernández JLC, González MJC, Galiana MA, Hernández EYR (2018) Síndrome metabólico, un problema de salud pública con diferentes definiciones y criterios. Revista Médica de la Universidad Veracruzana 17(2):7–24

Hotamisligil GS, Bernlohr DA (2015) Metabolic functions of FABPs—mechanisms and therapeutic implications. Nature reviews. Endocrinology 11(10):592-605

Ingelsson E, Hulthe J, Lind L (2008) Inflammatory markers in relation to insulin resistance and the metabolic syndrome. Eur J Clin Investig 38(7):502–509

Ishimura S, Furuhashi M, Watanabe Y, Hoshina K, Fuseya T, Mita T et al (2013) Circulating levels of fatty acid-binding protein family and metabolic phenotype in the general population. PLoS One 8(11):e81318

Jin R, Hao J, Yi Y, Sauter E, Li B (2021) Regulation of macrophage functions by FABP-mediated inflammatory and metabolic pathways. Biochimica et Biophysica Acta (BBA)-Mol Cell Biol Lipids 1866(8):158964

Katsiki N, Athyros VG, Karagiannis A, Mikhailidis DP (2014) Characteristics other than the diagnostic criteria associated with metabolic syndrome: an overview. Curr Vasc Pharmacol 12(4):627–641

Koh KK, Han SH, Quon MJ (2005) Inflammatory markers and the metabolic syndrome: insights from therapeutic interventions. J Am Coll Cardiol 46(11):1978–1985

Kralisch S, Ebert T, Lossner U, Jessnitzer B, Stumvoll M, Fasshauer M (2014) Adipocyte fatty acid-binding protein is released from adipocytes by a non-conventional mechanism. Int J Obes 38(9): 1251–1254

Kumari R, Kumar S, Kant R (2019) An update on metabolic syndrome: metabolic risk markers and adipokines in the development of metabolic syndrome. Diabetes Metab Syndr Clin Res Rev 13(4):2409–2417

Lau E, Marques C, Pestana D, Santoalha M, Carvalho D, Freitas P, Calhau C (2016) The role of I-FABP as a biomarker of intestinal barrier dysfunction driven by gut microbiota changes in obesity. Nutr Metab 13:1–7

Lemieux I, Després JP (2020) Metabolic syndrome: past, present and future. Nutrients 12(11):3501

Li M, Ishibashi T (1992) Reversible conformational changes of rat liver fatty acid binding protein following lipid binding: circular dichroic and nuclear magnetic resonance analysis. Biomed Res 13(5):335–341

Li JC, Wu DA, Hou JS, Subeq YM, Chen HD, Hsu BG (2016) High serum adipocyte fatty acid binding protein is associated with metabolic syndrome in patients with type 2 diabetes. J Diabetes Res 2016(1):8380279

Li B, Hao J, Zeng J, Sauter ER (2020) SnapShot: FABP functions. Cell 182(4):1066–1066

Li HL, Wu X, Xu A, Hoo RLC (2021) A-FABP in metabolic diseases and the therapeutic implications: an update. Int J Mol Sci 22(17):9386

Lin MH, Khnykin D (2014) Fatty acid transporters in skin development, function and disease. Biochimica et Biophysica Acta (BBA)-Mol Cell Biol Lipids 1841(3):362–368

Makowski L, Boord JB, Maeda K, Babaev VR, Uysal KT, Morgan MA et al (2001) Lack of macrophage fatty-acid–binding protein aP2 protects mice deficient in apolipoprotein E against atherosclerosis. Nat Med 7(6):699–705

Mita T, Furuhashi M, Hiramitsu S, Ishii J, Hoshina K, Ishimura S et al (2015) FABP4 is secreted from adipocytes by adenyl cyclase-PKA-and guanylyl cyclase-PKG-dependent lipolytic mechanisms. Obesity 23(2):359–367

Mohamed SM, Shalaby MA, El-Shiekh RA, El-Banna HA, Emam SR, Bakr AF (2023) Metabolic syndrome: risk factors, diagnosis, pathogenesis, and management with natural approaches. Food Chem Adv 3:100335

Nakamizo S, Honda T, Kabashima K (2019) Obesity and inflammatory skin diseases. Trends Immunother 3(1):50–57

Oda E (2018) Historical perspectives of the metabolic syndrome. Clin Dermatol 36(1):3–8
Pacia MZ, Mateuszuk L, Buczek E, Chlopicki S, Blazejczyk A, Wietrzyk J et al (2016) Rapid biochemical profiling of endothelial dysfunction in diabetes, hypertension and cancer metastasis by hierarchical cluster analysis of Raman spectra. J Raman Spectrosc 47(11):1310–1317
Pelsers MM, Namiot Z, Kisielewski W, Namiot A, Januszkiewicz M, Hermens WT, Glatz JF (2003) Intestinal-type and liver-type fatty acid-binding protein in the intestine. Tissue distribution and clinical utility. Clin Biochem 36(7):529–535
Rodriguez-Calvo R, Girona J, Alegret JM, Bosquet A, Ibarretxe D, Masana L (2017) Role of the fatty acid-binding protein 4 in heart failure and cardiovascular. J Endocrinol 233:R173–R184
Rodríguez-Calvo R, Girona J, Rodríguez M, Samino S, Barroso E, de Gonzalo-Calvo D et al (2019) Fatty acid binding protein 4 (FABP4) as a potential biomarker reflecting myocardial lipid storage in type 2 diabetes. Metabolism 96:12–21
Saito N, Furuhashi M, Koyama M, Higashiura Y, Akasaka H, Tanaka M et al (2021) Elevated circulating FABP4 concentration predicts cardiovascular death in a general population: a 12-year prospective study. Sci Rep 11(1):1–11
Saklayen MG (2018) The global epidemic of the metabolic syndrome. Curr Hypertens Rep 20(2): 1–8
Terra X, Quintero Y, Auguet T, Porras JA, Hernández M, Sabench F et al (2011) FABP 4 is associated with inflammatory markers and metabolic syndrome in morbidly obese women. Eur J Endocrinol 164(4):539–547
Thuijls G, van Wijck K, Grootjans J, Derikx JP, van Bijnen AA, Heineman E et al (2011) Early diagnosis of intestinal ischemia using urinary and plasma fatty acid binding proteins. Ann Surg 253(2):303–308
Tso AW, Xu A, Sham PC, Wat NM, Wang Y, Fong CH et al (2007) Serum adipocyte fatty acid–binding protein as a new biomarker predicting the development of type 2 diabetes: A 10-year prospective study in a Chinese cohort. Diabetes Care 30(10):2667–2672
Turkovic LF, Pizent A, Dodig S, Pavlovic M, Pasalic D (2012) FABP2 gene polymorphism and metabolic syndrome in elderly people of croatian descent. Biochem Med Zagreb 22(2): 217–224. https://doi.org/10.11613/bm.2012.024
Unger RH, Clark GO, Scherer PE, Orci L (2010) Lipid homeostasis, lipotoxicity and the metabolic syndrome. Biochimica et Biophysica Acta (BBA)-Mol Cell Biol Lipids 1801(3):209–214
Uysal KT, Scheja L, Wiesbrock SM, Bonner-Weir S, Hotamisligil GS (2000) Improved glucose and lipid metabolism in genetically obese mice lacking aP2. Endocrinology 141(9):3388–3396
Vekic J, Zeljkovic A, Stefanovic A, Jelic-Ivanovic Z, Spasojevic-Kalimanovska V (2019) Obesity and dyslipidemia. Metabolism 92:71–81
Weiss EP, Brown MD, Shuldiner AR, Hagberg JM (2002) Fatty acid binding protein-2 gene variants and insulin resistance: gene and gene-environment interaction effects. Physiol Genomics 10(3):145–157
Wells JM, Brummer RJ, Derrien M, MacDonald TT, Troost F, Cani PD et al (2017) Homeostasis of the gut barrier and potential biomarkers. American Journal of Physiology-Gastrointestinal and Liver Physiology 312(3):G171–G193
World Health Organization (2024a) https://www.who.int/diabetes/publications. Accessed July 2024
World Health Organization (2024b) https://www.who.int/health-topics/diabetes. Accessed July 2024
Xu A, Tso AW, Cheung BM, Wang Y, Wat NM, Fong CH et al (2007) Circulating adipocyte–fatty acid binding protein levels predict the development of the metabolic syndrome: a 5-year prospective study. Circulation 115(12):1537–1543
Yao F, Jiang DD, Guo WH, Guo LS, Gao MM, Bai Y et al (2020) FABP4 inhibitor attenuates inflammation and endoplasmic reticulum stress of the islet in leptin receptor knockout rats. Eur Rev Med Pharmacol Sci 24(24):12808
Zheng X, Lv G, Zhang Y, Lv X, Gao Z, Tang J, Mo J (2019) Rapid and non-invasive screening of high renin hypertension using Raman spectroscopy and different classification algorithms. Spectrochim Acta A Mol Biomol Spectrosc 215:244–248

Physical Activity and Its Impact on Cardiometabolic Disorders

J. Gustavo Vázquez-Jiménez and Tatiana Romero-García

Contents

Abstract

The significant concern about the incidence and prevalence of cardiometabolic disorders around the world continues to rise as this upward trend persists. As researchers intensify their search for underlying causes, there is a growing demand for effective methods of prevention and treatment. In this sense, technology dependence, high-calorie diets, and a shortage of opportunities, time, and interest in physical activity primarily drive the growth in sedentary behavior among the global population, which is strongly associated with the emergence

J. G. Vázquez-Jiménez
Facultad de Medicina y Nutrición, Universidad Autónoma de Baja California, Mexicali, Mexico

T. Romero-García (✉)
Facultad de Deportes Mexicali, Universidad Autónoma de Baja California, Mexicali, Mexico
e-mail: tatiana.romero@uabc.edu.mx

A. Rueda, M. Nieves-Cintrón (eds.), *Cardiovascular Alterations in Metabolic Diseases*, Handbook of Experimental Pharmacology 293,
https://doi.org/10.1007/164_2026_792

of cardiometabolic disorders. Thus, this chapter will highlight the importance of physical activity for metabolic and cardiovascular health through the revision of the various studies carried out around the world, highlighting the benefits at a molecular and physiological level for people who suffer from obesity, metabolic syndrome and, type 2 diabetes mellitus, as well as providing a general overview regarding the particularities in the prescription of exercise for people with these conditions.

Keywords

Cardiovascular disease · Exercise · Exerkines · Metabolic syndrome · Obesity · Sedentarism · Type 2 diabetes mellitus

1 Introduction

The rise of acquired metabolic disorders is linked to external factors, including unhealthy lifestyle habits, high caloric intake, and physical inactivity. Indeed, some research suggests that our lifestyle influences inherited epigenetic patterns, which in turn affect gene expression and protein activity, thereby contributing to the development of cardiometabolic diseases (Eckel et al. 2010). Thus, critical approaches against this growing global issue that cardiometabolic disorders represent include weight loss and maintaining at least a moderate level of physical activity, with medication being an additional option for managing some of these pathological conditions (Heal et al. 2009). Hence, the role of physical activity in improving people's well-being while reducing the incidence of non-communicable diseases (NCDs) is highly relevant. Consequently, worldwide public health priorities include improving health parameters to ensure longevity and quality of life, primarily through the promotion of physical activity and a healthful diet, which impacts both short-term and long-term health. In this respect, the *WHO Package of Essential Non-communicable Disease Interventions for Primary Health Care in Low-Resource Settings* highlights the importance of promoting physical activity, while providing guidelines to gradually increase physical activity until reaching the WHO's global recommendations.

Physical inactivity is a leading contributor to global mortality, also representing a significant financial challenge that costs over US$54 billion in direct health care. Several prevention initiatives have been implemented to mitigate poor dietary habits and physical inactivity, which are key factors that directly contribute to overweight and increase cardiovascular risk. For instance, the "*WHO Global Action Plan on Physical Activity and Health 2018–2030: More Active People for a Healthier World*" (GAPPA) was presented during the 71st Global Health Assembly to counteract physical inactivity by recommending a set of 20 evidence-based policy areas for improving the opportunities and environments for people of all region, ages, gender, and health conditions to become and maintain an active lifestyle (World

Health Organization 2020). This initiative aims to reduce physical inactivity by at least 15% by 2030; however, progress has been slow.

It is common to believe that physical activity is just sports or exercise. However, physical activity involves any movement of the human body promoted by the skeletal muscles at the expense of cellular energy expenditure. Therefore, the activities performed during a regular day, including walking, work, and domestic chores, could be considered physical activity. Nevertheless, the intensity and duration of the physical activity performed on a daily basis have proven to be a crucial factor for a person to be categorized as an active or a sedentary person, with all the cardiometabolic risks that this implies (Rodulfo 2022).

2 Sedentarism and Metabolic Disorders

A sedentary lifestyle is detrimental to several aspects of life quality, such as impaired fitness and cardiovascular health, excess adiposity, sleep duration, and behavioral conduct (Bull et al. 2020). During the last century, the time dedicated to physical activity has dramatically decreased. This trend keeps increasing, along with technological advances that promote sedentary activities that demand a low energy expenditure, such as watching television, playing video games, or browsing the Internet, which are activities associated with poorer fitness by generating an imbalance between calorie intake and expenditure that compromises cardiovascular health.

Insufficient physical activity combined with excessive intake of saturated fats, trans fats, and free sugars constitutes one of the main risks for cardiometabolic diseases emerging around the globe. The evidence concerning the inverse relationship between physical activity and cardiovascular mortality, cardiovascular incidence, and type 2 diabetes mellitus (T2DM) incidence is well established. Recent device-based data confirm that any level of any intensity of physical activity reduces the risk of all-cause mortality, cardiovascular disease (CVD), T2DM, and hypertension incidence (Ekelund et al. 2019).

Lack of physical activity contributes to weight gain and obesity, which is commonly accompanied by chronic low-grade inflammation and unfavorable changes in lipid levels, such as increased triglycerides and reduced HDL cholesterol that negatively impact cardiovascular health by promoting endothelial dysfunction, reducing heart rate variability, and increasing the risk of hypertension and coronary artery disease (Bull et al. 2020; Rodulfo 2022). Likewise, a sedentary lifestyle is a significant risk factor for metabolic syndrome (MetS), which is a cluster of conditions including high blood pressure, hyperglycemia, central obesity, and dyslipidemia that increase the risk of heart disease, stroke, and T2DM (Tune et al. 2017). As well, physical inactivity leads to reduced insulin sensitivity, which can induce insulin resistance, increasing the risk for T2DM by impairing glucose metabolism; notably, the incidence of T2DM is inversely correlated with higher volumes of physical activity regardless of body composition (Boyer et al. 2018).

It is calculated that if the physical inactivity prevalence remains unaltered, at least 500 million new cases of NCDs will emerge between 2020 and 2030, generating

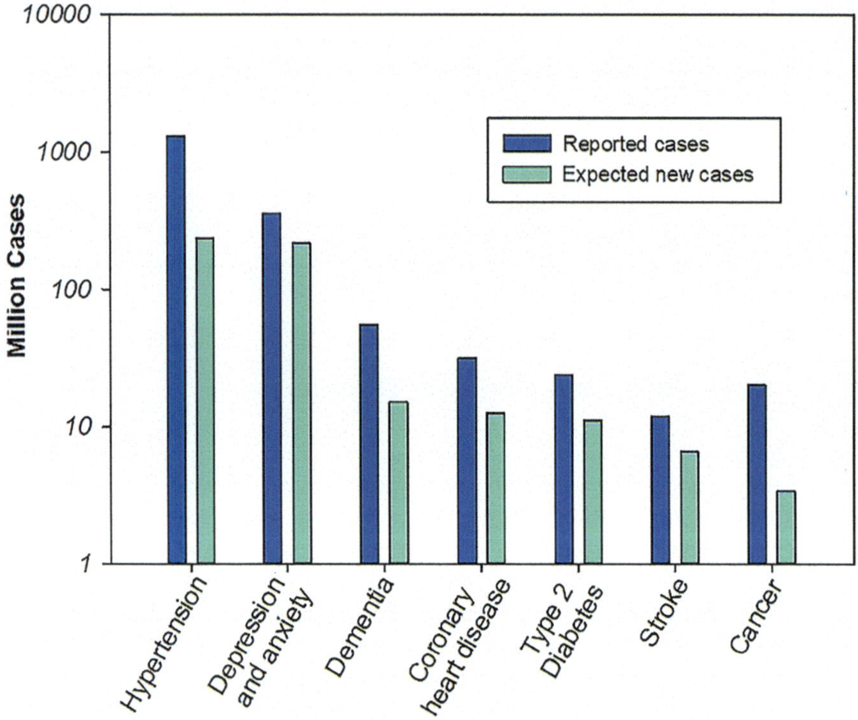

Fig. 1 Global current incidence and expected new cases by 2030 of non-communicable diseases and mental health conditions attributed to physical inactivity. (Adapted from Costa Santos et al. 2023)

high healthcare system costs, particularly in middle-income countries where most of the world's population is concentrated (Costa Santos et al. 2023; Katzmarzyk et al. 2022). Multiple studies have estimated the prevalence of physical inactivity in many regions to be about 27.5% by 2016, with no critical changes since 2001, although the pathway differed for each country (Guthold et al. 2018). However, more extensive and recent research identified that nearly one-third of the global population failed to reach the recommended physical activity levels, with significant disparities based on sex, age, region, and country. Insufficient physical activity prevalence increased in 52% of the countries analyzed, representing an increase of 26.4% from 2010, and it is calculated that if this trend continues, as shown in Fig. 1, the GAPPA 2030 objectives will not be achieved (Strain et al. 2024).

Interestingly, prevalence data also reveal that women are less likely to engage in physical activity than men across most countries, which constitutes a serious concern given that women present unique risk factors for cardiometabolic disorders such as pregnancy, polycystic ovary syndrome, gestational diabetes mellitus, pre-eclampsia, and menopause by the influence of sex hormones regulation, as well as by the gender differences on biochemical markers of risk like uric acid, IL-6, leptin, adiponectin, among others. These factors have an impact on the higher obesity and MetS prevalence in women compared to men (Gerdts and Regitz-Zagrosek 2019; Meloni et al. 2023).

Generally, sedentary behavior is evaluated by device-based assessments or physical activity questionnaires like IPAQ and GPAQ, which usually classify levels of physical activity based on intensity by applying the metabolic equivalent method (MET), where one unit corresponds to the level of energy expenditure at rest, and the physical activity is categorized as light intensity (<3 METs), moderate intensity (3–6 METs), and vigorous intensity (>6 METs), with some authors recommending that below 1.5 METs is defined as sedentary behavior (González et al. 2017).

3 Exercise and Cardiometabolic Health

Physical activity is defined as any movement involving the major muscle groups that elevates the basal metabolic rate, which represents the energy required to maintain the physiological processes at rest. Physical activity can be either unstructured, when it is a free, spontaneous recreational activity, or structured, when there is a precise aim in its practice (sports training, physical performance, physical fitness, control of a health condition, etc.); this is called exercise (World Health Organization 2020).

Based on the American College of Sports Medicine recommendations (American College of Sports Medicine 2013), physical activity should be performed considering these elements:

- Frequency refers to the number of times the activity is performed in a determined period.
- Duration refers to the length of time the activity is performed in a session.
- Volume refers to the total activity performed, usually expressed in terms of repetitions or series.
- Intensity refers to the magnitude of the effort needed to complete the activity or the rate of the exercise performed. Accordingly, the intensity is considered moderate when the activity implies an effort between 3 and 5.9 times above rest metabolic activity. At the same time, the intensity is considered vigorous when the activity implies an effort at least 6 times above rest metabolic activity.

The *Global Recommendations on Physical Activity for Health,* set out by the WHO, establish the proper frequency, duration, intensity, type, and total amount of physical activity to be considered a preventive component for NCDs; accordingly, physical inactivity is defined as not meeting these guidelines. The general recommendations suggest that adults should engage in at least 150 min of moderate-intensity or 75 min of vigorous aerobic physical activity each week, spread over different days, and include muscle-strengthening activities on two or more days (Bull et al. 2020). Beyond these recommendations, some reports suggest that any physical activity is better than none. For instance, the CARDIA study indicates that even modest increases in physical activity can lead to significant health improvements. Specifically, there is an improvement in cardiometabolic health when replacing sedentary time with light-intensity physical activity (LPA), as evidenced by changes in parameters such as waist circumference and insulin levels, as well as an increase in high-density lipoprotein (HDL) cholesterol over a 10-year period (Whitaker et al. 2019). Of course, it must be considered that for a sedentary person, the intensity, frequency, and duration of physical activity should increase gradually until reaching the recommended levels.

Likewise, physical activity can be classified into different types according to several features and modes of participation: aerobic (or endurance), resistance (or strength), balance, and flexibility. Aerobic exercise, also known as cardio, is characterized by an increase in respiratory and heart rates through prolonged activity executed at a moderate to low intensity. Resistance exercise is characterized by a short-term activity executed at vigorous intensity. Balance exercises are intended to enhance the ability to control the person's center of gravity by regulating body posture and movement, while flexibility exercises focus on stretching muscles while maintaining the full range of motion possible at a joint. Usually, the training routines are designed to include all four types of exercise, so pure aerobic or pure resistance exercise with no balance or flexibility abilities involved is scarce (Hughes et al. 2018). Although the outcomes of the different types of exercise training may differ, the combination maximizes health benefits induced by the adaptations to exercise. Table 1 summarizes some of the specific health benefits of each type of exercise.

3.1 Physiological and Metabolic Adaptations to Exercise

When physical activity starts, various metabolic responses are quickly triggered, leading to disruptions in cellular homeostasis. Exercise is a stressor agent that triggers responses after acute exposure and adaptations after chronic exposure. This is due to a temporary rise in stress hormones like cortisol and catecholamines, which results in increased blood flow and elevated heart and respiratory rates, increased oxygen consumption, as well as the activation of several enzymes involved in the oxidation of fatty acids and glucose, all together to meet the oxygen and energy demands of muscle (Lambert 2016).

Fundamentally, skeletal muscle requires sustained adenosine triphosphate (ATP) production to maintain muscular contraction and physical activity. After the nervous system generates a signal, an action potential is induced and transmitted to the muscle cells through a motor neuron in the neuromuscular junction. Once the motor neuron releases acetylcholine, this neurotransmitter bonds with its receptor on the muscle fiber's cell membrane, triggering the membrane depolarization and activating the calcium-dependent excitation-contraction coupling mechanism in the fiber's T-tubules. The increase in cytoplasmic calcium concentration accounts for actin-myosin cross-bridges, leading to muscular contraction mediated by the hydrolysis of an ATP molecule. Three different energy systems are responsible for maintaining muscle ATP demand. Energy for anaerobic high-intensity exercise derives from ATP-phosphocreatine (PC) and glycogen stores. In contrast, aerobic

Table 1 Comparison of the effects of types of exercise on health and fitness variables

Variable	Aerobic exercise	Resistance exercise	Balance exercise	Flexibility exercise
Body composition				
Bone mineral density	↑↑	↑↑	↑	↑
Muscular strength	↑↑	↑↑↑	↑	--
Body fat (%)	↓↓	↓	--	--
Metabolic parameters				
Basal metabolism	↑	↑↑	↑--	--
Basal insulin	↓	↓	↓ --	↓ --
Insulin sensitivity	↑↑	↑↑	↑ --	↑ --
Insulin response to glucose challenge	↓↓	↓↓	↓	↓
HDL cholesterol	↑↑	↑ --	--	--
LDL cholesterol	↓↓	↓ --	↓	↓
Cardiovascular parameters				
Resting heart rate	↓↓	--	--	--
Stroke volume	↑↑	--	--	--
Systolic pressure	↓↓	--	↓	--
Diastolic pressure	↓↓	↓ --	↓	--
Physiological resistance				
VO_{2max}	↑↑↑	↑	--	--
Endurance Time	↑↑↑	↑↑	--	--
Physical function	↑↑	↑↑↑	↑	↑

Adapted from Pollock and Evans (1999), World Health Organization (2010), Hamasaki (2024)
The number of arrows indicates the intensity of the effect. *HDL* High-density lipoprotein, *LDL* Low-density lipoprotein, VO_{2max} maximal oxygen consumption; ↑= increase; ↓ = decrease; -- = no effect; --↓↑ = the reports show inconsistent effects

moderate- to low-intensity exercise uses glycogen and triacylglycerols depending on the duration and intensity of the activity. Exercise has been proven to alter energy metabolism; for example, high-intensity interval training (HIIT) enhances the oxidative capacity of skeletal muscles, as evidenced by higher activity levels of mitochondrial enzymes such as cytochrome oxidase and citrate synthase, as well as a reduction in phosphagen and carbohydrate metabolism and a shift toward increased lipid oxidation after exercise (Gibala and Mcgee 2008).

Although responses to exercise training are temporary, constant exercise repetition leads to physiological adaptations in several body systems through protein synthesis upregulation, tissue remodeling, and altered regulation of molecular mechanisms. In fact, skeletal muscle is a tissue characterized by its plasticity and adaptability to exercise, including mechanical, physiological, and metabolic changes. For instance, resistance or anaerobic training increases muscle size and induces its remodeling, resulting from changes in muscle fiber composition; these adaptations, however, are influenced by factors such as the volume and intensity of the training. On the other hand, aerobic or endurance training enhances cardiac output, maximal oxygen consumption, blood flow, and mitochondrial biogenesis through proliferator-activated receptor gamma coactivator 1-alpha (PGC-1α) activation (Liu et al. 2020).

3.1.1 Cardiovascular Adaptations to Exercise

Cardiovascular function is altered during exercise training due to sympathetic molecular signaling acute responses, which increase heart rate and cardiac output, resulting in the rise of blood flow and blood pressure to distribute oxygen and nutrients to skeletal muscles effectively. Consequently, the heart of a physically active person undergoes cardiac remodeling as a response to an increased workload derived from the tenfold rise in its oxygen consumption that causes an increase in the size of the cardiomyocytes, hence inducing physiological cardiac hypertrophy and, unlike in a pathological context, this improves contractile function and mitochondrial energy metabolism. Studies performed in animal models have proved that exercise training upregulates several genes involved with cardiac hypertrophy, such as myonectin, arterial natriuretic peptides (ANP), alpha and beta myosin heavy chain (α-MHC and β-MHC, respectively), peroxisome proliferator-activated receptor alpha (PPAR-α), and PGC-1α, to mention a few. In addition, exercise increases the levels of cardiac insulin-like growth factor 1 (IGF-1), a hormone that constitutes a crucial molecular inductor of physiological cardiac hypertrophy by activating the PI3K/Akt pathway, causing impaired aortic constriction that, along with endothelial nitric oxide synthase (eNOS) activity upregulation, accounts for exercise-induced cardiac remodeling. Interestingly, hypertrophy resulting from exercise training increases by 10–20% the cardiac mass and is fully reversible and has no adverse effects, while cardiac hypertrophy due to heart disease progressively leads to a decline in normal cardiac function (Maillet et al. 2013; Burgos et al. 2017; Seo et al. 2020).

Besides hypertrophy, cardiometabolic adaptations to exercise focus on three axes: fatty acid metabolism, carbohydrate metabolism, and mitochondrial adaptation (Smith et al. 2018; Ashcroft et al. 2024). In this regard, exercise regulates the glucose-fatty acid cycle by enhancing fatty acid use through the upregulation of carnitine acyltransferase shuttles (CPT-1 and CPT-2) and control of phosphofructokinase activity (Gibb et al. 2017). Acute physical activity triggers several physiological responses, such as reactive oxygen species generation (ROS), AMP/ATP ratio shifts, increased catecholamine release, and increased intracellular calcium. These exercise outcomes are upstream mechanisms that ultimately lead to PGC-1α-induced mitochondrial biogenesis through the activation of pathways like tumor protein p53 (p53), AMP-activated protein kinase (AMPK), p38 mitogen-activated protein kinase (p38MAPK), and Ca^{2+}/calmodulin-dependent protein kinase (CaMK) (Sorriento et al. 2021). Mitochondrial biogenesis is a process in which the creation of new mitochondria is controlled to ensure adequate energy supply for the heart by balancing mitochondrial mass. PGC-1α regulates mitochondrial replication and transcription by interacting with several transcription factors, and its genetic deletion accelerates cardiac dysfunction (Dorn et al. 2015).

While not always harmful, ROS can have diverse physiological consequences based on their concentration. The heart is most vulnerable to oxidative alterations due to its high rate of oxidative metabolism and low levels of antioxidant activity. In this matter, aerobic training protects the heart against oxidative stress by stimulating the redox system and several antioxidant systems. Interestingly, the increased mitochondrial ROS production induced by high-intensity exercise provokes Ryanodine receptor (RyR) protein fragmentation in skeletal muscle, increasing the sarcoplasmic reticulum Ca^{2+} leak at rest, hence impairing force production, although there is no evidence if this is also the responsible mechanism operating on cardiac muscle–increased calcium release in the cytosol (Place et al. 2015). In this regard, it is well known that exercise promotes functional adaptations in the heart by enhancing cardiac performance and the contractile ability of cardiomyocytes. This improvement is achieved through the activation of RyR and the sarcoendoplasmic reticulum Ca^{2+} ATPase (SERCA), which accounts for increasing intracellular calcium levels, promoting CaMK activation, hence favoring the PGC-1α role (Kemi et al. 2008).

3.1.2 Other Metabolic Adaptations to Exercise

Beyond cardiac muscle, other metabolic-relevant organs and tissues undergo changes in response to exercise. Aerobic exercise improves nitric oxide bioavailability in vascular endothelium and facilitates blood flow dynamics, promoting unidirectional flow of high magnitude that enhances mitochondrial production in blood vessels. This stress improves mitochondrial networks and reduces glycolysis, enhancing mitochondrial lipid metabolism (Hong et al. 2022). Exercise also stimulates several ventilatory parameters, such as increased respiratory rate and tidal volume, and helps improve acid-base balance, pulmonary diffusion, and general ventilatory efficiency, improving aerobic capacity and oxidative metabolism (Leite De Prado et al. 2006).

The adaptations of the skeletal muscle depend on the type of exercise performed. Resistance training stimulates force development and promotes muscle hypertrophy by activating protein synthesis pathways while inhibiting protein degradation pathways, which augment the amount of the myofibrillar contractile proteins actin and myosin, with an increase in muscle cross-sectional area. In contrast, aerobic training promotes resistance to fatigue by enhancing mitochondrial biogenesis and capillary density, improving the body's capacity to transport and utilize oxygen for energy production, thereby postponing muscle fatigue during extended aerobic activities (Joyner and Coyle 2008).

Several molecular mechanisms have been identified as participants in the beneficial metabolic effects of exercise in skeletal muscle, including AMPK, the mammalian target of rapamycin (mTOR), and sestrin pathways. Sestrins are stress-inducible proteins essential for maintaining blood glucose and lipid homeostasis by inhibiting mTORC1 in an AMPK-dependent way. AMPK is activated during exercise-induced energy stress, influencing glucose and lipid metabolism via GLUT4 transcription. There are reports proving that exercise counters insulin resistance caused by a high-fat diet and reduces lipid buildup within muscle cells by activating AMPK signaling. On the other hand, mTOR, which regulates anabolic processes such as cell survival and cell growth by promoting protein synthesis, also mediates insulin sensitization and fatty acid oxidation during exercise (Liu et al. 2020).

Furthermore, white adipose tissue (WAT) is a crucial metabolic regulator that stores lipids, produces hormones, and supports immune functions. When WAT distribution is excessive in the visceral area, metabolic health is compromised, and the risks for dyslipidemia, T2DM, atherosclerosis, and insulin resistance are exacerbated. Exercise training promotes reductions in cell size and lipid content and redistribution of fat storage, reducing visceral fat content while favoring subcutaneous fat content. Exercise also increases mitochondrial biogenesis in this tissue via PGC-1α overexpression, improves glucose metabolism by increasing the expression of the GLUT4 transporter, and promotes the production of certain adipokines like leptin, adiponectin, interleukin-6 (IL-6), and TNFα (Stanford et al. 2015).

Indeed, the release of these chemical messengers is currently of great interest in the area of research into the health benefits associated with physical activity as a way to understand better the molecular mechanisms involved and search for potential therapeutic targets, which is why they have been grouped into a "new" cluster of endogenous substances known as exerkines through which biochemical and physiological adaptations to exercise occur.

3.2 Exerkines and Cardiometabolic Health

Besides endocrine glands, most tissues and organs with metabolic roles have been identified as contributors to endocrine response through the production and secretion of exercise-induced molecules known as exerkines (Jin et al. 2024). Exerkines relevance relies on their role as molecular transducers regardless of whether they are cytokines, hormones, peptides, lipids, nucleic acids, proteins, or metabolic products, participating in endocrine, paracrine, and autocrine responses. By the tissue/organ where the exerkines are produced, they could receive a specific denomination: myokine for the exerkines released from the skeletal muscle, adipokines for the exerkines released from the adipose tissue (there are also batokines for the specific exerkines excreted by the brown adipose tissue), cardiokines released from the heart, hepatokines released from the liver, and neurokines released from the nervous system (Chow et al. 2022).

There are several exercise-associated health benefits, but, specifically, those involved in cardiometabolic health are represented in Fig. 2. Among them, some stand out due to their involvement in molecular pathways that make them candidates for treating obesity, MetS, and T2DM complications. For instance, IL-6 is produced in different tissues, which allows this molecule to regulate different pathways. This myokine functions as an "energy sensor," promptly raising the release of energetic substrates from the liver and adipose tissue during exercise. Another relevant myokine is Musclin, a peptide homolog to natriuretic peptides secreted from skeletal muscle that improves cardiomyocyte contractility and promotes PGC-1α regulation, thus improving mitochondrial biogenesis (Robbins and Gerszten 2023).

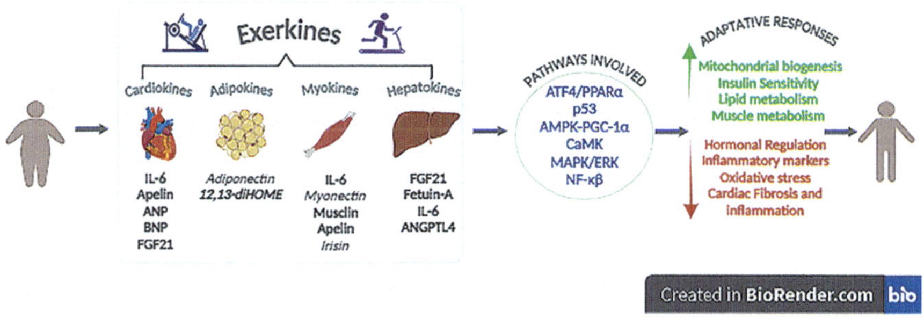

Fig. 2 Cardiometabolic disorders impair exerkines constitutive production and secretion. Some exerkines are upregulated (bold), while some exerkines are downregulated (italics) in cardiometabolic pathologies. Exercise regularizes its metabolic role and even enhances it, promoting the activation of several pathways that regulate adaptive responses to exercise, improving cardiometabolic health. 12,13-diHOME 12,13-Dihydroxy-9Z-octadecenoic acid, AMPK/PGC-1α AMP-activated protein kinase/proliferator-activated receptor gamma coactivator 1-alpha, ANGPTL4 angiopoietin-like protein 4, ANP atrial natriuretic peptide, ATF4/PPARα activating transcription factor 4/peroxisome proliferator-activated receptor alpha, BNP brain natriuretic peptide, CaMK Ca2+/calmodulin-dependent protein kinase, FGF21 fibroblast growth factor, IL-6 interleukin-6, AMPK/ERK Ras-Raf-MEK-ERK pathway, NF-Kβ nuclear factor kappa β, p53 tumor protein p53. (Created in BioRender.com)

12,13-Dihydroxy-9Z-octadecenoic acid (12,13-diHOME) is produced in brown adipose tissue as an oxidized linoleic acid metabolite that increases fatty acid uptake in skeletal muscle and heart as a response to both acute and chronic training also favoring insulin sensitivity and body mass index, although when chronically elevated is associated with metabolic dysregulation (Robbins and Gerszten 2023). Adiponectin, which is released from the WAT in response to acute and chronic training, enhances glucose and lipid uptake, diminishes oxidative stress, and, unlike other adipokines, maintains an inverse relationship with obesity and other metabolic disorders (Hoffstedt et al. 2004).

The role of the liver in the pathogenesis of cardiometabolic disorders is commonly underestimated; however, as it is a metabolically indispensable organ, it is important to mention the exerkines produced there. Fibroblast growth factor (FGF21) is a hepatokine directly associated with fatty liver as its expression increases to counteract the lipid accumulation damage; hence, it is commonly used as a biomarker of metabolic disease, and recent research underlines its potential effects as a treatment target improving lipid profile and fasting insulin in T2DM patients. Another example of a hepatokine, Fetuin-A, is a downregulated exerkine by regular exercise and is positively correlated with impaired glucose tolerance, insulin resistance, T2D, and liver fibrosis. Conversely, angiopoietin-like protein 4 (ANGPTL4) is increased during exercise, helping in the regulation of lipid and glucose metabolism, inhibiting lipolysis, and controlling fatty acid uptake to prevent lipid overload in heart and skeletal muscles (Ennequin et al. 2019).

Regarding the exercise characteristics that induce exerkines production and secretion, it has been determined that a more vigorous intensity of training accounts for a more pronounced release of exerkines than moderate-intensity training; likewise, a higher duration of the training helps to extend the exerkines release (Cullen et al. 2016). Exercise type also influences exerkines response and profile; for example, aerobic exercise promotes the production of certain exerkines such as IL-6 and adiponectin, favoring anti-inflammatory mechanisms and metabolic health, while resistance exercise induces the production of myokines like irisin and myonectin, thus facilitating muscle growth and metabolic regulation. Finally, the type and size of muscle groups stimulated during the exercise training could also affect exerkines production due to the difference in energetic substrate demand and physiological conformations (Chow et al. 2022). It is a fact that there is more to understand concerning the transient role of certain exerkines since the increase in their production does not necessarily affect their resting level permanently after repeated exercise sessions, or the changes may not be concordant, with permanent increases resulting in pathological outcomes and transient exercise-induced increases being beneficial to metabolic health (Robbins and Gerszten 2023).

Interestingly, exerkines production can be significantly disturbed due to cardiometabolic disorders, mitigating the responses and adaptations to exercise compared to physiological conditions. Certainly, obesity-derived conditions like inflammation and insulin resistance, which are present in most cardiometabolic disorders, are the key elements blunting the exerkines effect. The increased levels of inflammatory cytokines and hormonal imbalances disrupt some exerkines release and regulation pathways. In addition, individuals with a cardiometabolic disorder could present altered muscle composition or muscle atrophy, which further decreases exerkines production and overall reduces exercise capacity, falling into a vicious circle of physical inactivity (Robbins and Gerszten 2023; Jin et al. 2024).

3.3 Outcomes of Exercise on Cardiometabolic Diseases

As mentioned, the heart faces a significant workload, pumping blood to distribute oxygen and nutrients to the entire body, which implies large energy requirements. The metabolism of the heart is primarily maintained by the oxidation of fatty acids and glucose (approximately 70% and 30%, respectively). However, the myocardium exhibits some metabolic plasticity, and depending on several physiological changes, the proportion of ATP production sources can be modified. Notably, the variations in glucose and fatty acids availability and use determine the disturbances in cardiometabolic disorders in the heart. For instance, glucose metabolism is detrimentally affected due to impaired GLUT4 glucose-mediated uptake, which mediates the myocardial insulin resistance and forces an increased dependency on fatty acid consumption in the heart, establishing the early onset of diabetic cardiomyopathy (Nirengi et al. 2020). Glucose-derived buildup in the diabetic cardiac vessels has been associated with sustained O-GlcNAcylation, a post-translational modification that induces pathological states (Qin et al. 2017), and also with increased ROS production, increased intracellular calcium content, and decreased SERCA pump expression, which together contribute to mitochondrial and cardiac contractile dysfunction (Pereira et al. 2006). Although diabetic cardiomyopathy is a term used to indicate the cardiac dysfunction particularities in diabetic patients, several authors agree that patients with obesity, insulin resistance, and dyslipidemia may develop a form of cardiomyopathy linked to metabolism, even without diabetes; hence, obesity, MetS, and T2DM patients present similar characteristics for a "metabolic cardiomyopathy," just in different progress state (Nakamura and Sadoshima 2019).

Several treatments are implemented to manage diabetic cardiomyopathy complications, including pharmacological therapies for glucose or lipids control as well as management of body weight through caloric restriction and/or exercise, which contributes to the decrease in the risk of mortality related to heart failure with preserved ejection fraction (HFpEF), where weight loss has improved glycemic control to the same extent as antidiabetic drugs (Tsujimoto and Kajio 2017). Exercise is recognized as a non-drug intervention that enhances cardiovascular fitness in healthy and ill individuals, boosting exercise tolerance and improving overall quality of life. It has been proposed that the long-term impact of exercise on metabolic conditions is mainly due to a simultaneous reduction in abdominal fat, although this is not the sole factor (Carroll and Dudfield 2004).

A common factor in several cardiac pathologies involves mitochondrial dysfunction due to various proteins responsible for homeostasis and energy generation in the heart disturbed by post-translational modifications that affect their functionality, such as SUMOylation and phosphorylation in mitochondrial Rho GTPase (Miro2) and dynamin-related protein (DRP1), or alterations in the expression of mitofusin-2 (MFN2), mitochondrial dynamin-like GTPase (OPA1), and PGC-1α (Sorriento et al. 2021). In this regard, exercise triggers autophagy in the heart, constituting a protective mechanism against metabolic disorders. Various targeted strategies have been suggested to improve mitochondrial function in failing hearts, making physical exercise the most relevant non-pharmacological approach.

Although not all patients with cardiometabolic disease present hypertension, exercise also helps decrease diastolic pressure at rest in response to aerobic exercise by improving peripheral vascular resistance (Hegde and Solomon 2015). Another common complication among individuals with a cardiometabolic disorder that benefits from exercise is dyslipidemia. Several studies suggest that regular aerobic exercise enhances beneficial blood lipid levels, particularly HDL cholesterol, while lowering LDL cholesterol and triglycerides, where the exercise's duration determines the effect's size (Wewege et al. 2018).

The study of the most appropriate exercise characteristics to achieve cardiac and metabolic benefits is extensive. Some studies indicate that the intensity of exercise is a more crucial factor than the duration of exercise for health, recommending aerobic interval training, which involves periods of vigorous exercise followed by active recovery phases instead of complete rest (Wisløff et al. 2009). It is well known that aerobic training improves general cardiometabolic elements, contributing to the prevention and treatment of CVDs. Although the reports on resistance training benefits are scarcer, there is evidence supporting that this type of training also serves as an effective intervention for enhancing various aspects of cardiometabolic health, helping manage body weight, blood pressure, glycemic levels, and lipid profiles while also reducing the cardiovascular mortality risk by approximately 17% (Paluch et al. 2024). Indeed, the reports indicate that the best cardiovascular outcome is obtained from the combination of both types of exercise (Isath et al. 2023).

4 Exercise Recommendations for Cardiometabolic Diseases

4.1 Obesity and Exercise

Statistics concerning overweight and obesity around the world demonstrate the continuous increase in the prevalence of these disorders in all age populations, although with a more significant presence in some ethnic groups. In this context, exercise is expected to support weight loss by impairing the energy balance to an energy expenditure superior to the energy intake. Even a slight weight loss represents essential progress in countering CVD risk factors such as triglycerides and glucose blood levels, as long as the lost weight is not recovered (Jensen et al. 2014). Besides physical activity, effective weight loss requires the diminution of energy intake through dietary control, as obese individuals rarely reach the necessary fitness capacity to achieve the volume of physical activity needed (Liguori and American College of Sports Medicine (ACSM) 2021). A recent study demonstrates that a combination of diet and physical activity enhances glucose metabolism, insulin sensitivity, and maximal oxygen uptake while upregulating adiponectin production (Venojärvi et al. 2022).

Specifically, the goal of weight reduction is to decrease the fat mass content, particularly visceral fat, as it has been reported that the central role of this deposit is in the metabolic disturbances associated with obesity and the increased risk of developing MetS and T2DM. A higher proportion of lean body mass ensures a more significant resting energy expenditure and improved glucose homeostasis. Exercise also improves the lipid profile, usually altered in obese individuals, via lipoprotein lipase overactivation and the exchange of lipids over glycogen as the primary energy source in the skeletal muscle (Chomiuk et al. 2024). Table 2 summarizes the FIIT (frequency, intensity, time, type) principle for exercise prescription for individuals with obesity to optimize weight loss.

Resistance exercise alone does not significantly aid in weight loss; hence, its incorporation is advised to enhance muscular strength and physical function to augment the intensity and duration of aerobic physical activity progressively (Macfarlane et al. 2006).

4.2 Metabolic Syndrome and Exercise

According to the National Cholesterol Education Program (NCEP), Adult Treatment Panel III (ATP III) and the International Diabetes Federation (IDF) agree on three critical points for therapeutic intervention for MetS management, which are weight control, physical activity, and CVD risks treatment through dietary change and

Table 2 FITT recommendations for individuals with obesity

Exercise	Type	Frequency	Intensity	Time	Precautions
Aerobic	Prolonged rhythmic activities involving large muscle groups	≥ 5 days per week.	Moderate (40–59% HRR) or vigorous (≥ 60% HRR).	30–60 min per day (150–300 min per week)	*Care must be taken with symptoms like chest pain, joint pain, shortness of breath, dizziness, or excessive fatigue during exercise, and stop if they occur
Resistance	Resistance machines and/or free weights	2–3 days per week	60–70% of 1-RM with gradual increase	2–4 sets of 8–12 repetitions	*Begin with low- to moderate-intensity exercise to assess tolerance, gradually increasing intensity and duration
Flexibility	Static, dynamic, and/or PNF stretching	≥ 2–3 days per week	Stretch to the point of tightness or discomfort	Hold static stretch for 10–30 s; 2–4 repetitions of each exercise	

Adapted from Liguori and American College of Sports Medicine (ACSM) (2021)
1-RM one repetition maximum, *HRR* heart rate reserve, *min* minutes, *PNF* proprioceptive neuromuscular facilitation, *s* seconds

pharmacotherapy if necessary (National Cholesterol Education Program 2002; Alberti et al. 2006).

Regular exercise training ameliorates all MetS signs and may also help prevent or postpone the onset of T2DM in individuals with MetS, independently of weight loss due to its anti-inflammatory properties. The anti-inflammatory response induced by physical activity depends on the decrease in several inflammatory cytokine production, the increase in anti-inflammatory cytokines and myokines, and the antioxidant mechanisms associated with the regulation of nitric oxide intracellular pathways (Chomiuk et al. 2024). Interestingly, it is suggested that chronic inflammation linked to MetS may contribute to ongoing physical inactivity. Inflammatory states can diminish the motivation for physical activity, as demonstrated in studies that show that inflammation induces fatigue, reduced movement, and depressive symptoms (Matta et al. 2019). Conversely, stressor factors like exercise or caloric restriction can trigger anti-inflammatory responses and improve exercise capacity, promoting better overall fitness in MetS patients (Nunn et al. 2010).

FITT principle for individuals with MetS (Table 3) is consistent with the consensus public health recommendations for adults; however, given the variety of signs that patients with MetS may present, various parameters should be monitored before, during, and after exercise, such as blood pressure, glycemia, as well as all precautions for obese individuals (Liguori and American College of Sports Medicine (ACSM) 2021).

Table 3 FITT recommendations for individuals with metabolic syndrome

Exercise	Type	Frequency	Intensity	Time	Precautions
Aerobic	Exercises that involve large muscles continuously or intermittently	≥ 3 days per week	Moderate (40–59% HRR) Vigorous (60–89% HRR)	30–60 min per day (moderate), 20–60 min per day (vigorous), or a combination	*Changes in blood glucose during and after exercise should be taken care of to avoid hypoglycemia or hyperglycemia
Resistance	Multi-joint exercises with resistance machines, free or body weights	≥ 2 days per week	60–79% of 1-RM	Sets of 8–12 repetitions, progressing according to the level obtained	*Begin with low- to moderate-intensity exercise to assess tolerance, gradually increasing intensity and duration
Flexibility	Static (active, passive), dynamic, PNF	≥ 2–3 days per week	Stretch to the point of tightness or slight discomfort	Static: 10–30 s PNF: 3–6 s of voluntary contraction	*Care must be taken with symptoms like chest pain, shortness of breath, dizziness, or excessive fatigue during exercise, and stop if they occur

Adapted from Liguori and American College of Sports Medicine (ACSM) (2021)
1-RM one repetition maximum, *HRR* Heart rate reserve, *min* minutes, *PNF* proprioceptive neuromuscular facilitation, *s* seconds

While the fundamental role of aerobic exercise is recognized, reports have demonstrated that the prevalence of MetS can be reduced to a greater extent when resistance training is combined with aerobic training compared to aerobic training alone. In this sense, including resistance exercise also reduces the risk of developing dyslipidemia, IFG, prehypertension, and increased waist circumference—all components of the MetS cluster (Earnest et al. 2014).

4.3 Type 2 Diabetes Mellitus and Exercise

Severe blood glucose management therapy lowers the chance of progression to problems from T2DM in those with the illness. Thus, glycemic control is the primary objective of T2DM treatment, which involves a combination of diet, exercise, and, frequently, pharmacological prescription treatments, such as insulin, as well as the management of related comorbidities. In this sense, physical activity has been proven to benefit insulin resistance and T2DM progression, improving glucose tolerance, improving glucose uptake up to 48 h by insulin-dependent mechanisms, and reducing hemoglobin A1c (HbA1c) levels (Pan et al. 2018).

Also, individuals with T2DM are more likely to exhibit a higher prevalence of CVD risk factors, such as dyslipidemia and augmented inflammatory markers, than those without diabetes. mTOR overactivity in diabetic hearts leads to alterations in insulin sensitivity through molecular mechanisms that block PI3K/Akt signaling, which, in conjunction with diminished AMPK activation, accounts for cardiac dysfunction and heart failure. Additionally, diabetic cardiomyopathy involves disturbances in energy metabolism, where the diabetic heart utilizes fatty acid oxidation as the primary substrate for ATP production, ultimately leading to increased apoptosis, mitochondrial dysfunction, ROS accumulation, and activation of pro-inflammatory pathways (Suhara et al. 2017; Nirengi et al. 2020).

In this sense, exercise switches energy metabolism from fatty acid to glucose oxidation and enhances mitochondrial function by reducing ROS accumulation (Wang et al. 2020). Regarding the most appropriate type of exercise, a recent meta-analysis found no evidence that resistance exercise differs from aerobic exercise in its beneficial effects on several cardiovascular risk factors or safety in individuals with type 2 diabetes mellitus (T2DM). However, aerobic exercise increased cardiorespiratory fitness to a greater extent than resistance exercise, which is relevant because compromised cardiorespiratory fitness is one of the major predictors of mortality in patients with T2DM (Church et al. 2005; Yang et al. 2014).

Exercise prescription guidelines and recommendations for T2DM individuals take into account several precautions, particularly if the patient suffers from any CVD or is considered a sedentary individual. For instance, the American Diabetes Association (ADA) suggests previous exercise testing, especially if the programmed intensity would be vigorous, as well as medical clearance, including tests such as electrocardiogram stress testing, given that silent ischemia is often undetected in T2DM patients (Colberg et al. 2016; Liguori and American College of Sports Medicine (ACSM) 2021). Table 4 summarizes the FIIT principle for exercise prescription for individuals with T2DM.

Reports agree that combined aerobic and resistance training constitutes the best recommendation for individuals with T2DM to prevent injuries, reduce body weight, and enhance blood glucose levels and insulin action. Although flexibility and balance exercises are highly recommended, they should not be used as a substitute for aerobic or resistance training, given the limited evidence of their overall cardiometabolic benefits (Colberg et al. 2016). Special care must be taken with dehydration in individuals with T2DM due to its tendency to polyuria secondary to hyperglycemia, which can ultimately result in thermoregulation impairment and, hence, heatstroke (Liguori and American College of Sports Medicine (ACSM) 2021).

Table 4 FITT recommendations for individuals with type 2 diabetes mellitus

Exercise	Type	Frequency	Intensity	Time	Precautions
Aerobic	Prolonged activities using large muscle groups (e.g., walking, swimming or HIIT)	3–7 days per week (No more than 2 consecutive days without activity)	Moderate to vigorous	150–300 min per week	*Changes in blood glucose during and after exercise should be taken care of. It is essential to adjust the time of administration and dose of insulin and control carbohydrate consumption to avoid hypoglycemia
Resistance	Resistance machines, free or body weights, resistance bands.	A minimum of 2 non-consecutive days per week	Moderate (50–69% of 1-RM) Vigorous (70–85% of 1-RM)	At least 8–10 exercises with 1–3 sets of 10–15 repetitions to near fatigue per set early in training	*Exercise can increase the risk of foot injuries
Balance	Static, dynamic.	≥ 2–3 days per week	Light to moderate intensity	Any duration	*Begin with low- to moderate-intensity exercise to assess tolerance, gradually increasing intensity and duration as fitness improves
Flexibility	Yoga	≥ 2–3 days per week	Stretch to the point of tightness or slight discomfort	Hold static stretch for 10–30 s; 2–4 repetitions of each exercise	*Care must be taken with symptoms like chest pain, shortness of breath, dizziness, or excessive

(continued)

Table 4 (continued)

Exercise	Type	Frequency	Intensity	Time	Precautions
					fatigue during exercise, and stop if they occur

Adapted from Liguori and American College of Sports Medicine (ACSM) (2021)
1-RM one repetition maximum, *HIIT* high-intensity interval training, *min* minutes, *s* seconds

5 Final Considerations

Numerous studies emphasize the detrimental consequences of sedentary behavior on health and its undeniable association with the onset of cardiometabolic diseases. Physical activity is essential for preventing and managing cardiometabolic disorders like obesity, MetS, and T2DM. It enhances insulin sensitivity, improves lipid metabolism, reduces inflammation, lowers oxidative stress, regulates hormone levels, and increases muscle mass, thereby contributing to improved metabolic health. In addition to exercise, proper management of these disorders must include changes in the diet, psychological interventions, regular health monitoring, stress control techniques, and medications if needed. An effective approach that combines these strategies can significantly enhance health outcomes in individuals with cardiometabolic disorders (Sattar et al. 2020; Cosentino et al. 2023).

The ADA and the American Heart Association's (AHA) most recent recommendations agreed on the relevance of reducing sedentary behavior by engaging in light-intensity activities, progressively increasing the intensity until reaching at least 150 min of moderate-intensity aerobic activity throughout the week, including muscular strengthening for at least 2 days to enhance cardiometabolic health benefits (Jerome et al. 2023). Additionally, the ADA recommends personalizing the physical training according to the specific patient's condition and physical characteristics, promoting activities that help control blood glucose levels (Zhang and Yang 2024).

Indeed, engagement in physical activities involves some risks to cardiovascular health, such as atrial fibrillation when regular high-intensity or high-volume physical activity is performed, raised risk of sudden death, and acute myocardial infarction in individuals with underlying CVD after acute episodes of physical activity. However, physical activity is often a trigger more than a direct cause of these cardiac events (Isath et al. 2023). Therefore, it is essential to note that the risks associated with training should not overshadow the multiple health benefits.

Current research on the benefits of exercise for cardiometabolic disorders reveals several gaps. Many studies focus predominantly on specific populations (young adults, men, Caucasians), often neglecting gender, racial, and ethnic diversity, which limits insights into how exercise affects different groups based on their genetic features and geographical context. In this sense, there is a critical need to promote physical activity among underresourced populations to improve cardiovascular health equity and reduce health disparities associated with low activity levels (Jerome et al. 2023). There is also insufficient research on younger populations, which constitutes a relevant gap in fully understanding the implications of physical activity on the early stages of the pathogenesis of cardiometabolic disorders (Vázquez-Jiménez et al. 2025). Additionally, many studies do not consider comorbidities in the participants besides the cardiometabolic disorder, which can influence outcomes. While technology has the potential to promote physical activity, more rigorous studies are needed to assess the effectiveness of fitness-oriented apps and gadgets (DiPietro et al. 2020). Addressing these issues could improve the physical activity approach to prevent and manage cardiometabolic disorders.

References

Alberti K, Zimmet P, Shaw J (2006) Metabolic syndrome—a new world-wide definition. A consensus statement from the international diabetes federation. Diabet Med 23:469–480. https://doi.org/10.1155/2010/307409

American College of Sports Medicine (2013) ACSM'S guidelines for exercise testing and prescription. Lippincott Williams & Wilkins

Ashcroft SP, Stocks B, Egan B, Zierath JR (2024) Exercise induces tissue-specific adaptations to enhance cardiometabolic health. Cell Metab 36:278–300. https://doi.org/10.1016/j.cmet.2023.12.008

Boyer WR, Churilla JR, Ehrlich SF et al (2018) Protective role of physical activity on type 2 diabetes: analysis of effect modification by race–ethnicity. J Diabetes 10:166–178. https://doi.org/10.1111/1753-0407.12574

Bull FC, Al-Ansari SS, Biddle S et al (2020) World Health Organization 2020 guidelines on physical activity and sedentary behaviour. Br J Sports Med 54:1451–1462

Burgos JI, Yeves AM, Barrena JP et al (2017) Nitric oxide and CaMKII: critical steps in the cardiac contractile response to IGF-1 and swim training. J Mol Cell Cardiol 112:16–26. https://doi.org/10.1016/j.yjmcc.2017.08.014

Carroll S, Dudfield M (2004) What is the relationship between exercise and metabolic abnormalities? A review of the metabolic syndrome. Sports Med 34:371–418

Chomiuk T, Niezgoda N, Mamcarz A, Śliż D (2024) Physical activity in metabolic syndrome. Front Physiol 15:1365761

Chow LS, Gerszten RE, Taylor JM et al (2022) Exerkines in health, resilience and disease. Nat Rev Endocrinol 18:273–289. https://doi.org/10.1038/s41574-022-00641-2

Church TS, LaMonte MJ, Barlow CE, Blair SN (2005) Cardiorespiratory fitness and body mass index as predictors of cardiovascular disease mortality among men with diabetes. Arch Intern Med 165:2114–2120. https://doi.org/10.1001/archinte.165.18.2114

Colberg SR, Sigal RJ, Yardley JE et al (2016) Physical activity/exercise and diabetes: a position statement of the American Diabetes Association. Diabetes Care 39:2065–2079. https://doi.org/10.2337/dc16-1728

Cosentino F, Verma S, Ambery P et al (2023) Cardiometabolic risk management: insights from a European society of cardiology cardiovascular round table. Eur Heart J 44:4141–4156

Costa Santos A, Willumsen J, Meheus F et al (2023) The cost of inaction on physical inactivity to public health-care systems: a population-attributable fraction analysis. Lancet Glob Health 11: e32–e39. https://doi.org/10.1016/S2214-109X(22)00464-8

Cullen T, Thomas AW, Webb R, Hughes MG (2016) Interleukin-6 and associated cytokine responses to an acute bout of high-intensity interval exercise: the effect of exercise intensity and volume. Appl Physiol Nutr Metab 41:803–808. https://doi.org/10.1139/apnm-2015-0640

DiPietro L, Al-Ansari SS, Biddle SJH et al (2020) Advancing the global physical activity agenda: recommendations for future research by the 2020 WHO physical activity and sedentary behavior guidelines development group. Int J Behav Nutr Phys Act 17:1–11. https://doi.org/10.1186/s12966-020-01042-2

Dorn GW, Vega RB, Kelly DP (2015) Mitochondrial biogenesis and dynamics in the developing and diseased heart. Genes Dev:1981–1991. https://doi.org/10.1101/gad.269894

Earnest CP, Johannsen NM, Swift DL et al (2014) Aerobic and strength training in concomitant metabolic syndrome and type 2 diabetes. Med Sci Sports Exerc 46:1293

Eckel RH, Alberti KGMM, Grundy SM, Zimmet PZ (2010) The metabolic syndrome. Lancet 375: 181–183

Ekelund U, Tarp J, Steene-Johannessen J et al (2019) Dose-response associations between accelerometry measured physical activity and sedentary time and all cause mortality: systematic review and harmonised meta-analysis. BMJ 366:l4570. https://doi.org/10.1136/bmj.l4570

Ennequin G, Sirvent P, Whitham M (2019) Role of exercise-induced hepatokines in metabolic disorders. Am J Physiol Endocrinol Metab 317:11–24. https://doi.org/10.1152/ajpendo.00433.2018

Gerdts E, Regitz-Zagrosek V (2019) Sex differences in cardiometabolic disorders. Nat Med 25: 1657–1666

Gibala MJ, Mcgee SL (2008) Metabolic adaptations to short-term high-intensity interval training: a little pain for a lot of gain? Exerc Sport Sci Rev 36:58–63

Gibb AA, Epstein PN, Uchida S et al (2017) Exercise-induced changes in glucose metabolism promote physiological cardiac growth. Circulation 136:2144–2157. https://doi.org/10.1161/CIRCULATIONAHA.117.028274

González K, Fuentes J, Márquez JL (2017) Physical inactivity, sedentary behavior and chronic diseases. Korean J Fam Med 38:111–115

Guthold R, Stevens GA, Riley LM, Bull FC (2018) Worldwide trends in insufficient physical activity from 2001 to 2016: a pooled analysis of 358 population-based surveys with 1·9 million participants. Lancet Glob Health 6:e1077–e1086. https://doi.org/10.1016/S2214-109X(18)30357-7

Hamasaki H (2024) Effects of tai chi in diabetes patients: insights from recent research. World J Diabetes 15:1–10. https://doi.org/10.4239/wjd.v15.i1.1

Heal DJ, Gosden J, Smith SL (2009) Regulatory challenges for new drugs to treat obesity and comorbid metabolic disorders. Br J Clin Pharmacol 68:861–874

Hegde SM, Solomon SD (2015) Influence of physical activity on hypertension and cardiac structure and function. Curr Hypertens Rep 17:77. https://doi.org/10.1007/s11906-015-0588-3

Hoffstedt J, Arvidsson E, Sjölin E et al (2004) Adipose tissue adiponectin production and adiponectin serum concentration in human obesity and insulin resistance. J Clin Endocrinol Metab 89:1391–1396. https://doi.org/10.1210/jc.2003-031458

Hong SG, Shin J, Aldokhayyil M et al (2022) Mitochondrial and metabolic adaptations to exercise-induced fluid shear stress in endothelial cells. Exerc Sport Sci Rev 50:145–155. https://doi.org/10.1249/JES.0000000000000289

Hughes DC, Ellefsen S, Baar K (2018) Adaptations to endurance and strength training. Cold Spring Harb Perspect Med 8:1–17. https://doi.org/10.1101/cshperspect.a029769

Isath A, Koziol KJ, Martinez MW et al (2023) Exercise and cardiovascular health: a state-of-the-art review. Prog Cardiovasc Dis 79:44–52. https://doi.org/10.1016/j.pcad.2023.04.008

Jensen MD, Ryan DH, Apovian CM et al (2014) 2013 AHA/ACC/TOS guideline for the Management of Overweight and Obesity in adults. Circulation 129:S102–S138. https://doi.org/10.1161/01.cir.0000437739.71477.ee

Jerome GJ, Boyer WR, Bustamante EE et al (2023) Increasing equity of physical activity promotion for optimal cardiovascular health in adults: a scientific statement from the American Heart Association. Circulation 147:1951–1962. https://doi.org/10.1161/CIR.0000000000001148

Jin L, Diaz-Canestro C, Wang Y et al (2024) Exerkines and cardiometabolic benefits of exercise: from bench to clinic. EMBO Mol Med 16:432–444. https://doi.org/10.1038/s44321-024-00027-z
Joyner MJ, Coyle EF (2008) Endurance exercise performance: the physiology of champions. J Physiol 586:35–44
Katzmarzyk PT, Friedenreich C, Shiroma EJ, Lee IM (2022) Physical inactivity and non-communicable disease burden in low-income, middle-income and high-income countries. Br J Sports Med 56:101–106. https://doi.org/10.1136/bjsports-2020-103640
Kemi OJ, Ellingsen O, Smith GL, Wisloff U (2008) Exercise-induced changes in calcium handling in left ventricular cardiomyocytes. Front Biosci 13:356
Lambert MI (2016) General adaptations to exercise: acute versus chronic and strength versus endurance training. In: Exercise and human reproduction: induced fertility disorders and possible therapies. Springer, New York, pp 93–100
Leite De Prado DM, Dias RG, Credidio Trombetta I (2006) Clinical update cardiovascular, Ventilatory, and metabolic parameters during exercise: differences between children and adults. Arq Bras Cardiol 87:e92–e97
Liguori G, American College of Sports Medicine (ACSM) (2021) ACSM'S guidelines for exercise testing and prescription, 11th edn. Wolters Kluwer
Liu S, Niu Y, Fu L (2020) Metabolic adaptations to exercise training. J Sci Sport Exerc 2. https://doi.org/10.1007/s42978-019-0018-3
Macfarlane DJ, Taylor LH, Cuddihy TF (2006) Very short intermittent vs continuous bouts of activity in sedentary adults. Prev Med (Baltim) 43:332–336. https://doi.org/10.1016/j.ypmed.2006.06.002
Maillet M, van Berlo JH, Molkentin JD (2013) Molecular basis of physiological heart growth: fundamental concepts and new players. Nat Rev Mol Cell Biol 14:38–48. https://doi.org/10.1038/nrm3495
Matta J, Hoertel N, Kesse-Guyot E et al (2019) Diet and physical activity in the association between depression and metabolic syndrome: Constances study. J Affect Disord 244:25–32. https://doi.org/10.1016/j.jad.2018.09.072
Meloni A, Cadeddu C, Cugusi L et al (2023) Gender differences and Cardiometabolic risk: the importance of the risk factors. Int J Mol Sci 24:1588
Nakamura M, Sadoshima J (2019) Cardiomyopathy in obesity, insulin resistance and diabetes. J Physiol 598:1–17. https://doi.org/10.1113/JP276747
National Cholesterol Education Program (2002) Third report of the National Cholesterol Education Program (NCEP) expert panel on detection, evaluation, and treatment of high blood cholesterol in adults (Adult Treatment Panel III) final report. Circulation 106:3143–3421
Nirengi S, Valgas P, da Silva C, Stanford KI (2020) Disruption of energy utilization in diabetic cardiomyopathy; a mini review. Curr Opin Pharmacol 54:82–90. https://doi.org/10.1016/j.coph.2020.08.015
Nunn AV, Guy GW, Brodie JS, Bell JD (2010) Inflammatory modulation of exercise salience: using hormesis to return to a healthy lifestyle. Nutr Metab (Lond) 7:87. https://doi.org/10.1186/1743-7075-7-87
Paluch AE, Boyer WR, Franklin BA et al (2024) Resistance exercise training in individuals with and without cardiovascular disease: 2023 update: a scientific statement from the American Heart Association. Circulation 149:E217–E231. https://doi.org/10.1161/CIR.0000000000001189
Pan B, Ge L, Xun Y, qin et al (2018) Exercise training modalities in patients with type 2 diabetes mellitus: a systematic review and network meta-analysis. Int J Behav Nutr Phys Act 15:1–14. https://doi.org/10.1186/s12966-018-0703-3
Pereira L, Matthes J, Schuster I et al (2006) Mechanisms of [Ca2+]i transient decrease in cardiomyopathy of db/db type 2 diabetic mice. Diabetes 55:608–615
Place N, Ivarsson N, Venckunas T et al (2015) Ryanodine receptor fragmentation and sarcoplasmic reticulum Ca2+ leak after one session of high-intensity interval exercise. Proc Natl Acad Sci USA 112:15492–15497. https://doi.org/10.1073/pnas.1507176112

Pollock ML, Evans WJ (1999) Resistance training for health and disease: introduction. Med Sci Sports Exerc 31:10
Qin CX, Sleaby R, Davidoff AJ et al (2017) Insights into the role of maladaptive hexosamine biosynthesis and O-GlcNAcylation in development of diabetic cardiac complications. Pharmacol Res 116:45–56. https://doi.org/10.1016/j.phrs.2016.12.016
Robbins JM, Gerszten RE (2023) Exercise, exerkines, and cardiometabolic health: from individual players to a team sport. J Clin Invest 133. https://doi.org/10.1172/JCI168121
Rodulfo IA (2022) The Cardiometabolic burden of Sedentarism and its implications on health. Clin Med Res (NY) 11:95–101. https://doi.org/10.11648/j.cmr.20221104.12
Sattar N, Gill JMR, Alazawi W (2020) Improving prevention strategies for cardiometabolic disease. Nat Med 26:320–325. https://doi.org/10.1038/s41591-020-0786-7
Seo DY, Kwak HB, Kim AH et al (2020) Cardiac adaptation to exercise training in health and disease. Pflugers Arch 472:155–168
Smith RL, Soeters MR, Wüst RCI, Houtkooper RH (2018) Metabolic flexibility as an adaptation to energy resources and requirements in health and disease. Endocr Rev 39:489–517. https://doi.org/10.1210/er.2017-00211
Sorriento D, Di Vaia E, Iaccarino G (2021) Physical exercise: a novel tool to protect mitochondrial health. Front Physiol 12. https://doi.org/10.3389/fphys.2021.660068
Stanford KI, Middelbeek RJW, Goodyear LJ (2015) Exercise effects on white adipose tissue: Beiging and metabolic adaptations. Diabetes 64:2361–2368. https://doi.org/10.2337/db15-0227
Strain T, Flaxman S, Guthold R et al (2024) National, regional, and global trends in insufficient physical activity among adults from 2000 to 2022: a pooled analysis of 507 population-based surveys with 5·7 million participants. Lancet Glob Health 12:e1232–e1243. https://doi.org/10.1016/S2214-109X(24)00150-5
Suhara T, Baba Y, Shimada BK et al (2017) The mTOR signaling pathway in myocardial dysfunction in type 2 diabetes mellitus. Curr Diab Rep 17:38
Tsujimoto T, Kajio H (2017) Abdominal obesity is associated with an increased risk of all-cause mortality in patients with HFpEF. J Am Coll Cardiol 70:2739–2749. https://doi.org/10.1016/j.jacc.2017.09.1111
Tune JD, Goodwill AG, Sassoon DJ, Mather KJ (2017) Cardiovascular consequences of metabolic syndrome. Transl Res 183:57–70. https://doi.org/10.1016/j.trsl.2017.01.001
Vázquez-Jiménez JG, Casillas-Armenta OE, Oregel Cortéz MI, Romero-García T (2025) Comprehending metabolic syndrome in children and adolescents: cardiometabolic outcomes in response to exercise. Retos:122–131. https://doi.org/10.47197/retos.v62.108003
Venojärvi M, Lindström J, Aunola S et al (2022) Improved aerobic capacity and Adipokine profile together with weight loss improve glycemic control without changes in skeletal muscle GLUT-4 gene expression in middle-aged subjects with impaired glucose Toleranc. Int J Environ Res Public Health 19:1–18. https://doi.org/10.3390/ijerph19148327
Wang SY, Zhu S, Wu J et al (2020) Exercise enhances cardiac function by improving mitochondrial dysfunction and maintaining energy homoeostasis in the development of diabetic cardiomyopathy. J Mol Med 98:245–261. https://doi.org/10.1007/s00109-019-01861-2
Wewege MA, Thom JM, Rye K-A, Parmenter BJ (2018) Aerobic, resistance or combined training: a systematic review and meta-analysis of exercise to reduce cardiovascular risk in adults with metabolic syndrome. Atherosclerosis 274:162–171. https://doi.org/10.1016/j.atherosclerosis.2018.05.002
Whitaker KM, Gabriel KP, Buman MP et al (2019) Associations of accelerometer-measured sedentary time and physical activity with prospectively assessed cardiometabolic risk factors: the CARDIA study. J Am Heart Assoc 8. https://doi.org/10.1161/JAHA.118.010212
Wisløff U, Ellingsen Ø, Kemi OJ (2009) High-intensity interval training to maximize cardiac benefits of exercise training? Exerc Sport Sci Rev 37:139
World Health Organization (2010) Global recommendations on physical activity for health. World Health Organization

World Health Organization (2020) WHO Guidelines on physical activity and sedentary behaviour. World Health Organization
Yang Z, Scott CA, Mao C et al (2014) Resistance exercise versus aerobic exercise for type 2 diabetes: a systematic review and meta-analysis. Sports Med 44:487–499. https://doi.org/10.1007/s40279-013-0128-8
Zhang C, Yang J (2024) Personalizing physical activity for glucose control among individuals with type 2 diabetes: are we there yet? Diabetes Care 47:196–198

The manufacturer's authorised representative in the EU is Springer Nature Customer Service Centre GmbH, Europaplatz 3, 69115 Heidelberg, Germany. If you have any concerns regarding our products, please contact ProductSafety@springernature.com

Printed and bound by CPI Group (UK) Ltd, Croydon, CR0 4YY
16/09/2026
02217807-0002